DICTIONARY
OF
IMMUNOLOGY

DICTIONARY
OF
IMMUNOLOGY

FRED S. ROSEN
LISA STEINER
EMIL UNANUE

Elsevier
New York · Amsterdam · London

Elsevier Science Publishing Co., Inc.
655 Avenue of the Americas
New York, NY 10010

Sole distributors outside the United States and Canada:
THE MACMILLAN PRESS LTD
4 Little Essex Street, London WC2R 3LF

ISBN 0-444-01478-0

Printed in Great Britain

Contents

We dedicate this dictionary to the memory of our teachers John H. Humphrey, Irwin H. Lepow and Rodney R. Porter.

Introduction

This book contains definitions of terms that may be encountered in contemporary papers in immunology. It draws from the vocabulary of molecular biology, cell biology and genetics, as well as from immunology itself. For the immunologist or clinician, it may serve as a guide to these other disciplines; for the biologist with little background in immulogy, we hope it will clarify the complex terminology of this field. Many of the definitions are long and contain considerable, if not encyclopedic, detail. Usually, the first paragraph contains the overall meaning and the rest of the text, the fine details.

Whoever is so foolish as to write a dictionary can find wisdom, solace and sympathy in the writings of Samuel Johnson. His remark "the lexicographer can only hope to escape reproach" prompts us to encourage readers to bring errors to our attention so that they may be corrected in a future edition.

We are grateful to Julian B. Fleischman, William P. Girard, Richard A. Harrison, William P. Jencks, John W. Kimball, Roger K. Patient, David H. Raulet and Patricia Woo, who read large groups of definitions and provided helpful criticism.

We also thank colleagues who provided useful information and criticism: Chester A. Alper, David Baltimore, Timothy H. Bestor, Barbara K. Birshtein, Kurt J. Bloch, Bonnie Blomberg, David Botstein, John M. Buchanan, Steven J. Burakoff, Michael C. Carroll, Alvin E. Davis, III, Bernard D. Davis, Herman N. Eisen, George Feher, Sol H. Goodgal, W. Carey Hanley, Stephen C. Harrison, Nancy H. Hopkins, H. Robert Horvitz, Vernon M. Ingram, Fred Karush, Tomas Kirchhausen, Katherine L. Knight, Monty Krieger, Harvey F. Lodish, Rose G. Mage, Henry Metzger, Barbara Meyer, Marian R. Neutra, Alfred Nisonoff, Mary Lou Pardue, Jane R. Parnes, Andrew G. Plaut, Eileen Remold-O'Donnell, Uttam L. Rajbhandary, Linda S. Reidl, Phillips W. Robbins, Paul R. Schimmel, Milton J. Schlesinger, Sondra Schlesinger, Robert D. Schreiber, Ranjan Sen, Hee-Sup Shin, Steven L. Spitalnik, Ursula Storb, Eng M. Tan, Cox P. Terhorst, Anna Maria Torriani-Gorini, Philip W. Tucker, Jay C. Unkeless, Alexander Varshavsky, Thomas A. Waldmann, Robert A. Weinberg, Alexander S. Whitehead, Don C. Wiley and Diane J. Zezza.

Notes on use

The head words defined in the dictionary are placed in alphabetical order. This applies to the complete term regardless of spaces and hyphens. For example, **second-set rejection** comes after **secondary structure**.

Words in small capitals are terms defined in this dictionary.

Where a numeral occurs before the first letter of the head word, the entry will still be ordered under the first letter. For example **6-mercaptopurine** occurs before **metaproteranol**. Where the numeral immediately follows the first letter, they count as being first in the alpha ordering. For example **C9 deficiency** occurs immediately before **cachectin**.

Commonly Used Abbreviations

ABC – antigen binding capacity.
ADA – adenosine deaminase. *See*
ADENOSINE DEAMINASE DEFICIENCY.
ADCC – antibody-dependent cell-mediated
cytoxicity. *See* NATURAL KILLER CELLS.
AGN – acute post-streptococcal
glomerulonephritis.
AIDS – acquired immunodeficiency
syndrome.
ALS – anti-lymphocyte serum.
ANA – anti-nuclear antibody.
AP – alkaline phosphatase.
APC – antigen presenting cell.
ApoE – apolipoprotein E.
ARC – AIDS-related complex.
ASA – acetylsalicylic acid. *See* ASPIRIN.
AT – ataxia telangiectasia.
ATLL – adult T cell leukemia-lymphoma.
ATS – anti-thymocyte serum.
AZT – azidothymidine.*See* ZIDOVUDINE.
BCGF I – B cell growth factor I. *See*
INTERLEUKIN-4.
BCGF II – B cell growth factor II. *See*
INTERLEUKIN-5.
BiP – immunoglobulin heavy chain binding
protein.
BSF-1 – B cell stimulating factor-1. *See*
INTERLEUKIN-4.
BSF-2 – B cell stimulating factor-2. *See*
INTERLEUKIN-6.
C – complement.
C1 INH – C1 inhibitor.
C3NeF – C3 nephritic factor.
C4bp – C4 binding protein.
CALLA – common acute lymphocytic
leukemia antigen.
CD – cluster of differentiation.
CDR – complementarity-determining
region.
CGD – chronic granulomatous disease.
CLL – chronic lymphocytic leukemia.
cM – centiMorgan.
CMI – cell mediated immunity.
CR1 – complement receptor 1.

CR2 – complement receptor 2.
CR3 – complement receptor 3.
CR4 – complement receptor 4.
CRI – cross-reacting idiotype. *See* PUBLIC
IDIOTYPIC DETERMINANT.
CRP – C-reactive protein.
CTL – cytotoxic T lymphocyte.
CTLp – cytotoxic T lymphocyte precursor.
CVF – cobra venom factor.
CVI – common variable immunodeficiency.
DAF – decay antibody-accelerating factor.
DEC – dentritic epidermal cell.
DNP – dinitrophenyl.
DTH – delayed-typed hypersensitivity.
E – erythrocyte.
EAE – experimental allergic
encephalomyelitis.
EBV – Epstein–Barr virus.
EC – enzyme classification, International
Union of Biochemistry 1978.
E-LAM – endothelial–leukocyte adhesion
molecule.
ELISA – enzyme-linked immunosorbent
assay.
ER – endoplasmic reticulum.
ETAF – epithelial thymic-activating factor.
FACS – fluorescence-activated cell sorter.
GALT – gut-associated lymphoid tissue.
GVH – graft-*versus*-host disease.
HANE (or **HAE**) – hereditary
angioneurotic edema.
HIV – human immunodeficiency virus.
HMK – high molecular weight kininogen.
See KININOGEN.
HTLV – human T cell leukemia virus. *See*
ADULT T CELL LEUKEMIA-LYMPHOMA and
HUMAN IMMUNODEFICIENCY VIRUS.
ICAM-1 – intercellular adhesion
molecule-1.
ID – immunodeficiency.
IDDM – insulin-dependent diabetes
mellitus.
IdI – private idiotypic determinant.
IdX – public idiotypic determinant.

IEF – isoelectric focusing.
IEP – immunoelectrophoresis.
IFN – interferon.
Ii – invariant chain.
IK – immunoconglutination.
IL-1 – interleukin-1.
IL-2 – interleukin-2.
IL-3 – interleukin-3. *See* COLONY
STIMULATING FACTOR.
IL-4 – interleukin-4.
IL-5 – interleukin-5.
IL-6 – interleukin-6.
IL-2R – interleukin-2 receptor.
ISG – immune serum globulin.
ITP – idiopathic thrombocytopenic
purpura.
K – killer cell. *See* NATURAL KILLER CELL.
K – conglutinin.
K_A – association constant.
KAF – conglutination activation factor.
See FACTOR I.
kb – kilobase.
K_D – dissociation constant.
K_O – average association constant.
LAD – leukocyte adhesion deficiency.
LATS – long acting thyroid stimulator. *See*
GRAVE'S DISEASE.
LC – Langerhans cell.
LCM – lymphocytic choriomeningitis.
L-CA – leukocyte common antigen.
Leu 1 – *See* CD5.
Leu 2 – *See* CD8.
Leu 3 – *See* CD4.
Leu 4 – *See* CD3.
Leu 5 – *See* CD2.
Leu 6 – *See* CD1.
LFA-1 – lymphocyte function associated
antigen-1.
LFA-2 – lymphocyte function associated
antigen-2. *See* CD2.
LFA-3 – lymphocyte function associated
antigen-3.
LMK – low molecular weight kininogen.
See KININOGEN.
LPS – lipopolysaccharide.
LT – leukotriene.
LT – lymphotoxin.
MAC – membrane attack complex.
Mac1 – macrophage antigen 1. *See*
COMPLEMENT RECEPTOR 3.
MAF – macrophage activating factor.
MDP – muramyl dipeptide.
MHC – major histocompatibility complex.
MIF – migration inhibiting factor.
mIg – membrane immunoglobulin.
MLC – mixed lymphocyte culture.

MLR – mixed lymphocyte reaction.
Mo1 – monocyte antigen 1. *See*
COMPLEMENT RECEPTOR 3.
MPGN – membranoproliferative
glomerulonephritis.
6-MP – 6-mercaptopurine.
MPO – myeloperoxidase. *See*
MYELOPEROXIDASE DEFICIENCY.
NBT – nitroblue tetrazolium dye test.
NK – natural killer cell.
NZB – New Zealand black mouse. *See*
NEW ZEALAND MOUSE.
NZW – New Zealand white mouse. *See*
NEW ZEALAND MOUSE.
OAF – osteoclast activating factor.
ORF – open reading frame.
OT – old tuberculin.
P – properdin.
PA – pernicious anemia.
PAF – platelet-activating factor.
PCA – passive cutaneous anaphylaxis.
PFGE – pulsed field gradient gel
electrophoresis.
PGL – persistent generalized
lymphadenopathy. *See* HIV INFECTION.
P–K – Prausnitz-Küstner reaction.
PMA – phorbol myristate acetate. *See*
PHORBOL ESTER.
PMN – polymorphonuclear leukocyte.
PNP – purine nucleoside phosphorylase.
See PURINE NUCLEOSIDE PHOSPHORYLASE
DEFICIENCY.
PPD – purified protein derivative.
RA – rheumatoid arthritis.
RAST – radioallergosorbent test.
RES – reticuloendothelial system.
RFLP – restriction fragment length
polymorphism.
RI – recombinant inbred strain.
RIA – radioimmunoassay.
RIST – radioimmunosorbent test.
SAA – serum amyloid A component.
SAP – serum amyloid P component.
SCID – severe combined
immunodeficiency.
SDS–PAGE – polyacrylamide gel
electrophoresis in sodium dodecyl
sulfate.
sIg – secreted immunoglobulin.
SLE – systemic lupus erythematosus.
SpA – protein A.
SRS-A – slow reacting substance of
anaphylaxis.
T1 – *See* CD5.
T3 – *See* CD3.
T4 – *See* CD4.

T6 – *See* CD1.

T8 – *See* CD8.

T9 – *See* TRANSFERRIN RECEPTOR.

T11 – *See* CD2.

TdT – terminal deoxynucleotidyl transferase. *See* DNA NUCLEOTIDYLEXOTRANSFERASE.

T$_C$ – cytotoxic T lymphocyte.

TC2 – transcobalamin 2. *See* TRANSCOBALAMIN 2 DEFICIENCY.

TCGF – T cell growth factor. *See* INTERLEUKIN-2, INTERLEUKIN-4.

TcR – T cell receptor.

T$_H$ – helper T lymphocyte.

Ti – T cell idiotype. *See* T CELL RECEPTOR.

Ti/T3 – T cell idiotype/CD3. *See* CD3, T CELL RECEPTOR.

TNF – tumor necrosis factor.

TPA – tetradecanoylphorbol-13-acetate. *See* PHORBOL ESTER.

TRF – thymus replacing factor. *See* INTERLEUKIN-5.

T$_S$ – suppressor T lymphocyte.

URF – unidentified reading frame.

WAS – Wiskott–Aldrich syndrome.

XLA – X-linked agammaglobulinemia.

List of CD antigens*

CD1   T6, Leu 6, common thymocyte antigen

CD2   T11, Leu 5 LFA-2, E-rosette receptor

CD3   T3, Leu 4, (part of T cell receptor complex (Ti/CD3))

CD4   T4, Leu 3, ('helper/inducer' T cell subset)

CD5   T1, Leu 1, Ly1

CD6   T12 (M_r 100,000 molecules of all T lymphocytes)

CD7   Leu 9

CD8   T8, Leu 2, ('cytotoxic/suppressor' T cell subset)

CD9   BA2 (M_r 24,000 molecule of monocytes, pre-B cells, platelets)

CD10   **common acute lymphocytic leukemia antigen (CALLA)**

CD11a   Alpha chain of **lymphocyte function associated antigen-1** (LFA-1)

CD11b   Alpha chain of **complement receptor 3** (CR3), Mac1, Mo1

CD11c   Alpha chain of **p150,95**, LeuM 5

CD13   MY7

CD14   Leu M3, Mo3, My4

CD15   Leu M1, My1

CD16   **Fcγ receptor III**, Leu 11

CD18   Beta chain of LFA-1, CR3, **p150, 95**

CD19   Leu 12, B4 (M_r 95,000 molecule of B lymphocytes)

CD20   Leu 15, B1 (M_r 35,000 molecule of B lymphocytes)

CD21   **complement receptor 2** (CR2), B2

CD22   Leu 14 (M_r 135000 molecule of B lymphocytes)

CD23   **Fcε receptor II**

CD25   Tac, **interleukin-2 receptor**

CD28   **Tp44**

CD29   4B4 (*see* **inducer T lymphocyte**)

CD32   **Fcγ receptor II**

CD35   **complement receptor 1** (CR1)

CD38   T10, Leu 17 (M_r 45,000 molecule of precursor and mature T lymphocytes, natural killer cells, monocytes)

CD40   gpIIb/IIIa on platelets

CD41   gpIb on platelets

CD43   **sialophorin**

CD45   **common leukocyte antigen**, T200, Leu 18

* defined words or symbols are in bold type.

A

a allotype. Allotype associated with the VARIABLE REGIONS of most heavy chains of rabbit IMMUNOGLOBULINS. There are three alleles: *a1*, *a2* and *a3*; in a heterozygote, both alleles are expressed. A significant fraction (10–30 percent) of heavy chains of the immunoglobulins of every rabbit do not express any of the a allotypes, i.e., are 'a-negative'. There are a number of positions in the variable regions of rabbit heavy chains at which the a allotypes differ; these allotypes, therefore, are examples of COMPLEX ALLOTYPES. *See* b ALLOTYPE.

Abelson murine leukemia virus. Retrovirus that carries the v-*abl* ONCOGENE and causes leukemia, usually of B LYMPHOCYTE lineage in mice. This virus also can transform immature B lymphocytes (from fetal liver or adult bone marrow) in culture, yielding permanent cell lines representing PRE-B CELLS or earlier stages of the B-cell differentiation pathway. Studies of these cell lines have elucidated features of immunoglobulin differentiation, including assembly of heavy and light chain IMMUNOGLOBULIN GENES and immunoglobulin CLASS SWITCHING. Abelson virus is defective and cannot replicate without a co-infecting helper retrovirus.

ABO blood group. Carbohydrate ALLOANTIGENIC determinants on the membranes of human red blood cells and other cell types, as well as on soluble proteins of body fluids, that are detected by ALLOANTIBODIES (ISOAGGLUTININS) anti-A or anti-B. All individuals fall into one of four PHENOTYPES: A, B, AB and O. The blood groups can be distinguished by patterns of agglutination of red blood cells taken from one individual by normal serum taken from another individual. For example, people who are blood group A have A determinants on their red blood cells and anti-B antibodies in their serum (*see* Table). These antibodies agglutinate red blood cells of type B or type AB. Each individual normally synthesizes those antibodies that do not react with determinants on the red blood cells of that individual (e.g., someone of blood type A synthesizes anti-B, but not anti-A). Specific immunization is not required to raise anti-A and anti-B isoagglutinins, the relevant IMMUNOGENIC determinants presumably being encountered on naturally-occurring antigens. It is supposed that individuals who have endogenous A (or B) antigenic determinants cannot make anti-A (or anti-B) antibodies because they are tolerant to these determinants. Family studies have established that the inheritance of the ABO blood groups follows simple Mendelian principles, with A and B being the products of allelic genes that are co-expressed, and O being the lack of both genes. For example, about half the children of a type AB (genotype *AB*) father and a type O (genotype *OO*) mother will be type A (genotype *AO*), the remaining children being type B (genotype *BO*). The ABO locus is on chromosome 9.

Procedures of modern blood banking have virtually eliminated transfusion reactions due to ABO incompatibility. However, ABO mismatches can be a factor in tissue GRAFT REJECTION. The anti-A and anti-B isoagglutinins are mainly of the IgM class; IgG isoagglutinins are more abundant in type O individuals. Therefore, HEMOLYTIC DISEASE OF THE NEWBORN is much more common in the offspring of type O mothers than it is in the offspring of type A or type B mothers (IgG, but not IgM, crosses the placenta).

The ABO antigenic determinants reside on the terminal sugars of oligosaccharides that are the end-products of the sequential action of a series of glycosyl transferases. Four independent genes, acting on an oligo-

2 ABO blood groups

type 1 (secretions)

H   Gal $\xrightarrow{\beta1,3}$ GlcNAc $\xrightarrow{\beta1,3}$ Gal-R

     $\alpha1,2 \uparrow$ *Se*

     Fuc

A   GalNAc $\xrightarrow{\alpha1,3}$ Gal $\xrightarrow{\beta1,3}$ GlcNAc $\xrightarrow{\beta1,3}$ Gal-R

     A $\alpha1,2 \uparrow$ *Se*

     Fuc

B   Gal $\xrightarrow{\alpha1,3}$ Gal $\xrightarrow{\beta1,3}$ GlcNAc $\xrightarrow{\beta1,3}$ Gal-R

     B $\alpha1,2 \uparrow$ *Se*

     Fuc

Le^a Gal $\xrightarrow{\beta1,3}$ GlcNAc $\xrightarrow{\beta1,3}$ Gal-R

     $\alpha1,4 \uparrow$ *Le*

     Fuc

Le^b Gal $\xrightarrow{\beta1,3}$ GlcNAc $\xrightarrow{\beta1,3}$ Gal-R

     $\alpha1,2 \uparrow$ *Se* $\alpha1,4 \uparrow$ *Le*

     Fuc   Fuc

---

type 2 (red blood cells)

H   Gal $\xrightarrow{\beta1,4}$ GlcNAc $\xrightarrow{\beta1,3}$ Gal-R

     $\alpha1,2 \uparrow$ *H*

     Fuc

A   GalNAc $\xrightarrow{\alpha1,3}$ Gal $\xrightarrow{\beta1,4}$ GlcNAc $\xrightarrow{\beta1,3}$ Gal-R

     A $\alpha1,2 \uparrow$ *H*

     Fuc

B   Gal $\xrightarrow{\alpha1,3}$ Gal $\xrightarrow{\beta1,4}$ GlcNAc $\xrightarrow{\beta1,3}$ Gal-R

     B $\alpha1,2 \uparrow$ *H*

     Fuc

Gal, D-galactose; GalNAc, N-acetyl-D-galactosamine; GlcNAc, *N*-acetyl-D-glucosamine; Fuc, L-fucose saccharide precursor, are involved in the synthesis of these determinants, as well as in the synthesis of the Lewis (Le) antigenic determinants, which may occur on the same oligosaccharide moiety that expresses ABO. The four genes are: (1) A/B; (2) Se; (3) H; and (4) Le. The Se and H genes are tightly linked, and each encodes a distinct galactoside ($\alpha 1$–2) fucosyl transferase. There is no linkage between any other gene pair. The final ABO product can exist in a lipid-associated form (in cell membranes) or in water-soluble form (attached to a protein backbone in secretions). There are two types of precursors, designated type 1 and type 2.

type 1: Gal($\beta 1$–3)GlcNAc($\beta 1$–3)Gal–R
type 2: Gal($\beta 1$–4)GlcNAc($\beta 1$–3)Gal–R

The only difference between the two types is that the terminal galactose in linked to the penultimate N-acetylglucosamine in $\beta 1$–3 linkage in type 1 chains and in $\beta 1$–4 linkage in type 2 chains. Red blood cells possess mainly type 2 chains. Fucose is added in $\alpha 1$–2 linkage to the terminal galactose, a step that is catalysed by the transferase encoded by the Se or H genes. The Se gene is expressed in epithelial tissues and the corresponding enzyme acts preferentially on type 1 chains. The H gene is expressed in tissues of mesodermal origin; this enzyme acts preferentially on type 2 chains and is also found in serum. After the addition of fucose, the oligosaccharide is known as 'H substance'. Next, two different glycosyl transferases, encoded by the A or B genes, add N-acetylgalactosamine or galactose, respectively, to the terminal galactose of H substance, thereby forming the A or B blood group substances. The A or B determinant seems to consist of the terminal group of three or four sugars, not only the monosaccharide added by the A or B gene product.

Rare individauls lack gene H (are genotype hh); the corresponding fucosyl transferase cannot be detected in serum and fucose is not added to type 2 chains, so that H substance is not formed and the enzymes specified by the A and B genes do not have the appropriate substrate. Accordingly, the red blood cells of such individuals cannot express the A or B antigenic determinants. This condition is known as the Bombay phenotype. If the Se gene is present, A or B substances can be formed on type 1 chains and the corresponding determinant detected in secretions (the 'para-Bombay' phenotype).

The Le gene encodes a transferase that adds a fucose residue in $\alpha 1$–4 linkage to the penultimate N-acetylglucosamine of type 1 chains. (This enzyme cannot act on type 2 chains because the 4-position of the N-acetylglucosamine is preempted by the $\beta 1$–4 linkage to the galactose.) In the absence of Se activity (i.e., no fucose on the terminal galactose), the resulting antigenic determinant is known as Le^a. If the Le and Se genes act in concert, fucose is added to both the penultimate N-acetylglucosamine and to the terminal galactose, producing the Le^b antigenic determinant. Non-secretors (who lack the Se gene) cannot express the Le^b determinant, but may be Le^a. Since the enzyme encoded by the Le gene does not act on type 2 chains, the Lewis antigenic determinants are not endogenous to red blood cells. However, they may be detected on such cells due to passive ADSORPTION of glycolipid antigen from serum.

aboriginal mouse. Mouse that has never lived in close association with humans.

absorption. Removal of antibodies from an antiserum by addition of antigen or removal of antigens from a mixture by addition of antibodies. For example, this procedure can be used to render an antiserum specific for a

Blood group	Genotype	Antibodies in serum	Frequency (%)		
			Caucasian	Blacks	Orientals
A	AA or AO	anti-B	41	28	38
B	BB or BO	anti-A	11	17	22
O	OO	anti-A and -B	45	51	30
AB	AB	none	3	4	10

Modified from Stites, D. P., Stobo, J. D., Fudenberg, H. H., and Wells, J. V. Basic and Clinical Immunology, 5th edition, Lange Med. Pub., Los Altos, Ca (1984).

single antigen (or ANTIGENIC DETERMINANT) by removing antibodies to contaminants or to related antigens. Absorption refers to reactions between soluble antigens and antibodies. *See* ADSORPTION.

accessory cell.   Non-lymphocytic cell (DENDRITIC CELL, LANGERHANS CELL, MONONUCLEAR PHAGOCYTE) that helps in the induction of IMMUNE RESPONSES by presenting antigen to HELPER T LYMPHOCYTES. B LYMPHOCYTES can assume the function of accessory cells in ANTIGEN PRESENTATION.

acquired agammaglobulinemia. *See* COMMON VARIABLE IMMUNODEFICIENCY.

acquired C1 inhibitor deficiency.   Syndrome characterized by recurrent episodes of swelling of subcutaneous tissues, intestine and larynx. The symptoms are due to increased destruction of C1 INHIBITOR so that increased cleavage of C4 and C2 occurs when C1 is activated. A KININ-like peptide generated from C2b, which enhances vascular permeability, appears to cause the symptoms. Acquired C1 inhibitor deficiency occurs in patients with monoclonal proliferation of B LYMPHOCYTES or PLASMA CELLS (e.g., MULTIPLE MYELOMA, B cell LYMPHOMA, MACROGLOBULINEMIA OF WALDENSTRÖM) who also have ANTI-IDIOTYPIC ANTIBODIES to MEMBRANE IMMUNOGLOBULINS or to MYELOMA PROTEINS. The reaction of anti-idiotypic antibodies with the IDIOTYPE of the membrane immunoglobulin or myeloma protein leads to fixation of C1 and increased consumption of C4 and C2 and, for unknown reasons, increased consumption of C1 inhibitor. Acquired C1 inhibitor deficiency may also result from the reaction of C1 inhibitor with AUTOANTIBODIES. *See* HEREDITARY ANGIONEUROTIC EDEMA.

acquired immunodeficiency syndrome (AIDS).   Form of IMMUNODEFICIENCY that results from infection with a LYMPHOCYTOTROPIC virus, called HUMAN IMMUNODEFICIENCY VIRUS (HIV). HIV INFECTION can cause profound LYMPHOPENIA, primarily of the CD4 subset of T LYMPHOCYTES. Affected individuals have decreased or absent DELAYED-TYPE HYPERSENSITIVITY, extreme susceptibility to OPPORTUNISTIC INFECTIONS and may acquire certain unusual malignancies, such as KAPOSI'S SARCOMA or BURKITT'S LYMPHOMA. HIV also causes polyclonal expansion of B LYMPHOCYTES, leading to HYPERGAMMAGLOBULINEMIA. Despite the marked increase in amounts of IMMUNOGLOBULINS in serum, affected individuals are incapable of mounting a PRIMARY IMMUNE RESPONSE to newly encountered antigens. The syndrome has been recognized almost exclusively in 'at risk' groups, including homosexually active males, intravenous drug abusers, recipients of blood or blood products, and certain populations from Central Africa and the Caribbean. The syndrome has also been recognized in heterosexual partners of individuals in all 'at risk' groups and in infants of affected mothers. AIDS is almost invariably fatal. *See* AIDS-RELATED COMPLEX, HIV INFECTION, PEDIATRIC AIDS.

activated macrophage.   Macrophage (MONONUCLEAR PHAGOCYTE) that has increased microbicidal and tumoricidal activity compared to resting macrophages. Activated macrophages are approximately twice the size of resting macrophages, have an increased content of cytoplasmic organelles, especially lysosomes, tend to spread on wettable surfaces (e.g., glass) and develop ruffled borders. Macrophages are activated by lymphokines, especially by INTEFERON-GAMMA, which induces increased expression of CLASS II HISTOCOMPATIBILITY MOLECULES. Activated macrophages are essential in resistance to intracellular pathogenic microorganisms (e.g., Mycobacteria, Toxoplasma).

active immunity.   Immunity acquired as a result of stimulation with antigen after a natural infection or any other exposure to antigen. *See* PASSIVE IMMUNITY.

acute disseminated encephalomyelitis. INFLAMMATION of the brain following an acute viral infection usually of childhood (e.g., measles). It also may occur after smallpox vaccination or in recipients of rabies vaccine prepared in neural tissue. Patients develop headache, stiff neck, confusion and coma. The cerebrospinal fluid contains increased amounts of protein and mononuclear cells. There are perivascular infiltrates of NEUTROPHILS, LYMPHOCYTES and PLASMA CELLS. EXPERIMENTAL ALLERGIC

ENCEPHALOMYELITIS is a laboratory model for this disease.

acute phase reaction. Change in the rates of synthesis of certain serum proteins during inflammation. There is increased synthesis of C-REACTIVE PROTEIN, SERUM AMYLOID A COMPONENT, haptoglobin, ceruloplasmin, alpha-l antitrypsin and most of the COMPLEMENT components and decreased synthesis of SERUM ALBUMIN and transferrin. The acute phase reaction is induced by INTERLEUKIN-1, INTERLEUKIN-6 and TUMOR NECROSIS FACTOR. The acute phase reaction rapidly protects the host against microorganisms by bringing about an increase in proteins that are important in non-specific defense mechanisms (e.g., OPSONIZATION by complement components).

acute post-streptococcal glomerulonephritis (AGN). Benign form of IMMUNE COMPLEX DISEASE of the renal glomeruli, which occurs mainly in children 10–21 days following a streptococcal infection of the skin or pharynx. AGN is characterized by the sudden onset of hematuria (blood in the urine). Only infections with types 1, 4, 12 and 49 group A streptococci precede the nephritis, and hence these strains are called nephritogenic. Serum levels of C3 are decreased. IgG and C3, presumably complexed to streptococcal antigens, are deposited in the renal glomeruli, as demonstrated by IMMUNOFLUORESCENCE. See GLOMERULONEPHRITIS.

acute rheumatic fever. Febrile illness characterized by inflammation of connective tissue, the heart (carditis) and joints (arthritis), which usually follows a throat infection by group A streptococci. The arthritis is typically migratory, involving several joints in succession. The carditis can lead to scarring of the heart valves. Very high titers of antibodies to streptococcal antigens are found in the serum. Some of the antibodies (e.g., to the M protein of the streptococcal cell wall) cross-react with ANTIGENIC DETERMINANTS of human myocardium. In the heart tissues, massive deposition of IgG and COMPLEMENT has been found by IMMUNOFLUORESCENCE. Acute rheumatic fever is thought to be an AUTOIMMUNE DISEASE.

Addison's disease. Adrenal failure resulting from destruction of the adrenal cortex by infection (e.g., tuberculosis) or by AUTOIMMUNE DISEASE. The adrenal architecture is usually disrupted by a heavy infiltration of LYMPHOCYTES. The serum frequently contains AUTOANTIBODIES to adrenal cortical cells. Addison's disease is often associated with autoimmune disease of the thyroid, PERNICIOUS ANEMIA, INSULIN-DEPENDENT DIABETES MELLITUS and hypoparathyroidism.

adenosine deaminase deficiency. Form of SEVERE COMBINED IMMUNODEFICIENCY that results from the inheritance of mutant forms of adenosine deaminase (EC 3.5.4.4) (ADA). The immunodeficiency is caused by accumulation of metabolites that are toxic for T and B LYMPHOCYTES. ADA, which is present in all mammalian cells, catalyses deamination of adenosine and deoxyadenosine. ADA deficiency results in increased intracellular concentrations of adenosine, deoxyadenosine, adenosine triphosphate (ATP), deoxyadenosine triphosphate (dATP) and S-adenosyl homocysteine. dATP inhibits ribonucleoside-diphosphate reductase, an enzyme involved in DNA synthesis. Adenosine inhibits S-adenosyl homocysteine hydrolase, an enzyme involved in the S-adenosyl methionine-dependent pathway of DNA methylation. Precursors of B and T lymphocytes are more vulnerable to destruction by the accumulation of these metabolites than are other cells. ADA is relatively abundant in lymphoid tissue and is present in greatest concentration in THYMUS.

The gene encoding ADA has been mapped to chromosome 20q13-ter and encodes a single polypeptide chain (M_r 38,000) of 363 amino acid residues. In almost all cases of ADA deficiency, mRNA of normal size is present in normal or increased amounts. ADA deficiency is inherited as an autosomal recessive. Levels of ADA (usually measured in red blood cells) are half-normal in heterozygotes. ADA is absent from red blood cells of a few individuals who are not immunodeficient. In such cases, T lymphocytes contain mutant ADA with <10 percent of normal function but sufficient to prevent accumulation of toxic amounts of dATP.

ADA deficiency has been treated successfully with transplants of bone marrow cells or by intravenous infusion of ADA conjugated to polyethylene glycol. Recently, retrovirus VECTORS containing cDNA for

ADA have been transfected into bone marrow cells, with the aim of correcting ADA deficiency.

adherent cell. Cell that adheres to surfaces *in vitro*. The term is usually used to refer to MONONUCLEAR PHAGOCYTES. Since B and T LYMPHOCYTES are non-adherent, lymphocytes and macrophages can be separated on the basis of this property.

adjuvant. Substance that enhances, nonspecifically, the IMMUNE RESPONSE to an antigen. An adjuvant is usually administered with antigen, but may also be given before or after antigen. *See* FREUND'S ADJUVANT.

adjuvant disease. Form of arthritis induced in rats by injection of COMPLETE FREUND'S ADJUVANT. The disease is characterized by an acute sterile inflammation of several joints. Adjuvant disease is thought to be a laboratory model for RHEUMATOID ARTHRITIS.

adoptive transfer. Transfer of immunological reactivity by lymphocytes from a primed donor to an unprimed recipient. *See* ACTIVE IMMUNITY, PASSIVE IMMUNITY.

adsorption. Noncovalent binding of a molecule to a cell or particle: for example, antibodies are adsorbed to antigens on a surface. *See* ABSORPTION.

adult T-cell leukemia-lymphoma (ATLL). Rapidly progressive malignancy of mature T LYMPHOCYTES. The original cases were observed in southeastern Japan, but the disease has since been found in patients from the Caribbean Islands, parts of Africa and the southeastern United States. Lymphoma nodules are frequently present in the skin and LYMPH NODES and also in the SPLEEN and liver. Hypercalcemia is often present whether or not there are bone lesions. The causative agent of ATLL is usually the retrovirus HTLV-I (*see* HUMAN IMMUNODEFICIENCY VIRUS), although another retrovirus HTLV–II has been cultured from a few cases. The first isolate of HTLV–II was from a patient with hairy cell leukemia. The membrane phenotype of ATLL cells corresponds to that of a mature T lymphocyte bearing CD4 molecules. In addition, these cells bear receptors for INTERLEUKIN-2. There appears to be a longitudinal transmission of HTLV-I from mother to fetus. HTLV-I was the first retrovirus associated with cancer in humans. Its pathogenic effect *in vitro* is an uncontrolled proliferation of CD4+ T lymphocytes.

affinity. Measure of the reversible interaction between two molecules (e.g., an antibody and a LIGAND). In immunology, the term affinity is frequently used as a synonym for ASSOCIATION CONSTANT, although it is also used in a more qualitative sense. *See* AVIDITY, FUNCTIONAL AFFINITY, INTRINSIC ASSOCIATION CONSTANT.

affinity chromatography. Chromatographic procedure in which a mixture of substances is resolved by differential ADSORPTION to a matrix containing a determinant that reacts preferentially with one or more of these substances.

affinity labeling. Technique for specific covalent attachment of a LIGAND (HAPTEN or substrate) to the active site of an ANTIBODY or enzyme, respectively. The ligand contains a chemically reactive substituent (e.g., a diazonium group) capable of forming a covalent bond with an amino acid side chain. The ligand is specifically bound to the active site and forms a covalent bond with an amino acid residue in or near the site. To facilitate localization of the affinity-labelled residue, the ligand my be tagged, e.g., with a radioisotope.

agammaglobulinemia. Decreased amount of serum IMMUNOGLOBULIN. Immunoglobulins are not absent so the term hypogammaglobulinemia would be more accurate. Agammaglobulinemia may be primary (*see* ANTIBODY DEFICIENCY SYNDROME) due to decreased immunoglobulin synthesis, or secondary due to loss of immunoglobulin into the gut or through the skin as may occur in INFLAMMATORY BOWEL DISEASE or burns, respectively.

agar Complex acidic mucilaginous polysaccharide extracted from algae having the property of melting at 100°C and solidifying into a gel when cooled to approximately 45° C. The major components of agar are agaropectin (a sulfated polymer of D-galactose) and AGAROSE. Agar gels are used

for growing bacteria and for IMMUNODIFFU-
SION.

agarose. Linear polymer of alternating
D-galactose and 3,6-anhydrogalactose, the
major component of AGAR. Agarose gels are
used in IMMUNODIFFUSION and for ELECTRO-
PHORESIS of nucleic acids and proteins.

agglutination. Clumping of particulate
antigens (e.g., red blood cells, bacteria) as
by antibodies. Agglutination may be
observed grossly or microscopically, and
may be used as a test to measure antigen or
antibody.

agglutinin. ANTIBODY that agglutinates
cells or particles. At one time, it was thought
that the ability to bring about AGGLU-
TINATION was the property of a particular
antibody. It is now known that most antibodies can cause agglutination provided they
are directed to ANTIGENIC DETERMINANTS on
the surface of the cell or particle.

agglutinogen. Particulate antigen that is
agglutinated by antibodies (e.g., type A red
blood cell).

agranulocytosis. Marked decrease of
granulocytes, i.e., NEUTROPHILS, BASOPHILS
and EOSINOPHILS in the blood. *Synonym for*
granulocytopenia.

agretope. In ANTIGEN PRESENTATION, the
part of a protein antigen that interacts with a
CLASS II HISTOCOMPATIBILITY MOLECULE. It is
believed that different amino acid sequences
in a protein vary in their interaction with the
alleles of the class II histocompatibility
molecules. Agretope is derived from *a*ntigen
*r*estriction *e*lement. *See* DESETOPE, HISTO-
TOPE, RESTITOPE.

AIDS. *See* ACQUIRED IMMUNODEFICIENCY
SYNDROME.

AIDS-related complex (ARC). Conste-
lation of symptoms, including fever, night
sweats, swollen lymph nodes and weight loss
that occurs in some individuals following
infection with HUMAN IMMUNODEFICIENCY
VIRUS (HIV). ARC differs from full-blown
ACQUIRED IMMUNE DEFICIENCY SYNDROME
(AIDS) in that patients with ARC do not
have OPPORTUNISTIC INFECTIONS or malignan-

cies. In approximately 10 percent of cases,
ARC progresses rapidly (within 12 months)
to AIDS. *See* HIV INFECTION.

albumin. Protein that is characterized by
its solubility in water, as distinct from
GLOBULIN, which is insoluble or only sparingly soluble in water. Albumins are also
soluble in solutions of half-saturated ammonium sulfate. Examples of albumins are
SERUM ALBUMIN, the major protein component of SERUM, and ovalbumin, the major
protein in egg white.

Aleutian mink disease. Chronic fatal infection of mink and ferrets caused by a parvo-
virus. The infection results in a polyclonal
expansion of B LYMPHOCYTES and remark-
able HYPERGAMMAGLOBULINEMIA ($\sim$100 mg
IgG/ml). PLASMA CELLS and LYMPHOCYTES
infiltrate the viscera, and immune complexes
(*see* ANTIGEN–ANTIBODY COMPLEX) are deposited in the renal glomeruli. In severe forms
of the disease, the small and medium-sized
arteries of the heart, brain and kidney are
inflamed as a result of immune complex
deposition.

alexin. *Synonym for* COMPLEMENT.

alkaline phosphatase (AP). (EC 3.1.3.1).
Phosphomonoesterase that is active at alkaline pH. AP is a Zn^{2+} metalloenzyme
present in nearly all organisms, except some
plants. Human AP consists of three tissue-
specific forms (isozymes) encoded by at least
three genes. The different forms of AP are
found in placenta, intestine and liver/bone/
kidney. These APs are membrane-bound
glycoproteins consisting of a single polypeptide chain of approximately 500 amino acid
residues. The physiological role of AP is not
known, although it is thought to play a role
in bone mineralization.

   Alkaline phosphatase, usually from calf
intestine, is used for a variety of purposes in
immunological procedures and in molecular
cloning. It is widely used in enzyme-linked
immunoassays (*see* ELISA) and in IMMU-
NOBLOTTING. AP removes 5′-phosphate
groups from the ends of linear DNA. In the
preparation of DNA recombinants the
VECTOR, after cleavage with a RESTRICTION
ENDONUCLEASE, is usually treated with AP to
prevent recircularization, thereby reducing
the background of vector DNA. Genomic

DNA fragments that will be cloned are treated with the enzyme so that two or more fragments cannot ligate to each other. AP is also used to prepare 5'-[^{32}P]-end-labeled DNA or RNA fragments; the fragments are treated with the enzyme before incubation with POLYNUCLEOTIDE 5'-HYDROXYLKINASE in the presence of [γ-^{32}P]-ATP.

allele. Variant of a gene at a particular genetic locus.

allelic exclusion. Expression, in a single cell, of only one ALLELE at a particular locus. Allelic exclusion is characteristic of the expression of IMMUNOGLOBULIN GENES. Thus, in individuals who are heterozygous for ALLOTYPES at an IMMUNOGLOBULIN HEAVY or LIGHT CHAIN gene locus, individual PLASMA CELLS express only one or the other allele, but not both.

allergen. Antigen that induces ALLERGY. Common environmental allergens are globular proteins in pollens (from RAGWEED, grasses, trees), animal danders, insect venoms, and various foods. Certain individuals are prone to respond to allergens by producing antibodies of the IgE class. *See* ATOPY.

allergic bronchopulmonary aspergillosis. Form of ASTHMA due to pulmonary infection with fungi of the genus Aspergillus. The lung contains GRANULOMAS with many EOSINOPHILS. Patients have EOSINOPHILIA and elevated levels of IgE in the serum.

allergic contact dermatitis. Inflammation of skin that is a manifestation of a DELAYED-TYPE HYPERSENSITIVITY REACTION elicited by contact with a variety of low molecular weight (usually $M_r < 1,000$) chemicals. The sensitizing chemicals are usually hydrophobic and, after penetrating the intact skin, form covalent derivatives with skin proteins. Contact with the sensitizing chemical evokes redness and swelling of the skin beginning at about 12 hours and reaching maximal intensity in 24 – 48 hours. The affected skin develops blisters that may ooze and form crusts; the rash is intensely pruritic (itchy). The dermis is invaded by MONONUCLEAR PHAGOCYTES, LYMPHOCYTES and BASOPHILS; the blisters are filled with serum, NEUTROPHILS and mononuclear phagocytes. A great number of synthetic chemicals (e.g., drugs, cosmetics) as well as naturally occurring chemicals (e.g., catechols of poison ivy leaves) can be sensitizers. Reactive dinitrobenzene derivatives (e.g., DNFB, DNCB) have been used to elicit allergic contact dermatitis in humans and in experimental animals. *See* PATCH TEST.

allergic granulomatosis. Form of pulmonary VASCULITIS, frequently associated with ASTHMA. In addition to necrotizing vasculitis, GRANULOMAS form in the lung or in the walls of pulmonary vessels.

allergic orchitis. Experimental AUTOIMMUNE DISEASE induced in guinea-pigs by immunization with AUTOLOGOUS testicular extracts in COMPLETE FREUND'S ADJUVANT. After two to eight weeks, the guinea-pigs develop lymphocytic infiltrates in the testes and cytotoxic antibodies to sperm. Allergic orchitis may occur in men following vasectomy.

allergic rhinitis. IgE-mediated inflammation of the nasal mucosa. Patients experience nasal stuffiness, sneezing and rhinorrhea (runny nose). Nasal secretions from patients with allergic rhinitis contain elevated IgE concentrations. The disease may be seasonal, related to annual variations in the respiratory ALLERGENS. *Synonym for* hay fever.

allergy. Untoward reactivity to commonly encountered environmental antigens (e.g., pollen, food, insect venom). The term allergy was first used by von Pirquet in 1906. Environmental antigens that incite allergies are called ALLERGENS. *See* HYPERSENSITIVITY.

alloantibody. Antibody reacting with an ALLOANTIGEN.

alloantigen. Antigen found only in some members of a species (e.g., BLOOD GROUP SUBSTANCES).

allogeneic. Referring to genetic variants within a species.

allogeneic effect. Experimental phenomenon in which B LYMPHOCYTES specific for a hapten (e.g., DINITROPHENYL GROUP) make antibodies in the presence of allogeneic

T LYMPHOCYTES without requiring CARRIER-specific T lymphocytes. The allogeneic T lymphocytes upon reacting with CLASS II HISTOCOMPATIBILITY MOLECULES of the B lymphocytes, produce LYMPHOKINES that bring about the differentiation of the B lymphocytes to PLASMA CELLS.

allograft. GRAFT to a genetically different member of the same species. Allografts are rejected by virtue of an immunological response of T LYMPHOCYTES to histocompatibility antigens (*see* CLASS I and CLASS II HISTOCOMPATIBILITY MOLECULES). The time of rejection varies with the tissue grafted (e.g., seven to ten days with skin). *Synonym for* homograft.

allogroup. Group of ALLOTYPES, associated with different IMMUNOGLOBULIN CLASSES and subclasses, that tend to be inherited together. The heavy chains of the immunoglobulins in an allogroup are encoded by a set of closely-linked alleles. For example, one allogroup found frequently in Caucasians is G1m(1,17), G2m(23−), G3m(21), G4m(4a), A2m(1), reflecting the linkage of the associated heavy chain genes (i.e., $C_{\gamma 1}$, $C_{\gamma 2}$, $C_{\gamma 3}$, $C_{\gamma 4}$, $C_{\alpha 2}$). Although recombination within an allogroup is rare within families, some recombination has occurred during the course of human evolution, as the predominant allogroups of different races are genetically related to one another by recombinational events. An allogroup is an example of a HAPLOTYPE.

alloimmunization. IMMUNIZATION with an ALLOANTIGEN, such as occurs in HEMOLYTIC DISEASE OF THE NEWBORN.

allophenic mouse. Chimeric mouse resulting from the aggregation of two genetically different early (e.g., 8-cell) embryos. The cells form a single blastocyst, which is then transferred to the uterus of a pseudopregnant female (mated with a sterile male) and allowed to develop to term. Allophenic mice are also called tetraparental, as they have genetic material from four different parents. They have been used to study cell interactions and development and, in immunology, transplantation TOLERANCE.

allotope. ANTIGENIC DETERMINANT of an ALLOTYPE. *Synonym for* ALLOTYPIC DETERMINANT.

allotype. Set of ALLOTYPIC DETERMINANTS on an IMMUNOGLOBULIN HEAVY CHAIN or LIGHT CHAIN; alternatively, the chain (or IMMUNOGLOBULIN molecule) carrying these determinants. Allotypes are the products of allelic genes encoding immunoglobulin heavy or light chains. Because the allele encoding a given allotype segregates in a random-bred population, a given allotype is found in some, but not all, individuals of a species. Although the term allotype was introduced to describe allelic variation in immunoglobulins, it is now also used to describe similar variation in other proteins. *See* a ALLOTYPE, ALLOANTIGEN, ALLOTYPIC DETERMINANT, Am ALLOTYPE, b ALLOTYPE, COMPLEX ALLOTYPE, Gm ALLOTYPE, Km ALLOTYPE, SIMPLE ALLOTYPE.

allotypic determinant. ANTIGENIC DETERMINANT found on the IMMUNOGLOBULINS (or on other proteins) of some, but not all, individuals of a species. Allotypic determinants are the result of genetic POLYMORPHISM. Although an allotypic determinant typically reflects variations in the primary structure of either an IMMUNOGLOBULIN HEAVY or LIGHT CHAIN, the determinant (as measured by reaction with specific antisera) may or may not be expressed on an isolated chain; in some cases expression of the determinant may require association of heavy and light chains. Usually, a given allotypic determinant is IMMUNOGENIC in other individuals of the species, i.e., in those individuals that do not express that particular determinant on their immunoglobulins. *See* ALLOTYPE, Am ALLOTYPIC DETERMINANT, Gm ALLOTYPIC DETERMINANT, IDIOTYPIC DETERMINANT, ISOTYPIC DETERMINANT, Km ALLOTYPIC DETERMINANT. *Synonym for* allotope.

allotypy. Property, possessed by certain proteins such as IMMUNOGLOBULINS, of existing in several allelic forms or ALLOTYPES.

alpha-fetoprotein. One of the major serum proteins in the human fetus. Alpha-fetoprotein is a single polypeptide chain comprising 590 amino acid residues and is homologous (approximately 40 percent identity) to human serum albumin. It is synthesized by yolk sac and fetal liver cells, and is found in high concentrations in fetal serum and amniotic fluid; after birth, the concentration in serum drops rapidly to virtually undetectable levels. Alpha-fetoprotein is of interest in immunology because of its immunosuppressive effect (*see* IMMUNOSUPPRESSION), which may be important in neonatal TOLERANCE to antigens. In culture, alpha-fetoprotein decreases HELPER T LYMPHOCYTE reactivity and promotes SUPPRESSOR T LYMPHOCYTE activity. The concentration of alpha-fetoprotein is markedly increased in the serum of patients with cancer of the liver, and in some cases of tumors of the ovary or testis.

alpha heavy chain disease. Form of MYELOMATOSIS characterized by the presence in serum and urine of abnormal monoclonal IMMUNOGLOBULIN ALPHA CHAINS. The disease is found almost exclusively in the Near East and North Africa, and is almost always associated with gastrointestinal LYMPHOMA. Patients have malabsorption, weight loss, diarrhea, steatorrhea (fatty stools) and abdominal pains. Cells producing the alpha chains infiltrate the lamina propria of the intestine; unlike multiple myeloma, bone lesions are not seen. A few cases in children, both in Europe and in North America, have been associated with infiltration of the lung by cells producing alpha chains. The alpha chains have diverse internal deletions, no associated IMMUNOGLOBULIN LIGHT CHAINS, and are almost always alpha1, i.e., of the IgA1 subclass (*see* IgA and IMMUNOGLOBULIN ALPHA CHAIN). In most cases, the disease is fatal, although total remissions have been reported.

alpha-helix. Helical structure found in many polypeptides and proteins, characterized by a periodicity of 3.6 amino acid residues (0.54 nm) per turn of the helix. Thus, each residue is related to the next by a translation of 0.15 nm and a rotation of 100°. The peptide group and the alpha-carbon form the backbone of the helix. Hydrogen bonds nearly parallel to the long axis of the helix are formed between the carbonyl oxygen of each residue and the amide nitrogen of the fourth residue ahead (i.e., toward the carboxy terminus) in the linear sequence. Thus, all the –CO and –NH groups in the backbone are involved in hydrogen bonds. The side chains of the amino acid residues extend out from the helix. An alpha-helix can be either right- or left-handed, but all the alpha-helices in

proteins are right-handed. Segments of alpha-helix are prominent in many globular proteins (e.g., hemoglobin, lysozyme), but are not found in the IMMUNOGLOBULIN FOLD. Two or more alpha-helices can be wrapped around each other to form a coiled coil, as in keratin (of hair), myosin and tropomyosin (of muscle) and fibrin (of blood clots). *See* BETA-PLEATED SHEET, SECONDARY STRUCTURE.

alternative pathway of complement. One of two possible mechanisms (the other being the CLASSICAL PATHWAY OF COMPLEMENT) for the activation of C3. Unlike the classical pathway, activation of the alternative pathway, which is not well understood, is not dependent on antibodies. The proteins of the alternative pathway are C3b, FACTOR B and FACTOR D. C3b binds Factor B to form the complex, C3bB. Factor B in the complex is cleaved by Factor D into an active fragment, Bb, which remains bound to C3b, and an inactive fragment, Ba, which is released. C3bBb is the alternative pathway C3 CONVERTASE; the catalytic site of the enzyme lies in the Bb fragment. The cleavage of C3 into C3b and C3a by C3bBb generates more C3bBb; thus the alternative pathway is a positive feedback mechanism. The alternative pathway is inhibited by FACTOR I, which, in the presence of FACTOR H, cleaves the heavy chain of C3b, producing C3bi; C3bi cannot bind Bb and is therefore inactive in the alternative pathway. C3bBb is stabilized by PROPERDIN and by C3 NEPHRITIC FACTOR.

C3 ⟶ C3b + C3a
+
Factor B
↓
C3bB
↓ ← Factor D
C3bBb + Ba
↓
Factor H }⟶
Factor I }
C3bi + Bb + C3f

alternative pathway

alum-precipitated antigen. Antigen absorbed onto floccules of aluminum salts that act as an ADJUVANT. In practice, a protein antigen in solution is mixed with 1 percent potassium aluminum sulfate and increasing amounts of sodium hydroxide are added until floccules form. For primary IMMUNIZATION, diphtheria and tetanus TOXOIDS are administered as alum-precipitated antigens.

alveolar macrophage. MACROPHAGE in the alveoli of the lung. Alveolar macrophages are involved in the uptake of small air-borne particles.

Am allotype. Human IMMUNOGLOBULIN ALPHA CHAIN (or IgA molecule) carrying an Am ALLOTYPIC DETERMINANT. There are two allotypes of the IgA2 subclass, one carrying the A2m(1) and the other the A2m(2) determinant. These allotypes are the products of allelic genes at the *A2m* locus (the gene encoding the constant region of the alpha2 heavy chain).

Am allotypic determinant. ALLOTYPIC DETERMINANT of heavy chains of human IgA. A2m(1) and A2m(2) are allotypic determinants of the IgA2 subclass; these determinants reflect variations in primary structure of the alpha2 heavy chains. No allotypic determinants are known for the IgA1 subclass.

amboceptor. Antibodies that are used to sensitize sheep red blood cells for COMPLEMENT-mediated HEMOLYSIS. The term was introduced by Paul Ehrlich because he thought that these antibodies had one combining site for sheep red blood cells and another for complement. *See* FORSSMAN ANTIGEN.

aminophylline. *See* THEOPHYLLINE.

amyloidosis. Group of disorders that result from the deposition of amyloid in tissues leading to functional impairment of organs (e.g., kidneys, heart and gastrointestinal tract). The amyloid deposits consist of 4–6 nm protein filaments, which form long, twisting fibrils that stain metachromatically with toluidine blue or crystal violet, bind Congo red avidly, and give green birefringence with polarized light. Primary amyloidosis is associated with MULTIPLE MYELOMA and MACROGLOBULINEMIA OF WALDENSTRÖM. The deposits in this condition consist of IMMUNOGLOBULIN LIGHT CHAINS or portions of light chains and are found principally in the tongue, heart, skeletal muscle, skin, ligaments and gastrointestinal tract. Secondary amyloidosis can be associated with any chronic inflammatory disease (e.g., RHEUMATOID ARTHRITIS, INFLAMMATORY BOWEL DISEASE). The deposits in secondary amyloidosis infiltrate principally spleen, liver and kidney. They consist of two components: (1) fibrils of amyloid A protein (AA), a proteolytic fragment (M_r 8,000) derived from a serum alpha-globulin (SERUM AMYLOID A COMPONENT), which forms 85–90 percent of the deposits, and (2) discs of SERUM AMYLOID P COMPONENT, which form the remainder of the deposits. A form of amyloidosis is inherited as an autosomal dominant and is characterized by the deposition of a variant form of plasma prealbumin.

anamnestic response. *Synonym for* SECONDARY IMMUNE RESPONSE.

anaphylactoid shock. Phenomenon resembling ANAPHYLAXIS but induced by non-immunological means. For example, bee or certain snake venoms can induce systemic HISTAMINE release, thereby causing symptoms characteristic of anaphylaxis.

anaphylatoxin inactivator. Serum carboxypeptidase N. It cleaves carboxy-terminal arginine residues from C5a, C3a and C4a, thereby destroying their anaphylatoxic activity.

anaphylatoxin. Substance that is generated in serum following the addition of aggregated immunoglobulins, immune complexes or complex polysaccharides and that contracts smooth muscles. The three known anaphylotoxins C5a, C3a, and C4a are peptides cleaved from complement components C5, C3 and C4, respectively. Following injection of these peptides into the skin, MAST CELLS degranulate, HISTAMINE is released, and a wheal and flare reaction occurs. *See* URTICARIA.

anaphylaxis. Acute reaction that follows the rapid introduction of an antigen into an individual having pre-existing antibodies of the IgE class (or of the IgG1 subclass in some species). In systemic anaphylaxis, the reactions develop within seconds and are characterized by difficulty in breathing due to constriction of the larynx and bronchi and shock due to falling blood pressure. The symptoms vary in different species according to the tissue or organ that is primarily affected. The binding of antigen to IgE on MAST CELLS or BASOPHILS triggers the release of mediators. The primary (preformed) mediators of anaphylaxis are: HISTAMINE, SEROTONIN, EOSINOPHIL CHEMOTACTIC FACTORS, HEPARIN and a variety of enzymes (e.g., chymase, N-acetyl-β-glucosamini-dase). Secondary mediators (synthesized after antigen is bound and released more slowly) are: SLOW REACTING SUBSTANCE OF ANAPHYLAXIS (SRS-A), PLATELET-ACTIVATING FACTOR and BRADYKININ. In humans, the major causes of anaphylaxis are drugs (e.g., penicillin) or insect stings (e.g., bee venom).

Local anaphylactic reactions are acute inflammatory reactions caused by local contact with antigen, usually in the skin, nasal membranes or gastrointestinal tract. In cutaneous anaphylaxis, the reaction is a pale, elevated irregular wheal surrounded by a zone of redness (URTICARIA).

Systemic anaphylaxis can be mimicked by administration of antibodies to cell surface antigens – so-called cytotoxic anaphylaxis – or by aggregated IgG, which activates the COMPLEMENT system and releases ANAPHYLA-TOXINS.

anatoxin. *Synonym for* TOXOID.

anergy. Lack of an expected response of DELAYED-TYPE HYPERSENSITIVITY. This term is used in clinical medicine to describe the diminished delayed-type hypersensitivity found in some disease states (e.g., HODG-KIN'S DISEASE, SARCOIDOSIS). The anergy is usually demonstrated by skin tests with ubiquitous antigens (e.g., Monilia extracts).

angiogenesis factor. Protein that induces growth of vascular endothelial cells and that is important in the formation of new blood vessels, particularly in wound healing. Five distinct angiogenesis factors have been characterized. One of them, basic fibroblast growth factor, is secreted by MONONUCLEAR PHAGOCYTES and may be responsible for the formation of new blood vessels in DELAYED-TYPE HYPERSENSITIVITY reactions. Basic fibroblast growth factor consists of 146 amino acid residues.

ankylosing spondylitis. (Marie–Strümpel's disease). Inflammatory arthritis of the spine of young adult males. The disease affects the mobility of the vertebral column and may cause marked deformity of the back. Over 90 percent of patients are HLA-B27 (*see* HLA) The disease may result from an abnormal immune response to an as yet unidentified microorganism. A juvenile form of ankylosing spondylitis occurs in boys just after puberty and almost always involves the sacroiliac joints.

antibody. Protein that is produced in response to stimulation by ANTIGEN and that reacts specifically with that antigen. Antibodies are IMMUNOGLOBULINS. Antibodies are synthesized by B LYMPHOCYTES and PLASMA CELLS.

antibody binding site. *Synonym for* ANTI-BODY COMBINING SITE.

antibody combining site. Portion of an antibody molecule that makes physical contact with the corresponding ANTIGENIC DETERMINANT. It is formed by the VARIABLE REGIONS of the IMMUNOGLOBULIN HEAVY and LIGHT CHAINS. The size and shape of combining sites vary with specificity, according to the particular antigenic determinant bound; the site may be a cavity or an irregular flat surface. Residues in the HYPERVARIABLE REGION (i.e., the COMPLEMENTARITY-DETER-MINING REGION) are important in determining the structure of the combining site, although residues in the FRAMEWORK REGION may also participate in the site.

The term antibody combining site can also be used to describe the portion of an antigen that makes contact with the antibody. Which of the two meanings is intended is usually clear from the context.

antibody deficiency syndrome. Disease characterized by deficiency of one or more immunoglobulin classes or subclasses and associated with unusual susceptibility to recurrent PYOGENIC INFECTIONS. *See* PRIMARY IMMUNODEFICIENCY.

antibody-dependent cell-mediated cytotoxicity (ADCC) See NATURAL KILLER CELL.

antibody excess. Reaction of antigen and antibody in which antigen is saturated with antibody and some unreacted ANTIBODY COMBINING SITES are present. See PRECIPITIN CURVE.

anticodon. Triplet of contiguous nucleotides in tRNA that pair with complementary nucleotides (a CODON) in the mRNA.

anti-complementary. Attribute of any substance that inhibits COMPLEMENT FIXATION (e.g., HEPARIN).

antigen. Substance that can elicit an IMMUNE RESPONSE and that can react specifically with the corresponding antibodies or T CELL RECEPTORS. An antigen may contain many ANTIGENIC DETERMINANTS. See IMMUNOGEN, HAPTEN.

antigen excess. Reaction of antigen and antibody in which all ANTIBODY COMBINING SITES are occupied by antigen, and some ANTIGENIC DETERMINANTS are available for reaction with additional antibody. See PRECIPITIN CURVE.

antigen presenting cell (APC). See ACCESSORY CELL.

antigen presentation. Process whereby a cell expresses antigen on its surface in a form capable of being recognized by a T LYMPHOCYTE. The antigen must be associated with either CLASS II (for presentation to HELPER T LYMPHOCYTES) or CLASS I (for presentation to CYTOTOXIC T LYMPHOCYTES) HISTOCOMPATIBILITY MOLECULES that are also present on the cell surface. Cells that present antigen to helper T cells are ACCESSORY CELLS (e.g., MONONUCLEAR PHAGOCYTES) and B LYMPHOCYTES; cells that present antigen to cytotoxic T lymphocytes are various target cells (e.g., fibroblasts).

Antigen presentation by mononuclear phagocytes has been studied in some detail. Proteins are ingested by these cells and then degraded into peptides in acidic vesicles (endosomes). Chemicals, such as ammonium chloride and chloroquine, that raise the pH of these vesicles, inhibit antigen presentation. The peptides, usually consisting of eight to ten amino acid residues, bind to class II molecules on the cell surface in a saturable manner. The extent of binding of peptides to class II molecules varies depending on the allelic form of the class II molecules. Peptides, which bind, have the potential to be presented while those that bind weakly or not at all are not presented, and hence are not immunogenic (see IMMUNE RESPONSE GENE). Upon presentation of antigen to a helper T lymphocyte having an appropriate T CELL RECEPTOR, the T cell is activated, secretes INTERLEUKIN-2 and other LYMPHOKINES, and expresses an increased number of IL-2 RECEPTORS. The secreted lymphokines activate mononuclear phagocytes so that they become microbicidal, and they activate B lymphocytes so that they secrete antibody. Ordinarily (but not necessarily), protein antigens in their native form are recognized by B lymphocytes; after processing, the antigen is presented as a peptide to the T cell. Hence B and T lymphocytes usually recognize different forms of the same antigen (native and denatured or degraded, respectively). (see T–B CELL COLLABORATION).

antigen–antibody complex. Complex composed of antigen and antibody molecules. The molar ratio of antigen and antibody in such complexes can vary, according to the proportion of reactants. The complex may be soluble (usually containing excess antigen) or insoluble (precipitated). See PRECIPITIN CURVE.

antigen-binding capacity (ABC). Capacity of an antibody (or mixture of antibodies) to combine with antigen. See FARR TEST.

antigenic. Capable of being an antigen, i.e., of inducing an IMMUNE RESPONSE and of reacting with the corresponding antibodies or T CELL RECEPTORS. See IMMUNOGENIC.

antigenic competition. Decrease in the IMMUNE RESPONSE to one antigen due to a concurrent immune response to a different antigen. Antigenic competition is only found with proteins (THYMUS-DEPENDENT ANTIGENS). Antigenic competition can be explained in part by the fact that antigenic peptides compete for the single binding site ON CLASS II HISTOCOMPATIBILITY MOLECULES.

antigenic determinant. Portion of an antigen that makes contact with a particular antibody or T CELL RECEPTOR. In a typical protein antigen, it is likely that any residue accessible from the surface is part of one or another antigenic determinant. Most proteins probably have many determinants although, because of steric interference, only a limited number of antibodies can bind to the antigen at one time. A protein may have SEQUENTIAL and/or CONFORMATIONAL DETERMINANTS.

antigenic drift. Minor change in a surface antigen of a pathogenic microorganism. The phenomenon has been clearly described for the influenza A virus. Antigenic drift in this virus is presumably the result of mutation in the hemagglutinin and/or neuraminidase genes. The antigenic variants emerge by selection of mutants that are less susceptible to neutralization by the prevailing antibodies in the infected host.

antigenic modulation. Loss of detectable antigen from the surface of a cell after incubation with antibodies. Antibodies to a surface antigen either elicit specific clearance of that component from the membrane (e.g., by CAPPING) or remain bound, covering part of the antigen. In either case, the surface antigen is no longer available for reaction with other molecules of antibody.

antigenic shift. Abrupt major change in a surface antigen of a pathogenic microorganism. The phenomenon has been clearly described for influenza virus, type A; the major antigenic variants are called subtypes. Antigenic shifts in this virus result from changes in the hemagglutinin and possibly also in the neuraminidase antigens; these changes are not the result of a few mutations because peptide maps of hemagglutinins from distinct subtypes differ greatly. New antigens may be introduced into a 'human virus' by recombination with a virus found in an animal. When a major new variant of the influenza A virus appears, a new antigenic determinant is added but some of the original determinants are retained. The antibody response to a new influenza variant is predominantly directed against the cross-reacting antigens of the parental viral strain with which the individual had been previously infected ('doctrine of ORIGINAL ANTIGENIC SIN').

antigenic variation. Change in a surface antigen of a microorganism. Such changes, occurring in a pathogen, may enable the organism to evade destruction by host immunity. Recurrent epidemics of influenza occur because of antigenic variation in the flu virus (see ANTIGENIC DRIFT and ANTIGENIC SHIFT). Antigenic variation is also responsible for the ability of certain parasites, such as trypanosomes, to evade immune destruction by repeatedly changing the surface coat, the only parasite structure exposed to host antibodies. This is accomplished by translocation of a gene encoding a particular coat protein (called variant-specific surface glycoprotein or VSG). Translocation of genes also appears to account for antigenic variation in Borrelia (causative agent of relapsing fever) and in *Neisseria gonorrheae*.

antigenicity. Ability of an antigen to (1) induce an IMMUNE RESPONSE and (2) combine with specific antibodies and/or T CELL RECEPTORS.

antiglobulin test of Coombs. Method for detecting deposition of IgG antibodies or complement on red blood cells or for detecting the presence of circulating IgG antibodies to red blood cells. There are three different types of tests: (1) the direct test; red blood cells are thoroughly washed and then incubated with anti-human IgG. The degree of AGGLUTINATION of the red blood cells is related to the amount of IgG antibodies bound to the cell surface. (2) The indirect test; test serum is incubated with normal red blood cells, which are then washed and incubated with anti-human IgG. The degree of agglutination is related to the concentration of IgG antibodies in the test serum. (3) The 'non-gamma' test; red blood cells are incubated with antibodies to COMPLEMENT components C3 or C4. The degree of agglutination of the red blood cells is related to the amount of these complement components bound to the cell surface. The 'non-gamma' test is an indirect method for detecting IgM antibodies on the cell surface that have fixed complement. (IgM antibodies to antigens of the Rh BLOOD GROUP SYSTEM fix complement whereas IgG antibodies do not.)

antihistamine. Drug that binds to HISTAMINE receptors and blocks the action of

Diphenhydramine (an ethanolamine)

Chlorpheniramine (an alkylamine)

Pyrilamine (an ethylenediamine)

Chlorcyclizine (a piperazine)

H₁-blocking agents   Promethazine (a phenothiazine)

histamine. There are two types of histamine receptors (H_1 and H_2). Ethylamine derivatives block H_1 receptors, and thiourea derivatives (e.g., CIMETIDINE) block H_2 receptors.

anti-lymphocyte serum (ALS). Antiserum produced in one species against LYMPHOCYTES or thymocytes from another species. Intravenous administration of ALS induces severe LYMPHOPENIA resulting in IMMUNOSUPPRESSION. Antibodies in ALS bind to circulating lymphocytes, most of which are T LYMPHOCYTES; therefore, ALS mainly affects the responses of T lymphocytes. It is used clinically to suppress GRAFT REJECTION.

antimetabolite. Drug that interferes with cellular metabolic processes, particularly those involved in mitosis. Antimetabolites are used frequently to treat cancer, but are also used to achieve IMMUNOSUPPRESSION in AUTOIMMUNE DISEASE and in transplant recipients.

anti-nuclear antibody (ANA). Antibody to DNA, RNA, histone or non-histone proteins found in the serum of individuals with certain autoimmune diseases (e.g., SYSTEMIC LUPUS ERYTHEMATOSUS, SJÖGREN'S SYNDROME, POLYMYOSITIS, SYSTEMIC SCLEROSIS). To detect these antibodies, slices of mouse liver or kidney are incubated with the test serum followed by fluorescent antibody to human immunoglobulin. The autoantibodies stain the nuclei in various patterns of fluorescence depending on their specificity.

Disease	Anti-nuclear antibodies to
Systemic lupus erythematosus (SLE)	double-stranded DNA single-stranded DNA small ribonucleoproteins (Sm)
Discoid lupus	histones
Polymyositis and dermatomyositis	tRNA synthetase
Systemic sclerosis	DNA topoisomerase I
CREST syndrome	kinetochore proteins
Sjögren's syndrome	uridine-rich RNAs (SS-A/Ro) (SS-B/La)

antiserum. Serum containing antibodies against a known antigen.

anti-thymocyte serum (ATS). *See* ANTI-LYMPHOCYTE SERUM.

antitoxin. Antibodies to a toxin or ANTI-SERUM containing such antibodies. Before the introduction of antibiotics, antitoxin was commonly used to treat disease caused by toxigenic microorganisms (e.g., diphtheria, tetanus).

antivenom. Antibodies to a venom (e.g., of snakes or insects) or ANTISERUM containing such antibodies. Antivenom is used to treat victims of bites by poisonous snakes or insects.

Antrypol. *Synonym for* SURAMIN.

apolipoprotein E (ApoE). Plasma lipoprotein that binds very low-density lipids and high-density cholesterol esters. ApoE (M_r 33,000) is the major protein secreted by unstimulated MACROPHAGES. MONOCYTES, however, do not secrete ApoE, and macrophages secrete less after they are activated.

Arthus reaction. Immediate-type hypersensitivity reaction characterized by edematous, hemorrhagic lesions of the skin or viscera. Arthus reactions occur upon introduction of antigen into an individual with pre-existing IgG antibodies. Antigen–antibody complexes form in small blood vessels and activate COMPLEMENT. The generation of CHEMOTACTIC PEPTIDES (e.g., C5a) attracts NEUTROPHILS, which ingest the complexes and release lysosomal enzymes. Damage to blood vessel walls occurs with thrombus (clot) formation, hemorrhage, edema and NECROSIS. The Arthus reaction develops over the course of four hours and then subsides in about 12 hours at which time MONONUCLEAR PHAGOCYTES enter the lesion and clear up the debris. The passive cutaneous Arthus reaction is induced by intravenous injection of the antibodies into an unprimed recipient followed by injection of the antigen into the skin. The reverse passive cutaneous Arthus reaction is induced by injection of antibodies into the skin followed by injection of the antigen into the same site or intravenously. The passive Arthus reaction requires a large amount of antibody (100,000-fold more than is required for PASSIVE CUTANEOUS ANAPHYLAXIS). The Arthus reaction is an experimental model of IMMUNE COMPLEX DISEASE.

ascites. Exudate (fluid with inflammatory cells) in the abdominal cavity. In experimental animals, ascites may be formed by MYELOMAS or HYBRIDOMAS growing in this location and may contain high levels of myeloma proteins or specific antibodies. In clinical medicine, ascites may result from seeding of tumors in the peritoneum, obstruction to the portal circulation (e.g., cirrhosis of the liver) or hypoalbuminemia (e.g., in malnutrition).

asparagine-linked oligosaccharide. *See* N-LINKED OLIGOSACCHARIDE.

aspirin (ASA) (acetylsalicylic acid). Drug widely used for its anti-inflammatory, antipyretic and analgesic effects. Aspirin inhibits PROSTAGLANDIN synthesis.

aspirin

association constant (K_A). Constant that describes the equilibrium state of the reversible reaction between two molecular species: $A + B \rightleftharpoons AB$. The association constant $K_A = [AB]/[A][B]$ where [AB], [A] and [B] are the concentrations, at equilibrium, of the complex AB, and of free A and B, respectively; the units of K_A are liters/mole. A and B may be antibody and ligand, enzyme and substrate, cell surface receptor and virus, etc.

If A is an antibody with n binding sites for a univalent LIGAND L, then a series of association constants, K_i, describes the set of reactions between antibody molecules bearing differing numbers of bound ligands and additional ligand. When $i - 1$ sites of the antibody are occupied by ligand, the association constant, K_i for the binding of the next (i^{th}) site is given by:

$$K_i = [AL_i]/[AL_{i-1}] [L]$$

where $[AL_{i-1}]$ and $[AL_i]$ are the concentrations of all the species of antibody bearing, respectively, $i - 1$ and i molecules of bound ligand, and [L] is the concentration of free ligand. If all the ligand-binding sites on the antibody are equivalent and independent, each K_i is related to a constant, κ, that measures the binding of ligand to any single site:

$$K_i = \frac{n - i + 1}{i} \kappa$$

Chemists usually refer to κ as a microscopic association constant (because it refers to the binding of an individual site) and to K_i as a macroscopic association constant. Immunologists customarily refer to κ as an INTRINSIC ASSOCIATION CONSTANT.

For a BIVALENT antibody ($n = 2$), K_1 (the association constant for binding the first ligand) is 2κ and K_2 (the association constant for binding the second ligand) is $\kappa/2$. The difference between these two macroscopic constants (i.e., a factor of 4) is a statistical factor representing both the greater probability of association of the ligand to a molecule having two vacant sites and the greater probability of dissociation of the ligand from a molecule having both sites occupied. It is generally not possible to measure the concentrations of the individual species AL_i in an equilibrium mixture; hence the macroscopic constants, K_i, are not usually determined. Most experimental methods (e.g., EQUILIBRIUM DIALYSIS) yield the total amount of ligand bound, irrespective of its distribution among different antibody molecules. In such methods, the intrinsic association constant, κ, is determined from the concentrations of bound and free ligand. If all the ligand-binding sites are equivalent and independent, κ is defined uniquely and the individual macroscopic constants K_i can be calculated from the statistical factors.

The change in Gibbs free energy (ΔG) for the reaction $A + B \rightleftharpoons AB$ is:

$$\Delta G = \Delta G^\circ + RT \ln \frac{[AB]}{[A][B]}$$

where R is the gas constant (1.987 cal/mole.degree), T is the absolute temperature, and the quantities in brackets are the activities of the reactants, usually on the molar scale. In ideal solutions, the activity is equal to the concentration; in biological systems, solutions are usually dilute and concentrations are used directly, as an approximation, for both association constants and Gibbs energies*. ΔG°, the standard Gibbs energy change, is the free energy change for the formation of one mole of AB from one mole of A and one mole of B, when all of the reactants are maintained at a constant activity of 1 M (an artificial situation). At equilibrium, $\Delta G = 0$; therefore, it follows that:

$$\Delta G^\circ = - RT \ln \frac{[AB]}{[A][B]} = - RT \ln K_A$$

where the quantities in brackets are now activities (or concentrations) that exist under equilibrium conditions.
* Such constants are referred to as 'concentration equilibrium constants'; where practicable, it is suggested that these measurements be made at 25°C in 0.1 M KCl, with the lowest effective buffer concentration (see 'Recommendations for Measurement and Presentation of Biochemical Equilibrium Data', *Journal of Biological Chemistry* **251**: 6879 (1976)).

asthma. Symptom characterized by difficulty in breathing, with wheezing and shortness of breath, due to sudden constriction of bronchi with trapping of air in the lungs. This symptom is mediated by PROSTAGLANDINS D_2 and F_2 and LEUKOTRIENES C4, D4 and E4 which are released from MAST CELLS, BASOPHILS and NEUTROPHILS, and PLATELET-ACTIVATING FACTOR released from mast cells and basophils. These mediators incite INFLAMMATION and excessive secretions. Although HISTAMINE is also released, it is rapidly destroyed by HISTAMINASE in the lung and is not thought to play a role in causing asthma. Most asthma is triggered by the reaction of cell-bound IgE antibodies with respiratory ALLERGENS, so-called extrinsic asthma. In some patients, asthma accompanies respiratory infection, and there is no demonstrable allergen involved, so-called instrinsic asthma. Asthma may also be precipitated by fumes, exercise, emotional distress and exposure to cold. Asthma is treated with sympathomimetic amines (e.g., ISOPROTERENOL, METAPROTERENOL) and methylxanthines (e.g., THEOPHYLLINE) both of which dilate bronchi, and with inhibitors of mediator release (e.g., CROMOLYN) and CORTICOSTEROIDS.

ataxia telangiectasia (AT). Disease characterized by progressive cerebellar ataxia (unsteady gait) starting in the second year of life and telangiectasia (dilated capillaries) of the conjunctiva and skin that become prominent at 5–6 years of age. IgA deficiency is present in 70 percent of patients. The THYMUS is small and HELPER T LYMPHOCYTES have decreased function. Due to defective DNA repair mechanisms, cells of patients with AT have numerous chromosomal breaks, inversions and translocations and are extremely sensitive to the damaging effects of ionizing radiation and radiomimetic chemicals. The majority of the breaks have been mapped to the chromosomal regions that include T CELL RECEPTOR GENES and IMMUNOGLOBULIN GENES on chromosomes 7 and 14. As in other syndromes characterized by frequent chromosomal breaks, patients with AT have a high incidence of LYMPHOMA. ALPHA-FETOPROTEIN levels in serum are almost always elevated. AT is inherited as an autosomal recessive disorder.

atopic dermatitis. Chronic, itchy, eczematous skin eruption, occurring mainly in infants and children with a strong family history of ALLERGY. Most patients have elevated levels of IgE in serum (but it is not clear that this condition is mediated by these antibodies).

atopy. Heritable tendency towards IMMEDIATE HYPERSENSITIVITY reactions due to IgE antibodies. Manifestations of atopy are ASTHMA, ALLERGIC RHINITIS and URTICARIA. Approximately 10 percent of the population manifest one or another form of atopy.

attenuated vaccine. Vaccine composed of live microorganisms that have lost virulence but have retained the ability to induce ACTIVE IMMUNITY to pathogenic forms of the same microorganism (e.g., Bacille Calmette–Guérin (BCG), Sabin oral polio vaccine).

autoantibody. Antibody that reacts with an antigen that is a normal constituent of the body of the individual forming the antibody. *See* AUTOIMMUNITY.

autoantigen. Normal constitutent of the body that reacts with an autoantibody. *See* AUTOIMMUNITY.

autobody. IMMUNOGLOBULIN that binds to another immunoglobulin carrying the same IDIOTYPIC DETERMINANT. For example, anti-phosphorylcholine antibodies from BALB/c mice bearing the T15 idiotype bind to each other. The significance of this phenomenon is not known.

autograft. Graft taken from the same individual to whom it is applied.

autoimmune disease. Disease that is caused by antibodies or T lymphocytes reactive with antigenic determinants of self. In experimental animals, immunization with the appropriate tissue can evoke a response that is similar to the autoimmune disease; the responding animal develops pathological changes characteristic of the disease and the experimentally induced disease can be transferred to a normal recipient by serum or T lymphocytes (*see* AUTOIMMUNITY). The presence of autoantibodies and/or autoreactive T lymphocytes in many diseases does not in itself mean that these diseases are caused by the autoimmune response. In human autoimmune disease, the cause of autoantibody formation or formation of autoreactive T lymphocytes is generally not known. *See* AUTOIMMUNE HEMOLYTIC ANEMIA, CHRONIC LYMPHOCYTIC THYROIDITIS, EXPERIMENTAL ALLERGIC ENCEPHALOMYELITIS, GRAVES' DISEASE, MYASTHENIA GRAVIS, PEMPHIGUS, PERNICIOUS ANEMIA, SYSTEMIC LUPUS ERYTHEMATOSUS.

autoimmune hemolytic anemia. Accelerated destruction of red blood cells *in vivo* by AUTOANTIBODIES of the IgG class to an antigen on red blood cells, usually an Rh antigen (*see* Rh BLOOD GROUP). Red blood cells coated with autoantibodies are removed from the circulation by interaction of the autoantibodies with Fc RECEPTORS on the MACROPHAGES of the spleen and liver. The ANTIGLOBULIN TEST OF COOMBS is used in the diagnosis of autoimmune hemolytic anemia. *See* COLD AGGLUTININ SYNDROME.

autoimmunity. Immunological reaction to self components. Autoimmune reactions can produce severe inflammation or can be innocuous, as when directed to intracellular AUTOANTIGENS, which are not exposed to circulating antibodies or to T lymphocytes.

Autoimmunity can develop spontaneously or can be induced experimentally by IMMUNIZATION with autoantigens or antigens cross-reactive with autoantigens.

autologous. Derived from self. The term is used to describe self antigens or grafts taken from and returned to the same individual.

autoradiography. Technique for detecting radioisotopes by virtue of their effect on a radiation-sensitive medium, such as a photographic emulsion. Autoradiography is used in cell biology to localize particular substances in cells and tissues (e.g., DNA in the nucleus can be visualized after incorporation of [^{3}H]-thymidine). Autoradiography is also used to detect radioactive compounds in various analytical methods, such as RADIOIMMUNOELECTROPHORESIS and SOUTHERN BLOTTING.

autosome. Any chromosome other than the sex chromosomes X and Y.

average association constant (K_0). In the binding of a univalent ligand to a heterogeneous population of antibody combining sites, K_0 is usually defined as the reciprocal of the concentration of free ligand required for half-saturation of the sites. However, it should be noted that, in general, K_0 is not the mean ASSOCIATION CONSTANT and, only in special circumstances (symmetrical distributions), will it be the median value (see discussion under SIPS DISTRIBUTION). It would be more appropriate to define a term $K_{1/2}$ (or, in general, $K_{1/n}$) as the reciprocal of the free ligand concentration required for half (or $1/n$) saturation of the sites and not to designate this term as an average value of association constants.

avidin. Glycoprotein from egg white that has extremely high affinity for biotin. (Biotin, a water-soluble vitamin (vitamin H), is a cofactor in certain enzymes that catalyse carboxylation reactions, e.g., pyruvate carboxylase (EC 6.4.1.1), acetyl CoA carboxylase (EC 6.4.1.2).) Avidin consists of four identical subunits, each of which binds one molecule of biotin. Each subunit contains 128 amino acid residues, a single disulfide bridge, and one N-LINKED OLIGOSACCHARIDE. The isoelectric point of avidin is approximately pH 10. The ASSOCIATION CONSTANT for the binding of biotin is 10^{15} M^{-1}, one of the highest binding constants known.

The high affinity between avidin and biotin has been exploited in a variety of methods, utilizing appropriate indicator molecules (e.g., antibodies, enzymes, fluorescent dyes, electron-dense proteins) to localize specific macromolecules in cells, tissue sections, and blots. For example, in enzyme-linked immunosorbent assay (ELISA) techniques, an enzyme conjugated to avidin can be used to bind to biotinylated antibody. Alternatively, avidin can be used as the 'glue' that binds a biotinylated enzyme to a biotinylated antibody. Biotin-labeled polynucleotides, prepared by cross-linking biotin to nucleic acids or by enzymatic incorporation of biotin derivatives of nucleotides, can be used as specific MOLECULAR HYBRIDIZATION PROBES.

A similar but slightly smaller protein, streptavidin, isolated from *Streptomyces avidinii*, can be used in place of avidin. Streptavidin also consists of four identical subunits and has a similar affinity for biotin; however, it lacks carbohydrate and has an isoelectric point near pH 6. It is reported to have less non-specific binding and, therefore, a higher signal-to-noise ratio in assay procedures.

avidity. Descriptive term referring to the stability of complexes formed by MULTIVALENT antibodies with an antigen having many determinants to which these antibodies bind. Generally, the avidity of an antigen–antibody interaction is enhanced by: (1) a large number of binding sites on the antigen; (2) many binding sites on the antibody (e.g., IgM rather than IgG); (3) many different antibodies reacting with a variety of determinants on the antigen; and (4) high affinity of the reactions between individual antigen and antibody sites. Avidity as well as AFFINITY may also be affected by non-specific interactions between antigen and antibody (e.g., ionic and hydrophobic interactions). In contrast to affinity, avidity is not defined in thermodynamic terms, but by the particular assay used to measure the interaction (e.g., the dissociation of antigen–antibody complexes as a result of dilution). Multivalent binding can be described more precisely by determination of ASSOCIATION CONSTANTS (see FUNCTIONAL AFFINITY).

axenic. Not contaminated by or associated with any foreign organism. Axenic is used to describe pure cultures of microorganisms or GERM-FREE MICE (or other animals).

azathiorprine. (6-[(1-methyl-4-nitro-1H-imidazol-5-yl)thio]-1H-purine). Derivative of MERCAPTOPURINE widely used in the treatment of malignant disease and for IMMUNOSUPPRESSION. It is used to prevent graft rejection and to suppress the symptoms of RHEUMATOID ARTHRITIS and SYSTEMIC

azathioprine

LUPUS ERYTHEMATOSUS. Azathioprine is cleaved *in vivo* to the active form, 6-mercaptopurine.

azidothymidine. *See* ZIDOVUDINE.

B

b allotype. ALLOTYPE associated with rabbit IMMUNOGLOBULIN KAPPA CHAINS. These allotypes are the products of allelic genes at the κ*l* locus. There are four alleles in domestic rabbit populations: *b4, b5, b6* and *b9*. The kappa chains that are the products of these alleles differ in many amino acid residues of the CONSTANT REGION and are, therefore, examples of COMPLEX ALLOTYPES. *See* a ALLOTYPE.

B cell growth and differentiation factor. Factor that promotes the growth and/or differentiation of B LYMPHOCYTES *in vitro*, usually obtained from T CELL-CONDITIONED MEDIA. The number and function *in vivo* of B cell growth and differentiation factors are not known. Examples are INTERLEUKIN-4, INTERLEUKIN-5, INTERLEUKIN-6.

B cell growth factor I (BCGF I). *Synonym for* INTERLEUKIN-4.

B cell growth factor II (BCGF II). *Synonym for* INTERLEUKIN-5.

B cell stimulating factor-1 (BSF-1). *Synonym for* INTERLEUKIN-4.

B cell stimulating factor-2 (BSF-2). *Synonym for* INTERLEUKIN-6.

B complex. MAJOR HISTOCOMPATIBILITY COMPLEX (MHC) of the chicken. It appears to contain one locus *(B–F)* encoding CLASS I HISTOCOMPATIBILITY MOLECULES, another locus *(B–L)* encoding CLASS II HISTOCOMPATIBILITY MOLECULES, and a third locus *(B–G)* encoding uncharacterized red blood cell antigens. The degree of polymorphism of the B complex is not known.

B lymphocyte. LYMPHOCYTE that produces immunoglobulin. B lymphocytes constitute about one-half of all lymphocytes. In LYMPH NODES, B lymphocytes are localized mainly in the follicles, whereas T LYMPHOCYTES are found in the deep cortex. B lymphocytes are derived from STEM CELLS found abundantly in BONE MARROW and in fetal liver; these cells mature without passing through the thymus. In birds, B lymphocyte stem cells are found in the BURSA OF FABRICIUS.

The early steps in the development of B lymphocytes are not influenced by antigen. The first known stage of differentiation is the pre-B cell in which the genes for IMMUNOGLOBULIN MU CHAINS, but not for IMMUNOGLOBULIN LIGHT CHAINS, have been rearranged and immunoglobulin mu chains are found in the cytoplasm. Next, rearrangement of light chain genes occurs, resulting in the expression of MEMBRANE IMMUNOGLOBULIN (containing mu and either kappa or lambda chains), which acts as a receptor for antigen. The resulting cell is now known as a B lymphocyte. Subsequently, IgD is coexpressed with IgM in the membrane. Later events in B cell development are driven by antigen and T LYMPHOCYTES. Membrane IgD disappears. Some mature B lymphocytes express only IgM on their membranes, whereas others express an additional immunoglobulin class (IgA, IgG or IgE) (*see* CLASS SWITCHING). In the process of terminal differentiation of B lymphocytes into PLASMA CELLS, immunoglobulin disappears from the cell surface and the cell begins to synthesize large quantities of secretory immunoglobulin (several thousand immunoglobulin molecules per second). This immunoglobulin is identical to that last expressed on the B lymphocyte except that the heavy chain is the secreted rather than the membrane form. Some B lymphocytes do not undergo terminal differentiation to plasma cells but are thought to become long-lived memory B lymphocytes that retain membrane immunoglobulin and can respond to another encounter with the same antigen.

B lymphocytes are usually differentiated from T lymphocytes by the presence of membrane immunoglobulin, which can be detected with fluorescent-labeled anti-immunoglobulin antibodies. B lymphocytes, but not T lymphocytes, have COMPLEMENT RECEPTOR 2 on their surface. B lymphocytes also have CLASS II HISTOCOMPATIBILITY MOLECULES, which are not found on resting T lymphocytes. These class II molecules have an important role in ANTIGEN PRESENTATION by B lymphocytes.

B lymphocyte hybridoma. Clone resulting from the fusion of a B LYMPHOCYTE and a MYELOMA cell. To obtain such a clone, activated B lymphocytes (e.g., spleen cells from an immunized mouse) are mixed with a suspension of myeloma cells and cell fusion is induced (e.g., by polyethylene glycol). The cells are then plated into multi-well tissue culture dishes containg HAT MEDIUM, a selective medium in which only hybrids survive. (The myeloma cells used for this purpose are deficient in the enzyme hypoxanthine-guanine phosphoribosyl transferase and therefore cannot grow in HAT medium; spleen cells survive in suspension culture for only a few days.) Those wells containing hybridomas are screened for antibody production. The hybridomas that test positive must now be cloned (*see* CLONE). This is done either by limiting dilution (*see* LIMITING DILUTION ANALYSIS) or by cloning in soft AGAR. Hybridomas are expanded by propagation in tissue culture or by growth in the peritoneal cavities of mice (*see* ASCITES) of the same strain as the cells.

B lymphocyte hybridomas combine the specificity of the B lymphocyte with the capacity for unlimited replication that is characteristic of a myeloma cell. As hybridomas can be maintained in culture indefinitely, they are said to be 'immortal'. B lymphocyte hybridomas are the major source of MONOCLONAL ANTIBODIES.

B mouse. Mouse selectively deprived of T LYMPHOCYTES. This is usually accomplished by THYMECTOMY followed by lethal irradiation and reconstitution with bone marrow cells. Such mice are used in experimental work to study the responses of B LYMPHOCYTES to THYMUS-INDEPENDENT ANTIGENS.

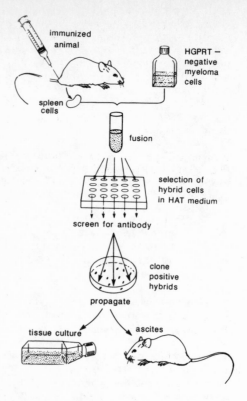

immunized animal

HGPRT — negative myeloma cells

spleen cells

fusion

selection of hybrid cells in HAT medium

screen for antibody

clone positive hybrids

propagate

tissue culture   ascites

B lymphocyte hybridoma

bactericidin. Antibody or other substance that kills bacteria.

bacteriolysin. Antibody that lyses bacteria in the presence of COMPLEMENT.

bacteriolysis. LYSIS of bacteria. In immunology bacteriolysis usually means lysis by ANTIBODIES and COMPLEMENT.

bacteriophage lambda. *See* LAMBDA BACTERIOPHAGE.

balanced polymorphism. A POLYMORPHISM that is stable over time. A balance of selective forces can give rise to a stable polymorphism. This may be the result of HETEROZYGOUS ADVANTAGE, a situation in which the fitness (in natural selection) of a heterozygote is greater than the fitness of either homozygote. Balance between the occurrence of a deleterious mutation and selection against it can also give rise to balanced polymorphism.

bas. MUTATION in rabbits resulting in greatly reduced expression of the major type of IMMUNOGLOBULIN KAPPA CHAIN (κ1). Most immunoglobulins in rabbits having the bas mutation bear lambda light chains (*see* IMMUNOGLOBULIN LAMBDA CHAIN), but a small proportion have light chains of the κ2 ISOTYPE. The bas mutation has been shown to result from a mutation in an acceptor site for mRNA splicing.

basophil. Type of POLYMORPHONUCLEAR LEUKOCYTE, characterized by SECONDARY GRANULES that stain blue with basophilic dyes (as in Wright or Giemsa stains). These granules contain HEPARIN, HISTAMINE, PLATELET-ACTIVATING FACTOR and other vaso-active amines, which are important mediators of IMMEDIATE HYPERSENSITIVITY. Basophils constitute 2 percent of white blood cells. Although similar in function, basophils are distinct from MAST CELLS. They both have high affinity Fcε RECEPTORS. Upon contact with antigen, granules are released from the basophils by EXOCYTOSIS.

BB rat. Mutant strain of rat, characterized by the development of several autoimmune diseases, the most prominent of which is INSULIN-DEPENDENT DIABETES MELLITUS. B/B rats are lymphopenic (*see* LYMPHOPENIA) and have deficiencies of T LYMPHOCYTES. Drugs that are toxic for lymphocytes prevent or delay the onset of insulin-dependent diabetes mellitus in B/B rats.

BCG. (Bacille Calmette–Guérin). Attenuated strain of bovine *Mycobacterium tuberculosis* used as a vaccine to protect against tuberculosis (and leprosy). It is named after the two French workers who first cultivated the organism.

Behçet's disease. Chronic disease of young adult males characterized by recurrent painful ulcers of the mouth and genitalia, bilateral iritis and joint pains. Histopathologically, the disease is characterized by perivascular infiltrates of LYMPHOID CELLS. Immune complexes are present in the serum, and AUTOANTIBODIES to oral mucous membrane can be demonstrated by IMMUNOFLUORESCENCE. The disease is presumed to have an immunologic cause; it is associated with HLA-B5 (*see* HLA) in Middle-Eastern populations and in the Japanese, but not in Caucasians.

beige mouse. Mouse of a mutant strain characterized by abnormalities in pigmentation. The *bg* mutation is inherited as an autosomal recessive. These mice resemble humans with the CHEDIAK–HIGASHI SYNDROME in that they have poor NATURAL KILLER CELL activity and a high incidence of malignancies.

Bence-Jones protein. Protein in urine of patients with MULTIPLE MYELOMA that precipitates when heated to 45–60°C and redissolves on further heating. A Bence-Jones protein is the light chain (monomers and/or dimers) of the MYELOMA PROTEIN found in the serum of the same patient. It was named after Henry Bence-Jones, the British physician who first reported the unusual behaviour upon heating of the urine from a patient with multiple myeloma.

benign monoclonal gammopathy. Presence in 'normal' serum of MONOCLONAL IMMUNOGLOBULIN of the IgG, IgA, IgD, or IgE class. The concentration of monoclonal immunoglobulin is usually less than 20 mg/ml. The BONE MARROW is not infiltrated with PLASMA CELLS, and there are no bone lesions. Some (less than 20 percent) individuals with benign monoclonal gammopathy develop MULTIPLE MYELOMA.

beta-2 microglobulin. Light chain of CLASS I HISTOCOMPATIBILITY MOLECULES. Beta-2 microglobulin resembles an IMMUGLOBULIN DOMAIN in that it consists of 99 amino acid residues, including a pair of half-cystines (position 25 and 80) that are joined in a disulfide bridge. The amino acid sequence of beta-2 microglobulin resembles (up to 30 percent identity) that of immunoglobulin constant domains. It is a member of the IMMUNOGLOBULIN SUPERFAMILY. Beta-2 microglobulin was discovered in the urine of patients with impaired reabsorption in the kidney tubules. It is found in large quantities in urine immediately following kidney transplantation and in individuals with advanced AIDS. The gene for beta-2 microglobulin has been mapped to chromosome 15q21-22 in humans and to chromosome 2 in mice.

beta-pleated sheet. Structure composed of extended polypeptide chains in which hydrogen bonds are formed between carbonyl oxygen and peptide nitrogen groups in neighboring chains. The axial distance between adjacent amino acid residues is 0.35 nm. A beta-pleated sheet can be parallel (amino termini of adjacent strands at same end) or antiparallel (amino termini at opposite ends). An extended polypeptide chain folding back on itself results in an antiparallel arrangement. Antiparallel beta-pleated sheets are found in silk fibroin and are important structural features of the IMMUNOGLOBULIN FOLD. *See* ALPHA-HELIX, SECONDARY STRUCTURE.

binding constant. *See* ASSOCIATION CONSTANT, EQUILIBRIUM CONSTANT.

binding protein (BiP). *Synonym for* IMMUNOGLOBULIN HEAVY CHAIN BINDING PROTEIN.

Birbeck granule. Small, round cytoplasmic vesicle, found characteristically in the LANGERHANS CELLS of the skin. It is 10–30 nm in diameter and contains electron-dense material at its center.

bivalent. Having two binding sites.

blast cell. Larger (greater than 8 μm) cell of any lineage with a prominent nucleus and cytoplasm rich in RNA. Blast cells are active in DNA synthesis.

blocking antibody. Antibody that inhibits the reaction between antigen and other antibodies or sensiᶻed T LYMPHOCYTES (e.g., antibodies of e IgG class that compete with IgE antibodies for antigen, thereby blocking an allergic response). Blocking antibodies that inhibit agglutination reactions by other antibodies were at one time thought to be univalent, but it is now thought that the inhibition is due to the reaction of the antibodies with ANTIGENIC DETERMINANTS on the same particle. (*See* MONOGAMOUS BINDING.) Blocking antibodies that bind to tumors and prevent destruction of tumor cells by CYTOTOXIC T LYMPHOCYTES have also been called enhancing antibodies.

blood group substance. Alloantigenic determinant of red blood cells. *See* ABO BLOOD GROUP, Rh BLOOD GROUP, DUFFY BLOOD GROUP, KELL–CELLANO BLOOD GROUP, KIDD BLOOD GROUP, LUTHERAN BLOOD GROUP, MNSs BLOOD GROUP.

Common blood groups

Blood group	Common alleles
ABO	A,B,O
Rh	C,D,E,c,d,e
Kell–Cellano	K,k
Lutheran	Lu^a, Lu^b
Duffy	Fy^a,Fy^b
Kidd	Jk^a,Jk^b
MNSs	M,N,S,s

bm-12 mouse. Mutant mouse derived from the inbred strain C57BL/6. Bm-12 mice are characterized by altered IMMUNE RESPONSES to certain proteins that are under IMMUNE RESPONSE GENE control. For example, these mice cannot make antibodies to pork insulin, whereas mice of the parental strain can make such antibodies. The *bm-12* mutation results in changes in three amino acid residues in the beta chain of CLASS II HISTOCOMPATIBILITY MOLECULES.

Bombay phenotype. *See* ABO BLOOD GROUP.

bone marrow. Soft tissue within the cavities of bones. The bone marrow contains hematopoietic cells in different stages of maturation to red blood cells, LEUKOCYTES and PLATELETS.

bone marrow cell. Mature or immature cell from BONE MARROW including STEM CELLS from which all the formed elements of the blood are derived (i.e., red blood cells, LEUKOCYTES and PLATELETS). Bone marrow is rich in B LYMPHOCYTES and precursors of T LYMPHOCYTES. Bone marrow is used as a source of B lymphocytes and of pluripotential stem cells for long-term reconstitution of an irradiated host. Transplants of bone marrow cells are used to treat patients with leukemias, aplastic anemia and certain immunodeficiencies. AUTOGRAFTS of bone marrow cells are used to replenish the bone marrow of patients who have received high doses of irradiation.

booster. Secondary antigenic stimulus to induce a SECONDARY IMMUNE RESPONSE weeks, months or years after the primary stimulus.

bradykinin. Nonapeptide cleaved by plasma KALLIKREIN from KININOGENS of the plasma that causes increased vascular permeability, local extravasation of leukocytes and pain, as well as hypotension. The sequence of bradykinin is Arg–Pro–Pro–Gly–Phe–Ser–Pro–Phe–Arg. Lysyl-bradykinin (kallidin), cleaved by tissue kallikreins from kininogens has, in addition, a lysine residue at the amino-terminus. The term, bradykinin, derives from the fact that it contracts smooth muscle more slowly than HISTAMINE does. Because increased amounts of bradykinin can be detected in ANA-PHYLAXIS and ENDOTOXIC SHOCK, it is presumed to play a role in the pathogenesis of these conditions. Joint fluid from patients with arthritis contains bradykinin.

Bruton's agammaglobulinemia. *Synonym for* X-LINKED AGAMMAGLOBULINEMIA.

Bruton's disease. *Synonym for* X-LINKED AGAMMAGLOBULINEMIA.

Burkitt's lymphoma. Distinctive B cell LYMPHOMA that occurs frequently in African children and sporadically elsewhere in the world. Burkitt's lymphoma is distributed geographically in areas where malaria is endemic, but it has also frequently been observed in patients with ACQUIRED IMMUNO-DEFICIENCY SYNDROME and in recipients of bone marrow transplants who have been immunosuppressed (*see* IMMUNOSUPPRES-SION). Although the tumor has a predilection for the jaw and facial bones, it may become widespread and affect all the viscera. EPSTEIN–BARR VIRUS is found in the tumor cells. In these cells, there frequently are reciprocal rearrangements between one copy of the chromosome bearing c-*myc* and the chromosomes bearing immunoglobulin heavy chain genes.

bursa of Fabricius. Sac-like lympho-epithelial organ of birds, derived from a dorsal diverticulum of the cloaca. The bursa is the primary lymphoid organ of B lymphocytes in birds; it is composed mainly of primary follicles. Removal of the bursa at the time of birth results in a failure of B lymphocyte development and consequently a failure to make antibodies (i.e., AGAMMA-GLOBULINEMIA). In other vertebrates there is no known equivalent to the bursa, and it appears that antigen-independent B lymphocyte differentiation takes place in the yolk sac and liver of the fetus, and the bone marrow of adults. The bursa involutes at sexual maturity; the involution can be accelerated by the administration of testosterone. B lymphocytes are so-called because, in birds, these cells mature in the bursa. The bursa resembles the THYMUS in that both organs develop from epithelial invaginations of the endoderm that become infiltrated with lymphoid STEM CELLS and that involute at pubescence. The bursa of Fabricius is named after its discoverer, Hieronymus Fabricius, a 17th century Italian anatomist.

busulfan. (1,4-butanediol dimethanesulfonate). Alkylating agent that is used to destroy BONE MARROW CELLS in prospective recipients of bone marrow transplants.

$$H_3C-\overset{\overset{O}{\|}}{\underset{\underset{O}{\|}}{S}}-O-CH_2-CH_2-CH_2-CH_2-O-\overset{\overset{O}{\|}}{\underset{\underset{O}{\|}}{S}}-CH_3$$

busulfan

BXSB mouse. Mouse from a recombinant inbred strain, derived from a cross between C57BL/6J and SB/Le and characterized by enlarged LYMPH NODES and SPLEEN, HEMOLY-TIC ANEMIA, polyclonal HYPERGAMMAGLO-BULINEMIA and many AUTOANTIBODIES. The disease of BXSB mice resembles SYSTEMIC LUPUS ERYTHEMATOSUS, except that it is much more severe in males.

C

c allotype. ALLOTYPE associated with the LAMBDA LIGHT CHAIN of rabbit immunoglobulins. Two such allotypes have been identified: c7 and c21.

C gene segment. Segment of DNA encoding the CONSTANT REGION of an IMMUNOGLOBULIN or T CELL RECEPTOR polypeptide chain. *C* gene segments include one or several exons (*see* IMMUNOGLOBULINE GENES and T CELL RECEPTOR GENES).

C_α. CONSTANT REGION of an IMMUNOGLOBULIN ALPHA CHAIN. In humans there are two ISOTYPES of such constant regions designated $C_{\alpha 1}$ and $C_{\alpha 2}$; $C_{\alpha 1}$ and $C_{\alpha 2}$ denote the corresponding gene segments.

C_γ. CONSTANT REGION of an IMMUNOGLOBULIN GAMMA CHAIN. In humans there are four isotypes of such constant regions designated $C_{\gamma 1}$, $C_{\gamma 2}$, $C_{\gamma 3}$ and $C_{\gamma 4}$; $C_{\gamma 1}$, $C_{\gamma 2}$, $C_{\gamma 3}$ and $C_{\gamma 4}$ denote the corresponding gene segments.

C_δ. CONSTANT REGION of an IMMUNOGLOBULIN DELTA CHAIN, C_δ denotes the corresponding gene segment.

C_ϵ. CONSTANT REGION of an IMMUNOGLOBULIN EPSILON CHAIN, C_ϵ denotes the corresponding gene segment.

C_κ. CONSTANT REGION of an immunoglobulin kappa chain; C_κ denotes the corresponding gene segment.

C_λ. CONSTANT REGION of an IMMUNOGLOBULIN LAMBDA CHAIN; C_λ denotes the corresponding gene segment. In humans and in mice, there are several isotypes of C_λ (e.g., $C_{\lambda 1}$, $C_{\lambda 2}$ and $C_{\lambda 3}$ in mice).

C_μ. CONSTANT REGION of an IMMUNOGLOBULIN MU CHAIN; C_μ denotes the corresponding gene segment.

C1. First component of COMPLEMENT. C1 is a complex of proteins, C1q, C1r and C1s, which are responsible for the initiation of the CLASSICAL PATHWAY OF COMPLEMENT activation. Erythrocytes (E) coated with antibody (A) are converted by C1 from EA to EAC1. In the presence of Ca^{2+} each C1 molecule is composed of one molecule of C1q, two molecules of C1r, and two molecules of C1s (C1q–C1r$_2$–C1s$_2$) with a sedimentation constant of 16 S.

C1 deficiencies. Rare genetic deficiencies of C1q, C1r, or C1r and C1s, which are inherited as autosomal recessive traits. Isolated C1s deficiency has not yet been described. Most affected individuals have less than 1 per cent of the normal amount of the C1 subcomponent(s) in serum. However, approximately 50 percent of individuals with C1q deficiency have normal or near normal amounts of mutant, nonfunctional C1q in serum. Individuals with C1 subcomponent deficiencies are at a greater risk than normal individuals for the development of IMMUNE COMPLEX DISEASE. It is difficult to detect heterozygotes and they are clinically normal.

C1 inhibitor (C1 INH). Serum protein that inhibits the activation of C1r, the cleavage of C1s by C1r and the cleavage of C4 and C2 by C1s. C1 INH is a single polypeptide chain containing 478 amino acid residues. It has six N-LINKED OLIGOSACCHARIDES attached to asparagine residues at positions 3, 47, 59, 216, 231 and 330 and at least seven O-linked oligosaccharides attached to serine at position 42 and threonines at positions 26, 49, 61, 66, 70 and 74. C1 INH is the most highly glycosylated protein in serum (~ 50 percent is carbohydrate). C1 INH also inhibits plasmin, KALLIKREIN and Factors XIa and XIIa of the clotting system. C1 INH is a serine

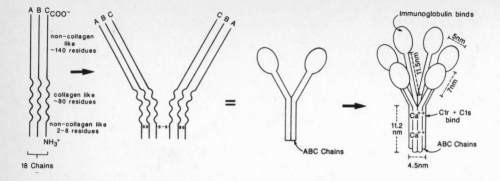

C1q

protease inhibitor (serpin); it has approximately 30 percent amino acid sequence identity with other serpins (e.g., alpha-1 antitrypsin, anti-thrombin III). The serine proteases cleave an arginine–threonine bond at position 444–445 of C1 INH. The amino-terminal segment (444 residues) of the inhibitor remains bound to the enzyme and a covalent bond between the two is formed; the carboxy-terminal segment (34 residues) is released. After C1 INH complexes with C1r and C1s, these C1 subcomponents dissociate from C1q. C1 INH has been mapped to chromosome 11 in humans. Its synthesis is defective in HEREDITARY ANGIONEUROTIC EDEMA and its catabolism is increased in ACQUIRED C1 INHIBITOR DEFICIENCY.

C1q. Subcomponent of the C1 complex that binds to IMMUNOGLOBULIN and thereby initiates COMPLEMENT activation by the CLASSICAL PATHWAY. C1q is composed of 18 polypeptide chains of three types: A, B and C (each of $M_r \sim 25,000$). The A chain consists of 224 amino acid residues, the B chain of 226 residues and the C chain of 222 residues. Each A chain is linked to a B chain by a disulfide bridge, and each C chain is linked by a disulfide bridge to another C chain. Each chain has a collagen-like sequence with glycine in every third position and containing hydroxyproline and hydroxylysine residues: about 80 percent of the hydroxylysine residues are glycosylated with the disaccharide glucosyl-galactose. A triple-stranded helix is formed by the collagen-like regions of one A, one B and one C chain; the remaining portions of the three chains form a 'globular head'. One C1q molecule is

composed of six such units; the triple helices are aligned in parallel for half their length and then diverge into the six globular head regions. Thus, it has been said that the C1q molecule resembles a bunch of tulips. The globular heads bind to immunoglobulin molecules. The collagen-like portion binds C1r and C1s. The genes encoding the C1q A and B chains have been mapped to chromosome 1p in humans. The gene encoding the B chain contains two EXONS of which one encodes a SIGNAL SEQUENCE of 29 amino acid residues and the amino-terminal 35 residues; the other exon encodes residues 36–226. The two exons are separated by an INTRON of 1.1 kilobases.

C1r (EC 3.4.21.41). One of two serine esterases that are part of the C1 complex, the other being C1s. Two molecules of C1r are bound by Ca^{2+} to the collagen-like stalk of C1q. C1r is a single chain (M_r 83,000). Upon activation, which is autocatalytic, C1r is cleaved. The amino-terminal fragment becomes the alpha (or A) chain of 463 amino acid residues and the carboxy-terminal fragment becomes the beta (or B) chain of 243 residues, which contains the active site. C1r cleaves an arginine–isoleucine bond in C1s, which is thereby activated. The carboxy-terminal portion of the alpha chain of C1r contains two short homologous repeats of approximately 60 amino acid residues, found in proteins that bind to C3 and/or C4. See CONSENSUS SEQUENCE OF c3/c4 BINDING PROTEINS. A segment of the alpha chain (positions 115–176) has extensive homology with epidermal growth factor; at position 150, there is an unusual amino acid, erythro-β-hydroxyaspa-ragine, which is characteristic of epidermal growth factor-like domains and is believed to be involved in the binding of Ca^{2+}. There are four sites for attachment of N-LINKED OLIGOSACCHARIDES, two on the alpha and two on the beta chain.

In humans, the gene encoding C1r has been mapped to chromosome 12p13-ter and is linked to the gene encoding C1s.

C1s (EC 3.4.21.42). One of two serine esterases that are part of the C1 complex, the other being C1r. Two molecules of C1s are bound by Ca^{2+} to the collagen-like stalk of C1q. C1s is a single chain (M_r 85,000) which, on activation, is cleaved by C1r into an alpha (or A) chain of 431 amino acid residues and a beta (or B) chain of 243 residues, which contains the active site. C1s cleaves an arginine–alanine bond in C4 and an arginine–lysine bond in C2. The primary structure of C1s, insofar as has been deter-mined, resembles that of C1r.

C2. Second component of COMPLEMENT. It actually reacts third in sequence following fixation of C1 and C4b to ANTIGEN–ANTIBODY COMPLEXES. C2 is a single polypeptide chain of 732 amino acids. When C2 associates with the complex of C1 and C4b, an arginine–lysine bond (position 223–224) in C2 is cleaved by C1s to form C2b, which is released, and C2a, which remains associated with the complex. In the CLASSICAL PATHWAY OF COMPLEMENT fixation, erythrocytes (E) coated with antibody (A), C1 and C4b are converted by C2a in the presence of Mg^{2+} to EAC14b2a. The active site of the classical pathway C3 CONVERTASE (C4b2a) resides in C2a. The structural gene for C2 has been mapped to the major histocompatibility complex (MHC) on the short arm of the sixth chromosome (6p) in humans and to the S REGION of chromosome 17 in the mouse. C2 is polymorphic. Three alleles of C2 in humans are: *C2A* (acidic), *C2B* (basic) and *C2C* (common).

C2 deficiency. Rare genetic deficiency inherited as an autosomal recessive. Affected individuals have less than 1 percent of the normal amount of C2 in serum and are at greater risk than are normal individuals for the development of IMMUNE COMPLEX DISEASE, particularly SYSTEMIC LUPUS ERY-THEMATOSUS. By SOUTHERN BLOTTING the gene encoding C2 appears to be normal in C2 deficient individuals; no mRNA for C2 is detected. Heterozygotes have half-normal amounts of C2 in serum and are clinically normal. They constitute 1 percent of the Caucasian population. The gene for C2 defi-ciency occurs in the EXTENDED HAPLOTYPE (HLA-B18, HLA-DR2, COMPLOTYPE SO42).

C2a. Major product of C2 cleavage by C1s. C2a consists of the 509 carboxy-terminal amino acid residues of C2. C2a has six sites for attachment of N-LINKED OLIGOSACCHARIDES. The carboxy-terminal sequence (287 residues) of C2a, which con-tains the catalytic site for the cleavage of C3 and C5, is homologous to other serine pro-teases. C2a associates with C4b to form the classical pathway C3 CONVERTASE (C4b2a).

C2b. Minor product of C2 cleavage by C1s. C2b consists of the 223 amino-terminal residues of C2. C2b contains three short homologous repeats of approximately 60 amino acid residues found in proteins that bind to C3 and/or C4 (*see* CONSENSUS SEQUENCE OF C3/C4 BINDING PROTEINS); it has two sites for attachment of N-LINKED OLIGO-SACCHARIDES. Plasmin or trypsin cleave a peptide from the carboxy-terminus of C2b. This peptide may play an important role in edema formation in patients with HEREDI-TARY ANGIONEUROTIC EDEMA. The residual protein (188 residues) is designated C2b'.

C3. Third component of COMPLEMENT. It actually reacts fourth in sequence following fixation of C1, C4b and C2a to antigen–antibody complexes. C3 is composed of two polypeptide chains: alpha and beta, cross-linked by a disulfide bridge. An arginine–serine bond (position 77–78) of the alpha chain is cleaved by C3 CONVERTASES to form C3a, which is released, and C3b, which binds to antigen–antibody–complement complexes. In the CLASSICAL PATHWAY OF COMPLEMENT, erythrocytes (E) coated with antibody (A) and C1, C4b and C2a are converted by C3b to EAC14b2a3b. One EAC14b2a site may result in the deposition of up to 500 molecules of C3b on the red blood cell surface.

C3 is synthesized as a single chain (*see* PRO-C3) of 1,663 amino acid residues, con-sisting of a signal sequence (22 residues), the beta chain (645 residues), a connecting pep-tide (Arg–Arg–Arg–Arg) and the alpha chain (992 residues). There is an internal thiolester at residues 1010–1013 in the C3d (or C3dg) segment of the alpha chain. When C3 is cleaved by C3 convertase the thiolester is hydrolysed and a reactive acyl group can form a bond with amino or hydroxyl groups on cell surfaces.

In humans, the gene for C3 has been mapped to chromosome 19. C3 is polymorphic. There are two common alleles in humans: *C3S* (for slow electrophoretic mobility) and *C3F* (for fast electrophoretic mobility). In addition, there are several rare alleles (< 1 percent in the population).

C3 is the most abundant of the complement proteins in serum (1–2 mg/ml). Upon cleavage of its internal thiolester, it can bind covalently to amino or hydroxyl groups of bacteria, red blood cells and other particles. It is the principal OPSONIN of the blood. The several biological activities of C3 are enumerated in the definitions of its various

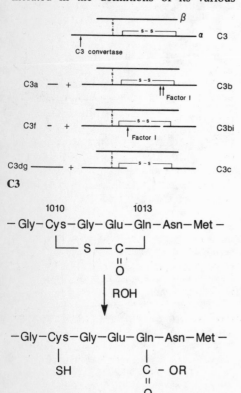

internal thiolester

fragments: C3a, C3b C3bi (iC3b), C3dg, C3e. *Synonym for* beta-1C globulin.

C3 convertase. Enzyme complex of the CLASSICAL PATHWAY (C4b2a) (EC 3.4.21.43) or of the ALTERNATIVE PATHWAY OF COMPLEMENT (C3bBb) (EC 3.4.21.47) that cleaves C3 into C3b and C3a. The alternative pathway convertase triggers a positive feedback amplification loop (*see* ALTERNATIVE PATHWAY OF COMPLEMENT). Both enzymes are unstable and their components dissociate rapidly unless stabilized by C3 NEPHRITIC FACTOR in the case of the classical or alternative pathway or properdin in the case of the alternative pathway. The catalytic sites are in C2a or in Bb.

C3 deficiency. Very rare genetic deficiency inherited as an autosomal recessive. Affected individuals have less than 1 percent of the normal amount of C3 in serum and are susceptible to recurrent PYOGENIC INFECTIONS. Heterozygotes have half-normal amounts of C3 in serum and are clinically normal. C3 deficiency also occurs in dogs; C3-deficient dogs have increased susceptibility to pyogenic infections and an increased incidence of MEMBRANOPROLIFERATIVE GLOMERULONEPHRITIS.

C3 nephritic factor (C3NeF). OLIGOCLONAL IgG autoantibodies of the alternative pathway C3 CONVERTASE (C3bBb) or less commonly of the classical pathway C3 convertase (C4b2a). The antibodies to C3bBb are found in the sera of patients with MEMBRANOPROLIFERATIVE GLOMERULONEPHRITIS and PARTIAL LIPODYSTROPHY; they stabilize C3bBb. The antibodies to C4b2a are found in patients with SYSTEMIC LUPUS ERYTHEMATOSUS; they stabilize C4b2a. In both cases, there is accelerated cleavage of C3 *in vivo*.

C3a. Minor product of C3 cleavage by the C3 CONVERTASES: C4b2a or C3bBb. C3a is a peptide consisting of the 77 amino-terminal residues of the alpha chain of C3; C3a has anaphylatoxin activity (i.e., releases HISTAMINE from MAST CELLS and contracts smooth muscle).

C3a receptor. Membrane protein that acts as a receptor for the ANAPHYLATOXIN C3a derived from C3. It is found on mast cells and basophils mediates HISTAMINE release. Its structure has not yet been determined.

C3b. Major product of C3 cleavage by the C3 CONVERTASES: C4b2a or C3bBb. C3b consists of the residual C3 after C3a has been released by proteolysis. C3b binds FACTOR B to form the ALTERNATIVE PATHWAY C3 convertase (C3bBb); C3b also binds to C4b2a to form the CLASSICAL PATHWAY C5 convertase (C4b2a3b). In the presence of Factor H, two arginine–serine bonds (positions 1303–1304 and 1320–1321) in C3b are cleaved by FACTOR I to form C3bi (iC3b), releasing a peptide, C3f. C3b bound to particles binds to COMPLEMENT RECEPTOR 1.

C3b inactivator. *See* FACTOR I.

C3bi (iC3b). Major product of C3b cleavage by FACTOR I. In the presence of FACTOR H or COMPLEMENT RECEPTOR 1 an arginine–glutamic acid bond (position 954–955) in C3bi is cleaved by Factor I to form C3c and C3dg. The reaction of particle-bound C3bi with COMPLEMENT RECEPTOR 3 on monocytes and NEUTROPHILS enhances PHAGOCYTOSIS. C3bi binds CONGLUTININ of bovine serum, and this reaction also appears to enhance phagocytosis.

C3c. Major product of C3bi cleavage by FACTOR I (in the presence of FACTOR H or COMPLEMENT RECEPTOR 1). It is composed of an intact beta chain bound to two fragments of the alpha chain (M_r 27,000 and 43,000) by disulfide bonds. C3c has no known function.

C3d. Carboxy-terminal 301 amino acid residues of C3dg (M_r 33,000). C3d reacts with COMPLEMENT RECEPTOR 2 found on B LYMPHOCYTES. C3d is a growth factor for B lymphocytes. The thiolester of the C3 alpha chain is located in C3d. C3d is produced by cleavage of a lysine–histidine bond (position 1001–1002) in C3dg with proteolytic enzymes (e.g., trypsin). This cleavage is not known to occur *in vivo*.

C3dg (α_{2d}). Minor product of C3bi cleavage by FACTOR I (in the presence of FACTOR H or COMPLEMENT RECEPTOR 1). C3dg (M_r 41,000) consists of 349 amino acid residues

(positions 955–1303). There is a receptor for C3dg on NEUTROPHILS (COMPLEMENT RECEPTOR 4) and on B LYMPHOCYTES, (COMPLEMENT RECEPTOR 2).

C3e. Nonapeptide from the alpha chain of C3c (amino acid positions 946–954) that induces leukocytosis. C3e is Thr–Leu–Asp–Pro–Glu–Arg–Leu–Gly–Arg. A putative receptor on leukocytes for C3e has been described but has not been characterized.

C3f. Peptide of 17 amino acid residues (positions 1304–1320) cleaved from the alpha chain of C3b by FACTOR I (in the presence of FACTOR H or COMPLEMENT RECEPTOR1). It has no known biological function.

C3g. Amino-terminal 47 amino acid residues of C3dg (M_r 8,000). C3g has no known biological function. C3g is produced by cleavage of C3dg with proteolytic enzymes (e.g., trypsin).

C3H/HeJ mouse. Mouse of a mutant strain, derived from C3H, characterized by a depressed response of B LYMPHOCYTES and MACROPHAGES to stimulation with LIPOPOLYSACCHARIDES. The C3H/HeJ mutation (*lps*) is inherited as an autosomal dominant and has been mapped to chromosome 4. Macrophages of C3H/HeJ mice fail to secrete INTERLEUKIN-1 and TUMOR NECROSIS FACTOR after exposure to lipopolysaccharide. C3H/HeJ mice have increased susceptibility to certain microorganisms.

C4. Fourth component of COMPLEMENT. It actually reacts second in sequence following fixation of C1 to antigen–antibody complexes. C4 is composed of three polypeptide chains: alpha, beta and gamma, cross-linked by disulfide bridges. An arginine–alanine bond (position 76–77) in the alpha chain of C4 is cleaved by C1s to form C4a, which is released, and C4b, which remains bound to C1. In the CLASSICAL PATHWAY OF COMPLEMENT, erythrocytes (E) coated with antibody (A) and C1 are converted by C4b to EAC14b.

C4 is synthesized as a single chain (*see* PRO-C4) of 1722 amino acid residues, consisting of the beta chain (656 residues), a connecting peptide (Arg–Lys–Lys–Arg), the alpha chain (767 residues), a second connecting peptide (Arg–Arg–Arg–Arg) and finally the gamma chain (291 residues). After translation of pro-C4, three tyrosine residues (positions 1395, 1398 and 1400) are sulfated. After cleavage of connecting peptides in pro-C4, and secretion of the C4 molecule, 26 amino acid residues (positions 1406–1431) are cleaved from the newly exposed carboxy-terminus of the alpha chain. C4 contains an internal thiolester, which is located at residues 991–994 in the C4d segment of the alpha chain.

C4 is encoded by two closely linked genes in the MAJOR HISTOCOMPATIBILITY COMPLEX on the short arm of human chromosome 6 (6p) or on mouse chromosome 17. The genes for human C4, *C4A* and *C4B*, and for mouse C4, *Slp* and *Ss*, are highly polymorphic. *Synonym for* beta-1E globulin.

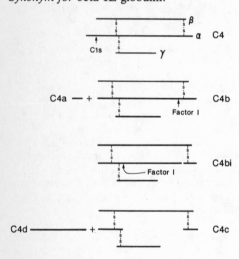

C4

C4 binding protein (C4bp). Serum protein that binds to C4b, thereby impairing the association of C2a with C4b and enhancing the dissociation of C4b2a into C4b and C2a. C4bp is required for the cleavage of C4b to C4bi and of C4bi to C4c and C4d by FACTOR I. C4bp is composed of seven identical polypeptide chains, each of 540 amino acid residues, linked by disulfide bonds. The amino-terminal 491 residues are composed of eight short homologous repeats of approximately 60 residues, found in proteins that bind to C3 and/or C4 (*see* CONSENSUS SEQUENCE OF C3/C4 BINDING PROTEINS). In humans the gene encoding C4bp has been mapped to chromosome 1q3.2. *See* RCA LOCUS.

C4 deficiency. Rare genetic deficiency inherited as an autosomal recessive. Affected individuals, who do not express either of the *C4A* or *C4B* genes, have less than 1 percent of the normal amount of C4 in serum and are at very great risk for the development of fatal IMMUNE COMPLEX DISEASE. Their parents have half-normal amounts of serum C4.

It has been found in population surveys that approximately 30 percent of all Caucasians do not transcribe one or two of the four C4 genes. Deletions of *C4B* alleles may include deletions of a gene for cytochrome P-450 21-hydroxylase, which is located 1.5 kilobases from the 3'-end of the *C4B* gene. In homozygotes, this results in congenital adrenal hyperplasia. Because the 21-hydroxylase gene 3' to the *C4A* gene is not transcribed in humans (i.e., it is a PSEUDOGENE) congenital adrenal hyperplasia does not occur when this gene is deleted. C4 deficiency also occurs in inbred strains of guinea-pigs.

C4A. Product of the *C4A* gene. C4A is highly polymorphic. Almost all C4A molecules bear the Rodgers antigen (*see* CHIDO RODGERS ANTIGEN). SLP (sex-limited protein) is the product of this gene in mice. C4A is hemolytically less active than is C4B. C4A is 100 times more reactive with amino groups than is C4B and 10 times less reactive with hydroxyl groups. The only differences between C4A and C4B are four amino acid residues at positions 1101, 1102, 1105 and 1106 in the C4d segment of the alpha chain.

C4A Pro–Cys–Pro–Val–Leu–Asp
C4B Leu–Ser–Pro–Val–Ile–His

C4a. Minor product of C4 cleavage by C1s. C4a is a peptide consisting of the 76 amino-terminal residues of the alpha chain of C4; C4a has anaphylatoxin activity (i.e., releases HISTAMINE from MAST CELLS and contracts smooth muscle) but it is a 100-fold less active than is C3a or C5a.

C4B. Product of the *C4B* gene. C4B is polymorphic, but less so than C4A. Almost all C4B molecules bear the Chido antigen (*see* CHIDO RODGERS ANTIGENS). The Ss PROTEIN is the product of this gene in mice. C4B is hemolytically more active than is C4A. C4B is 10 times more reactive with hydroxyl groups than is C4A but 100-fold less reactive with amino groups. *See* C4A for amino acid differences between C4A and C4B.

C4b. Major product of C4 cleavage by C1s. C4b consists of the residual C4 after C4a has been released by proteolysis. C4b associates with C2a to form the CLASSICAL PATHWAY C3 convertase (C4b2a). In the presence of the C4 BINDING PROTEIN, an arginine–asparagine bond (position 1318–1319) in C4b is cleaved by FACTOR I to form C4bi. Particle-bound C4b interacts with COMPLEMENT RECEPTOR 1.

C4b inactivator. *See* FACTOR I.

C4bi (iC4b). Major product of C4b cleavage by FACTOR I, which (in the presence of the C4 binding protein) cleaves an arginine–threonine bond (position 937–938) in the alpha chain to form C4c and C4d.

C4c. Major product of C4bi cleavage by FACTOR I (in the presence of the C4 BINDING PROTEIN). C4c (M_r 145,000) is composed of C4 beta and gamma chains and two fragments of the alpha chain, linked together by disulfide bonds. C4c has no known function.

C4d. Minor product of C4bi cleavage by FACTOR I (in the presence of the C4 BINDING PROTEIN). C4d (M_r 45,000) contains the internal thioester of the C4 alpha chain. The difference between Chido and Rodgers antigens (*see* CHIDO RODGERS ANTIGENS) resides in C4d.

C5. Fifth component of COMPLEMENT. It reacts fifth in sequence following fixation of C1, C4b, C2a and C3 to antigen–antibody complexes. C5 is composed of two polypeptide chains: alpha and beta, cross-linked by disulfide bridges. An arginine–leucine bond (position 74–75) in the alpha chain is cleaved by C5 CONVERTASES to form C5a, which is released, and C5b which remains bound.

Mouse C5 is synthesized as a single chain (*see* PRO-C5). The beta chain is amino-terminal (634 residues) followed by a connecting peptide (Arg–Pro–Arg–Arg) and the carboxy-terminal alpha chain (1,002 residues).

In mice the gene for C5 has been mapped to chromosome 2. In humans C5 exhibits very little POLYMORPHISM.

C5 convertase. Complex of the CLASSICAL PATHWAY (C4b2a3b) (EC 3.4.21.43) or the ALTERNATIVE PATHWAY OF COMPLEMENT (C3bBb3b) (EC 3.4.21.47) that cleaves C5 into C5a and C5b. As in the C3 CONVERTASES, the catalytic sites are in C2a or Bb.

C5 deficiency. Very rare genetic deficiency inherited as an autosomal recessive. Affected individuals have less than 1 percent of the normal amounts of C5 in serum and are susceptible to recurrent neisserial infections. Heterozygotes have half-normal amounts of C5 in serum and are clinically normal. C5 deficiency is common in mice.

C5a. Minor product of C5 after cleavage by C5 CONVERTASES: C4b2a3b or C3bBb3b. C5a is a peptide consisting of the 74 amino-terminal residues of the alpha chain of C5; C5a has anaphylatoxin activity (e.g., releases HISTAMINE from MAST CELLS and contracts smooth muscle) and is potent in CHEMOTAXIS and degranulation of NEUTROPHILS. C5a increases expression of COMPLEMENT RECEPTOR 3 and p150,95 in the membranes of neutrophils; C5a increases superoxide production in neutrophils. *See* C5a$_{74desarg}$.

C5a$_{74desarg}$. Cleavage product of C5a after the carboxy-terminal arginine is removed by ANAPHYLOTOXIN INACTIVATOR. It is active in chemotaxis but 100-fold less active than is C5a.

C5a receptor. Membrane protein that is a receptor for C5a, the ANAPHYLATOXIN derived from C5 of NEUTROPHILS, MAST CELLS, BASOPHILS, T LYMPHOCYTES, EOSINOPHILS and PLATELETS. The receptor on mast cells and basophils mediates histamine release and that on neutrophils induces superoxide production and chemotaxis.

C5b. Major product of C5 cleavage by C5 CONVERTASES. C5b consists of the residual C5 after C5a has been released by proteolysis. C5b has a metastable binding site for C6. Complexes of C5b and C6 initiate the formation of the MEMBRANE ATTACK COMPLEX of complement, which results in membrane damage and lysis of cells.

C6. Sixth component of COMPLEMENT. It is composed of a single polypeptide chain (M_r

124,000). C6 forms part of the MEMBRANE ATTACK COMPLEX. C6 is polymorphic; two common alleles, *C6A* and *C6B*, have been defined.

C6 deficiency. Very rare genetic deficiency inherited as an autosomal recessive. Affected individuals have less than 1 percent of the normal amount of C6 in serum and they are susceptible to recurrent neisserial infections. Heterozygotes have half-normal amounts of C6 in serum and are clinically normal. C6 deficiency is common in rabbits.

C6–7 deficiency. Genetic disorder that has been observed in one family. It is inherited as an autosomal recessive. The genes for C6 and C7 are linked, but no chromosomal assignment has yet been made.

C7. Seventh component of COMPLEMENT. C7 binds to complexes of C5b and C6 to form C5b67. These complexes appear, under the electron microscope, like a leaf on a stalk, approximately 25 nm in length. The stalk is composed of C6 and C7 and the leaf of C5b. When C7 binds to the complex C5b6, a hydrophilic–amphiphilic transition occurs and the stalk of the C5b67 becomes embedded in a cell membrane without forming a transmembrane channel (C8 is required to form such channels). Membrane-bound C5b67 enables the binding of C8 and C9 to target membranes (*see* MEMBRANE ATTACK COMPLEX). When complexes of C5b67 form in the fluid phase they polymerize with each other to form rosettes.

C7 consists of a single polypeptide chain of 843 amino acid residues, including a signal sequence of 22 residues. It has two sites for attachment of N-LINKED OLIGOSACCHARIDES (asparagine at positions 180 and 732). The amino-terminal 524 residues have approximately 25 percent sequence identity with the alpha and beta chains of C8 and C9. C7 exhibits very little POLYMORPHISM in Caucasians, but is highly polymorphic in Orientals.

C7 deficiency. Very rare genetic deficiency inherited as an autosomal recessive. Affected individuals have less than 1 percent of the normal amount of C7 in serum and they are susceptible to recurrent neisserial infections. Heterozygotes have half-normal amounts of C7 in serum and are clinically normal.

C8. Eighth component of COMPLEMENT. It is composed of three polypeptide chains: alpha (M_r 64,000), beta (M_r 64,000) and gamma (M_r 22,000). The alpha and gamma chains are linked by disulfide bond(s) and are joined to the beta chain by non-covalent forces. The beta chain of C8 binds to C5b of complexes of C5b, C6 and C7; thereupon two segments of the alpha chain undergo conformational changes from BETA-PLEATED SHEETS to ALPHA HELIXES. The complex forms a transmembrane channel. The alpha chain of C8 can bind one C9 molecule; this binding initiates the polymerization of C9 (*see* MEMBRANE ATTACK COMPLEX).

The three chains of C8 are encoded in genes at three separate loci; there is extensive genetic polymorphism of the alpha and beta chains of C8. The alpha chain consists of 583 amino acid residues including a signal sequence of 30 residues and the beta chain consists of 590 residues including a signal sequence of 54 residues. The alpha chain has two sites for attachment of N-LINKED OLIGOSACCHARIDES (asparagine at positions 13 and 397); the beta chain has three such sites (asparagine at positions 47, 189 and 498). Residues 224 to 234 and 317 to 327 in the alpha chain appear to be candidates for the alpha helical transmembrane domains. There is 33 percent identity of amino acid sequence between the alpha and beta chains of C8; they both have approximately 25 percent identity with C7 and C9.

C8 deficiency. Very rare genetic deficiency inherited as an autosomal recessive. The deficiency of the alpha and gamma chains of C8 has been observed mainly in Blacks and of the beta chain of C8 mainly in Caucasians. Both types of deficiency result in susceptibility to recurrent neisserial infections. It is difficult to detect heterozygotes and they are clinically normal.

C9. Ninth component of COMPLEMENT. It is the terminal component of the MEMBRANE ATTACK COMPLEX. Following its reaction with membrane-bound complexes of C5b, C6, C7 and C8 (C9 actually binds to the alpha chain of C8), C9 undergoes a major conformational change: it doubles in length and hydrophobic structures, capable of interacting with the lipid bilayer of cell membranes, are exposed. In the presence of Zn^{2+}, 12 or more molecules of C9 polymerize to form cylinders of 100 nm in diameter, which insert into cell membranes and form transmembrane channels. Cells thus attacked become permeable to ions and other low molecular weight substances; the cells rapidly imbibe sodium and water, swell and burst (LYSIS).

C9 consists of a single chain of 535 amino acid residues. C9 has approximately 25 percent amino acid sequence identity with C7 and the alpha and beta chains of C8. It is structurally related to PERFORIN. The gene encoding C9 is located on human chromosome 5. C9 is not polymorphic. See S PROTEIN.

C9 deficiency. Rare genetic deficiency inherited as an autosomal recessive. Affected individuals have less than 1 percent of the normal amount of C9 in serum and the deficiency appears to have no clinical consequences. Heterozygotes have half-normal amounts of C9 in serum. C9 deficiency is common in the Japanese population, in which one in 40 persons is heterozygous for the deficiency.

cachectin. See TUMOR NECROSIS FACTOR.

capping. Ligand-induced redistribution of membrane proteins to one pole of the cell. The first step in this redistribution is the formation of patches as a result of the reaction of bivalent or multivalent ligands with membrane proteins (see PATCHING). Next, in the capping step, the antigen–antibody aggregates in the patches flow to and accumulate at one pole of the cell, where they form a large mass – the cap – which may then be internalized (ligand-induced ENDOCYTOSIS). Unlike the formation of patches, which is a passive phenomenon, capping is an energy-dependent process that may require participation of microfilaments (see CYTOSKELETON) attached to the cytoplasmic side of the membrane. The process of capping has been studied in detail in LYMPHOCYTES, but it also takes place in many other cells. See CO-CAPPING.

carcinoembryonic antigen (CEA). Glycoprotein antigen (M_r 200,000) of the membrane of gastrointestinal tract epithelial cells. CEA is present in large amounts on colorectal carcinoma cells and in lesser amounts on normal fetal colon cells. Serum CEA levels may rise in colorectal cancer, pancreatitis, INFLAMMATORY BOWEL DISEASE and cirrhosis of the liver. Measurement of serum CEA levels is useful in detecting the recurrence and severity of colon cancer. CEA is a member of the IMMUNOGLOBULIN SUPERFAMILY. It is composed of a single polypeptide chain with six constant region-like domains and a single variable region-like domain at the amino terminus. See ONCOFETAL ANTIGEN.

carrier. Protein to which a HAPTEN becomes attached in vitro or in vivo, thereby rendering the hapten IMMUNOGENIC.

CBA/N mouse. Mutant CBA mouse, characterized by an inability to make an immune response to certain THYMUS-INDEPENDENT ANTIGENS (e.g., linear polysaccharides). The mutation (xid) is inherited as an X-linked recessive trait. CBA/N mice have B LYMPHOCYTES that are either immature or abnormal. They lack a subpopulation of B lymphocytes that bear the Lyb3, Lyb5 and Lyb7 ALLOANTIGENIC DETERMINANTS normally found in adult mice but not in newborn mice. CBA/N mice also respond poorly to THYMUS-DEPENDENT ANTIGENS; the levels of IgG in serum are low. The cause of the immunological defect in CBA/N mice is not known.

CD1 (T6, Leu6). Membrane glycoprotein of thymocytes defined in the human with mouse monoclonal antibodies, anti-T6 or anti-Leu6. CD1 is first expressed during the intermediate stage of THYMUS CELL DIFFERENTIATION and is found on more than 95 percent of thymocytes. It is a single polypeptide chain (M_r 46,000). CD1 may be associated with BETA-2 MICROGLOBULIN or it may form disulfide-linked HETERODIMERS with CD8. CD1 is found on both medullary and cortical thymocytes, but it is associated with CD8 only in the latter. The function of CD1 is not known. The gene(s) for CD1 have been mapped to human chromosome 1. CD1 is composed of 229 amino acid residues – a stretch of 10 residues at the amino-terminus, two domains of 93 residues, a connecting peptide of five residues, a putative transmembrane segment of 22 residues and a cytoplasmic segment of six residues; it has four sites for attachment of N-LINKED OLIGO-SACCHARIDES. CD1 is a member of the IMMU-NOGLOBULIN SUPERFAMILY. The carboxy-terminal domain of the extracellular portion of CD1 is homologous with constant region-like domains.

CD2   (T11, Leu5). Membrane glycoprotein of T LYMPHOCYTES and thymocytes defined in humans by mouse monoclonal antibodies, anti-T11 or anti-Leu5. CD2 was first described as the receptor for sheep erythro-cytes (E). CD2 is a single polypeptide chain (M_r 50,000–58,000). Three ANTIGENIC DETER-MINANTS of CD2 are detected by different mouse monoclonal antibodies and are called $T11_1$, $T11_2$ amd $T11_3$. $T11_1$ and $T11_2$ are detected only on resting T lymphocytes and thymocytes, whereas $T11_3$ is detected only on MITOGEN–activated T lymphocytes. Anti-bodies to $T11_1$ inhibit the formation of E ROSSETTES. Antibodies to $T11_2$ induce the appearance of $T11_3$. The simultaneous addition of antibodies to $T11_2$ and $T11_3$ activates T lymphocytes and brings about increased expression of INTERLEUKIN-2 RECEPTORS and CLASS II HISTOCOMPATIBILITY MOLECULES. The activation of T lymphocytes by antibodies to $T11_2$ and $T11_3$ mimics the effects of antibodies to CD3 or to the T CELL RECEPTOR and has, therefore, been called the alternative pathway of T cell activation.

CD2 is one of two markers for early cells of T lineage (the other is CD7) in the THYMUS (*see* THYMUS CELL DIFFERENTIATION). CD2 on CYTOTOXIC T LYMPHOCYTES binds to LYMPHOCYTE FUNCTION ASSOCIATED ANTIGEN-3 on target cells; this interaction promotes adhesion of lymphocytes to target cells and may be important in the killing of the target cells. CD2 is composed of 360 amino acid residues including a signal sequence of 24 residues, two extracellular domains (185 residues), a putative transmembrane seg-ment of 26 residues and a cytoplasmic domain of 125 residues. There are four sites for N-LINKED OLIGOSACCHARIDES in the extra-cellular domains. CD2 is a member of the IMMUNOGLOBULIN SUPERFAMILY. The two extracellular domains are homologous to constant region-like domains. The gene encoding CD2 has been mapped to chromo-some 1p13 in humans.

CD3   (T3, Leu4). Complex of at least five polypeptides in the membranes of mature human and mouse T lymphocytes that is non-covalently associated with the T CELL RECEPTOR. Human CD3 was first identified by its reaction with mouse monoclonal anti-bodies, anti-T3 and anti-Leu4. The CD3 polypeptides are T3γ (M_r 25,000), T3δ (M_r 20,000), T3ε (M_r 20,000) and a dimer of T3ζ (M_r 16,000). Mouse monoclonal antibodies to CD3 induce the CO-CAPPING of the CD3 polypeptides and the T cell receptor, acti-vate T lymphocytes and bring about their cell division. CD3 is thought to be important for signal transduction when the T cell receptor interacts with antigen plus major histocompatibility molecules.

The gene encoding the T3δ polypeptide has five exons contained within approxi-mately 4 kilobases. The exons encode: (1) 18 of the 21 amino acid residues of the signal sequence; (2) the remainder of the signal sequence and a segment of 70 residues; (3) a segment of 44 residues including a putative transmembrane segment; (4) and (5) 36 amino acid residues that constitute the intra-cellular domain. The *T3δ* gene has been mapped to human chromosome 11q23-ter. The mouse *T3δ* gene has a similar organi-zation and encodes a homologous protein. It has been mapped to mouse chromosome 9.

The structure for T3ε has been deduced from an analysis of a cDNA clone. It is composed of an amino-terminal hydrophilic domain of 104 amino acid residues, a putative transmembrane segment of 26 resi-dues and a cytoplasmic domain of 81 resi-dues. The gene for T3ε is linked to the gene for T3δ.

The structure for T3γ has also been deduced from a cDNA clone. It is composed of an amino-terminal hydrophilic domain of 89 amino acid residues, a putative transmembrane segment of 27 residues and a cytoplasmic domain of 44 residues. T3ε, unlike T3δ and Tγ, is not glycosylated. T3δ and T3γ have two sites for N-LINKED OLIGO-SACCHARIDES (asparagine residues 30 and 70 for T3γ and 16 and 52 for T3δ).

The structure for T3ζ has been deduced from a mouse cDNA clone. It is composed of a signal sequence of 21 amino acid resi-dues, an amino-terminal extracellular segment of 9 residues, a putative transmem-brane segment of 21 residues and a cytoplas-mic domain of 44 residues. T3ζ, like

T3ε, is not glycosolated. T3ζ forms disulfide-linked homodimers.

T3δ and T3ε contain an aspartic acid residue and T3γ a glutamic acid residue in the transmembrane segment. These negatively charged residues are thought to form salt bridges with the lysine residue in the transmembrane segments of the alpha and beta chains of the T cell receptor. These ionic interactions may account for the association of CD3 and T cell receptor, and hence the co-capping of the complex. Serine residues at position 126 in T3δ and position 113 and T3γ are thought to be potential sites for phosphorylation by protein kinase C. T3ζ has six sites for tyrosine phosphorylation.

During biosynthesis of CD3 molecules, a chain, T3ω (M_r 28,000), is associated with the T3γ, T3δ and T3ε chains. T3ω dissociates from the complex during the final stages of assembly and is not expressed in the membrane.

CD4 (T4, Leu3, L3T4). Membrane glycoprotein of a subset of T LYMPHOCYTES, thymocytes and MACROPHAGES. CD4 is also found on the surfaces of some B LYMPHOCYTES, MONONUCLEAR PHAGOCYTES and brain cells. CD4 in humans is detected by mouse monoclonal antibodies, anti-T4 and anti-Leu3. CD4 in mice is called L3T4. CD4 is expressed on T lymphocytes that react with antigen presented in association with CLASS II HISTOCOMPATIBILITY MOLECULES. The CD4 subset constitutes approximately 70 percent of mature T lymphocytes and contains HELPER T LYMPHOCYTES and INDUCER T LYMPHOCYTES. Some CD4+ lymphocytes are cytotoxic for target cells bearing class II histocompatibility molecules. CD4 is expressed in approximately 90 percent of human thymocytes (see THYMUS CELL DIFFERENTIATION). CD4 is the receptor for HUMAN IMMUNODEFICIENCY VIRUS.

Human CD4 is a single polypeptide chain composed of 459 amino acid residues, including a signal sequence of 23 residues, an amino-terminal domain of 110 residues, a long sequence of 265 residues, a transmembrane segment of 21 residues and a cytoplasmic domain of 40 residues. The amino-terminal domain and the middle portion of the long sequence of 265 residues have approximately 30 percent sequence identity with variable regions of IMMUNOGLOBULIN

LIGHT CHAINS (see IMMUNOGLOBULIN SUPERFAMILY). The carboxy-terminal portion of the long sequence of 265 residues contains a domain that is constant region-like. In the 265-residue segment, there are two sites for attachment of N-LINKED OLIGOSACCHARIDES. The gene for CD4 is encompased in 33 kilobases. *CD4* has been mapped to chromosome 12p12-ter in humans.

Mouse CD4 is also a single polypeptide chain of 457 amino acid residues, including a signal sequence of 22 residues, an amino-terminal domain of 110 residues, a long sequence of 262 residues, a transmembrane segment of 25 residues and a cytoplasmic domain of 38 residues. In the 262-residue segment, there are four sites for N-glycosylation. Mouse and human CD4 have approximately 60 percent sequence identity.

CD5 (T1, Leu1, Ly1). Membrane glycoprotein of all T LYMPHOCYTES, plus a small proportion of B LYMPHOCYTES. Human CD5 is detected by mouse monoclonal antibodies, anti-T1 or anti-Leu1; it is a single polypeptide chain (M_r 65,000). Mouse CD5 is detected by alloantibodies to Ly1. CD5 is expressed at higher levels on HELPER T LYMPHOCYTES than on CYTOTOXIC T LYMPHOCYTES or SUPPRESSOR T LYMPHOCYTES, and anti-Ly1 antibodies preferentially kill mouse helper T lymphocytes in the presence of COMPLEMENT. This was important in the initial characterization of helper T lymphocytes, but this population is now better defined by antibodies to CD4. The gene for CD5 in mice has been mapped to chromosome 19; there are two allelic forms, $Ly1^a$ and $Ly1^b$, which specify the Ly1.1 and Ly1.2 ALLOANTIGENS, respectively. Most inbred strains are $Ly1^b$. Only CBA, C3H, DBA/1 and DBA/2 inbred strains are $Ly1^a$. The function of CD5 is not known, but anti-CD5 antibodies stimulate cell division in the presence of small amounts of LECTINS (see Ly1 B CELL).

CD5 in mice is composed of 495 amino acid residues including a signal sequence of 24 residues, an extracellular region of 347 residues, a putative transmembrane segment of 30 residues and a cytoplasmic domain of 94 residues. There are three sites for N-LINKED OLIGOSACCHARIDES in the extracellular region. CD5 in humans consists of 471 amino acid residues. There is 63 percent amino acid sequence identity between mouse and human CD5.

CD7 (TP-40). Membrane glycoprotein of human T LYMPHOCYTES and thymocytes detected by mouse MONOCLONAL ANTIBODY, anti-Leu9. CD7 was first found in T cell acute lymphocytic leukemia. It is one of the two markers for early cells of T lineage (the other is CD2) in the THYMUS (*see* THYMUS CELL DIFFERENTIATION). CD7 is present on 75 percent of T lymphocytes; its function is not known. CD7 is composed of 240 amino acid residues, including a signal sequence of 25 residues, an extracellular domain of 155 residues, a transmembrane segment of 21 residues and a cytoplasmic region of 39 residues; there are two sites for N-LINKED OLIGOSACCHARIDES. The amino-terminal 102 amino acid residues form a V region-like domain, making CD7 a member of IMMUNOGLOBULIN SUPERFAMILY.

CD8 (T8, Leu2, Lyt2,3, MRC Ox8). Membrane glycoprotein of some thymocytes and a subset of T LYMPHOCYTES. CD8 in humans is detected by mouse monoclonal antibodies, anti-T8 and anti-Leu2. CD8 in mice is detected by alloantibodies anti-Lyt2 and anti-Lyt3 and in rats by mouse monoclonal antibodies anti-MRC Ox8. CD8 is expressed on T lymphocytes that are cytotoxic for TARGET CELLS bearing CLASS I HISTOCOMPATIBILITY MOLECULES. The CD8 subset constitutes approximately 30 percent of mature T lymphocytes and contains all SUPPRESSOR T LYMPHOCYTES and most CYTOTOXIC T LYMPHOCYTES. Mature T lymphocytes bearing CD8 are usually negative for CD4 and vice versa. CD8 is a member

of the IMMUNOGLOBULIN SUPERFAMILY; each CD8 chain has a variable region-like domain of approximately 110 amino acid residues.

CD8 molecules consist of two disulfide-linked chains: alpha (Lyt2 in mice) and beta (Lyt3 in mice). The two chains are encoded by closely linked genes that, in humans and mice, are also linked to the genes encoding IMMUNOGLOBULIN KAPPA CHAINS (*see* IMMUNOGLOBULIN GENES).

cDNA (complementary DNA). DNA that is synthesized from an RNA template by retroviral RNA-DIRECTED DNA POLYMERASE (reverse transcriptase). The reaction requires all four deoxynucleoside triphosphates and a primer that is base-paired with the template and bears a free 3'-OH group. For cloning purposes, the single-stranded cDNA can be converted into a double-stranded molecule by several procedures. In one method, the RNA template is destroyed by alkaline hydrolysis; synthesis of the second DNA strand is initiated from a hairpin loop at the 3'-end of the first DNA strand and catalysed by DNA-DIRECTED DNA POLYMERASE I from *E. coli* and/or reverse transcriptase, the first DNA strand serving as template. The hairpin loop and any single-stranded DNA at the other end of the cDNA molecule are then removed by treatment with the single-strand-specific S1 NUCLEASE. The resulting fully double-stranded cDNA can be cloned and thereby becomes a stable, renewable representation of a population of mRNA molecules.

CD8	Human	Alpha Mouse*	Rat	Human	Beta Mouse	Rat
No of amino acid residues/chain	198	247	218	210	213	236
Signal sequence	21	27	21	21	21	26
Extracellular domain	113	104	113	102	103	110
Connecting peptide	12	64	38	41	43	51
Transmembrane segment	25	25	27	27	27	23
Cytoplasmic segment	27	27	19	19	19	26
No. of N-linked ogliosaccharides**	1	4	3	1	1	1
Approx $M_r \times 10^{-3}$	30	38	37	30	29	32

*In mice the alpha' chain differs from the alpha chain in that the cytoplasmic segment consists of five amino acid residues.

**Variable amounts of O-linked saccharides comprise up to 30 percent of the M_r.

cell-mediated immunity (CMI). Immunological reactions initiated by T LYMPHOCYTES and mediated by effector T lymphocytes and MACROPHAGES (e.g, DELAYED-TYPE HYPERSENSITIVITY, GRAFT REJECTION, GRAFT-*VERSUS*-HOST DISEASE).

cellular immunity. *Synonym for* CELL-MEDIATED IMMUNITY.

centiMorgan (cM). Unit of distance in a genetic linkage map, as measured by recombination frequency. One cM corresponds to a recombination frequency of 1 percent (1 percent of the products of meiosis are recombinant). Usually, genetic distances are roughly proportional to physical distances on a chromosome, but occasionally this is not the case due to local variations in the frequency of recombination. In the HLA region, 1 cM is approximately equivalent to 1000 to 2000 kilobases. This unit was named in honor of the geneticist, Thomas Hunt Morgan.

central lymphoid organ. *See* PRIMARY LYMPHOID ORGAN.

C_H. CONSTANT REGION of an IMMUNOGLOBULIN HEAVY CHAIN; C_H denotes the corresponding gene segment.

C_H1. First constant domain of an IMMUNOGLOBULIN HEAVY CHAIN; C_H1 denotes the corresponding gene segment (exon).

C_H2. Second constant domain of an IMMUNOGLOBULIN HEAVY CHAIN; C_H2 denotes the corresponding gene segment (exon).

C_H3. Third constant domain of an IMMUNOGLOBULIN HEAVY CHAIN; C_H3 denotes the corresponding gene segment (exon).

C_H4. Fourth constant domain of an IMMUNOGLOBULIN HEAVY CHAIN, found in IMMUNOGLOBULIN MU and EPSILON CHAINS. C_H4 denotes the corresponding gene segment (exon).

CH_{50}. Quantity of COMPLEMENT required for 50 percent lysis of 5×10^8 optimally sensitized sheep red blood cells in one hour at 37°C. Complement TITERS are expressed as the number of CH_{50} contained in 1 ml of undiluted serum. This is usually determined by plotting $\log y/1-y$ (where y is percent lysis) against the log of the amount of serum. This plot is linear near $y/1-y = 1$ (50 percent lysis). In the example shown, the serum contains 280 CH_{50}/ml.

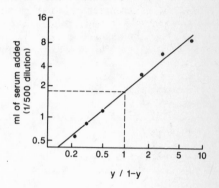

CH_{50}

challenge. Administration of an antigen to ascertain the state of IMMUNITY to a previous immunization or to immunity acquired naturally.

Charcot–Leyden crystal. Bipyramidal crystal found in the sputum of patients with ASTHMA. The crystals are composed of lysophospholipase (M_r 13,000) that is derived from the cell membranes of EOSINOPHILS.

Chediak–Higashi syndrome. Disease characterized by partial albinism and susceptibility to pyogenic infections. NEUTROPHILS contain abnormal, large granules, which may result from fusion of PRIMARY and SECONDARY GRANULES. Delayed killing of bacteria in the neutrophils results from failure of normal phagolysosome formation (*see* PHAGOCYTOSIS). Neutrophils also have defective mobility and capping due to an ill-defined defect in the cytoskeleton. In addition, patients have a marked decrease in the number of NATURAL KILLER CELLS. Lymphomas frequently occur in Chediak–Higashi disease. It is inherited as an autosomal recessive trait. Heterozygotes have not been detected. *See* BEIGE MOUSE.

chemiluminescence.   Generation of light by a chemical reaction. The phenomenon of chemiluminescence is used in the study of PHAGOCYTOSIS. Light is emitted from oxidants generated in NEUTROPHILS and MONOCYTES during the respiratory burst that occurs during phagocytosis. To detect chemiluminescence, Luminol (5-amino-2, 3-dihydro-1,4-phthalazinedione) is fed to phagocytes. When Luminol becomes oxidized, it amplifies intracellular luminescence. Chemiluminescence is used in the diagnosis of CHRONIC GRANULOMATOUS DISEASE.

chemotactic peptide.   Peptide that induces directed migration of cells (e.g, C5a, FORMYL-METHIONYL–LEUCYL–PHENYLALANINE).

chemotaxis.   Reorientation and migration of cells in response to chemical stimuli. In chemotaxis, the cells recognize a gradient of chemical stimulant and migrate toward or away from the zone of highest concentration. Chemotaxis is thought to be essential for NEUTROPHILS and MONOCYTES to migrate into areas of INFLAMMATION and infection. Chemotaxis can be tested in cell culture by a device consisting of two chambers separated by a filter (Boyden chamber). The cells are placed in one chamber and the chemical in the other. The cells migrating towards the chamber containing the chemical stimulant are counted on the filter. Several agents chemotactic for neutrophils have been identified (e.g., C5a, leukotriene B5).

Chido Rodgers antigens.   Antigenic determinants of C4d fragments bound to red cells and formerly thought to be BLOOD GROUP SUBSTANCES. Usually, the Chido antigenic determinant is present on C4d derived from C4B and the Rodgers antigenic determinant on C4d derived from C4A. The antigenic determinant of the Chido antigen is Ala–Asp–Leu–Arg; that of the Rodgers antigen is Val–Asp–Leu–Leu. These residues occupy positions 1188–1191 in the C4d segment of the alpha chain of C4.

chimera.   Coexistence in a single individual of tissues or cells of different genotype. For example, the recipient of a bone marrow transplant from a genetically different individual has blood cells of donor origin as well as AUTOLOGOUS cells. The term is derived

from Greek mythology: a monster with a head of a lion, a body of a goat and a tail of a dragon or a serpent.

chimerism.   Condition of being a CHIMERA.

chlorambucil   (4-[bis(2-chloroethyl)amino-phenylbutyric acid). Nitrogen mustard derivative used to achieve IMMUNOSUPPRESSION and in the treatment of MACROGLOBULINEMIA OF WALDENSTRÖM. The mechanism of action of chlorambucil is similar to that of CYCLOPHOSPHAMIDE.

$$HOOC-CH_2-CH_2-CH_2- \left\langle \bigcirc \right\rangle -N \Big\langle \begin{array}{c} CH_2-CH_2-Cl \\ CH_2-CH_2-Cl \end{array}$$

chlorambucil

chromosome walking.   Method for identifying cloned sequences flanking a particular segment of cloned DNA. Terminal fragments from one or both ends of the original CLONE (for unidirectional and bidirectional walking, respectively) are used as hybridization probes (*see* MOLECULAR HYBRIDIZATION PROBE) for screening a library of genomic DNA. Clones that overlap and therefore extend beyond the original DNA segment are identified. Terminal fragments from the non-shared end of the new clone can then be used to repeat the process for further extension. Contiguous fragments spanning several hundred kilobases have been obtained. Recent technical advances involving use of PULSED FIELD GRADIENT GEL ELECTROPHORESIS and 'chromosome jumping' allow the linking of fragments spanning thousands of kilobases.

chronic active hepatitis.   Focal NECROSIS of the liver with infiltrates of LYMPHOCYTES and PLASMA CELLS in the portal areas leading ultimately to cirrhosis of the liver. One form of the disease occurs predominantly in teenage females who develop jaundice, anorexia (loss of appetite), abdominal pain and enlargement of the liver and spleen. There are increased amounts of IMMUNOGLOBULIN of all ISOTYPES including numerous AUTOANTIBODIES such as ANTI-NUCLEAR ANTIBODIES, RHEUMATOID FACTOR, antibodies to smooth muscle, etc. The disease is associated with HLA-B8 (*see* HLA).

chronic granulomatous disease (CGD). Group of disorders, characterized by increased susceptibility to certain bacterial and fungal infections, due to a genetically determined deficiency of killing of the organisms within PHAGOCYTES. In CGD, there is decreased production of hydrogen peroxide and superoxide radicals during PHAGOCYTOSIS. Because certain ingested microorganisms cannot be killed and therefore persist intracellularly, abscess formation and GRANULOMAS occur. The abscesses and granulomas may occur in any organ, but are most prominent in LYMPH NODES, skin, lung and liver. CGD may be inherited as an autosomal or X-linked recessive trait. The X-linked form may be associated with the MCLEOD PHENOTYPE. Diagnosis is made by a NITROBLUE TETRAZO-LIUM DYE TEST or by demonstrating decreased CHEMILUMINESCENCE.

The gene for X-linked CGD has been mapped to Xp21.1 and encodes a protein of M_r 90,000, which associates with a protein of M_r 22,000 whose gene has been mapped to chromosome 16, thereby forming the phagocyte-specific b-cytochrome HETERO-DIMER. The catalytic site of this enzyme is in the M_r 22,000 polypeptide chain. Mutations in the gene for the M_r 90,000 subunit may lead to X-linked CGD and mutations in the gene for the M_r 22,000 subunit may lead to one of two types of autosomal recessive CGD. The genetic basis of a second type of autosomal recessive CGD is not known.

X-linked CGD has been successfully treated with INTERFERON-GAMMA.

chronic lymphocytic leukemia (CLL). Leukemia of B LYMPHOCYTES, characterized by progressive accumulation of long-lived, small lymphocytes in BONE MARROW, SPLEEN, LYMPH NODES, blood and other tissue. In over 95 percent of cases, CLL cells have surface MONOCLONAL IMMUNOGLOBULIN. Since these B lymphocytes do not function normally, patients with CLL frequently have HYPOGAMMAGLOBULINEMIA and develop clinical problems associated with B lymphocyte deficiency, such as recurrent PYOGENIC INFECTIONS. CLL runs a benign course and patients with CLL may survive for more than 30 years.

chronic lymphocytic thyroiditis. AUTOIMMUNE DISEASE of the thyroid, characterized by a heavy infiltration of LYMPHOCYTES, PLASMA CELLS and MACROPHAGES with destruction of the normal follicular architecture of the gland. The thyroid is enlarged (goiter), and thyroid function is diminished (hypothyroidism). The disease is much more common in women than in men. The sera of patients contain antibodies to peroxidase (M_r 107,000) in thyroid microsomes, to thyroglobulin and to the receptor for thyrotropin. A similar disease can be induced in animals by immunization with thyroid extracts. *Synonym for* Hashimoto's disease, autoimmune thyroiditis.

chrysotherapy. *See* GOLD THERAPY.

cimetidine. Antagonist of the HISTAMINE H_2-receptor (*see* ANTIHISTAMINE). Cimetidine inhibits acid secretion by the stomach and for this reason is used to treat peptic ulcers. It has been used successfully in the treatment of COMMON VARIABLE IMMUNODE-FICIENCY; its effect is thought to be due to inhibition of SUPPRESSOR T LYMPHOCYTES.

$$CH_4 \quad CH_2SCH_2CH_2N = CNHCH_3$$
$$HN-N\equiv C$$
$$HN \quad N$$

cimetidine

circulating anticoagulant. Antibody with specificity for one or another coagulation (clotting) factor. These antibodies are found in three clinical situations: (1) SYSTEMIC LUPUS ERYTHEMATOSUS, (2) following therapy with penicillin, isoniazid or streptomycin, (3) in hemophilia A or B after therapy with Factor VIII or Factor IX. These antibodies are usually IgG4 (*see* IMMUNOGLOBULIN SUBCLASS).

cisterna chyli. *See* THORACIC DUCT.

C_L. Constant domain of an IMMUNOGLOBULIN LIGHT CHAIN; C_L denotes the corresponding gene segment.

class I histocompatibility molecules. One of the two classes of cell membrane glycoproteins (the other being CLASS II HISTOCOMPATIBILITY MOLECULES) that mediate cellular interactions of the immune system. Class I molecules are found on all nucleated cells (except sperm and trophoblasts) but in especially high concentration on lymphocytes. T lymphocytes that are CD8+

recognize ANTIGENIC DETERMINANTS of foreign class I histocompatibility molecules or antigen associated with self class I molecules.

Class I molecules of mouse and humans are heterodimers consisting of a polymorphic heavy or alpha chain of approximately 340 amino acid residues (M_r 44000), which spans the cell membrane, and a noncovalently associated invariant light or beta chain, BETA-2 MICROGLOBULIN. The alpha chains are encoded by genes in the major histocompatibility complex (humans HLA-A, -B, -C, -E and in mice, H-2K, D, L). In mice, other class I molecules are encoded in the Tla complex adjacent to H-2. The alpha (α) chains consist of five domains. Three of these, α_1, α_2 and α_3, each composed of approximately 90 residues, are external to the cell surface, the α_1 being amino-terminal. There is also a transmembrane region of 20 residues and a cytoplasmic domain of approximately 40 residues. The α_2 and α_3 domains have intrachain disulfide bonds spanning approximately 60 amino acid residues. The α_1 and α_2 domains pair with each other. The α_3 domain pairs with beta-2 microglobulin and these two domains are proximal to the membrane. Soluble forms of class I molecules can be prepared by digestion with papain, which cleaves between the α_3 domain and the transmembrane segment.

In primary and three dimensional structure, the α_3 domain and beta-2 microglobulin resemble constant region-like domains (*see* immunoglobulin superfamily); the α_1 and α_2 domains do not resemble immunoglobulin structures. There are two N-LINKED OLIGOSACCHARIDES, one in the α_1 and one in the α_2 domain. Most of the sequence diversity of class I molecules lies in the α_1 and α_2 domains; there is very little sequence diversity in the α_3 domain. A class I gene contains eight exons, spread over 4 to 5 kilobases: one exon encodes the signal sequence, three others the α_1, α_2 and α_3 domains, another the transmembrane segment, three the cytoplasmic domain and the 3' untranslated region.

The α_1 and α_2 domains have an amino-terminal region of approximately 50 amino acid residues consisting of four strands of a BETA-PLEATED SHEET and a carboxy terminal region of approximately 40 residues containing ALPHA HELICES. The eight beta strands of the α_1 and α_2 domains form a platform structure that is the floor of the peptide binding site. The alpha helices lie on top of the beta-pleated sheets and form the sides of the site. The helical region of the α_1 domain is more diverse in sequence than the helical region of the α_2 domain, whereas the beta-stranded region of α_1 is somewhat less diverse than that of the α_2. Most of the positions of highest variability are in the peptide binding site.

class II histocompatibility molecules. One of the two classes of cell membrane glycoproteins (the other being CLASS I HISTOCOMPATIBILITY MOLECULES) that mediates cellular interactions of the immune system. Class II histocompatibility molecules are found on ACCESSORY CELLS and B LYMPHOCYTES. T LYMPHOCYTES that are CD4+ recognize ANTIGENIC DETERMINANTS of foreign class II histocompatibility molecules or antigens associated with self class II molecules. These T cells subsequently divide and secrete LYMPHOKINES, which are important for B cell growth and differentiation and activation of MACROPHAGES and CYTOTOXIC T LYMPHOCYTES.

The genes that encode class II molecules are in the MAJOR HISTOCOMPATIBILITY COMPLEX (in humans, in the HLA-D REGION and in mice, in the I REGION). Class II molecules of mouse and humans, also called Ia antigens, are HETERODIMERS consisting of a heavy or alpha (α) chain (M_r 30,000–34,000) noncovalently associated with a light or beta (β) chain (M_r 27,000–29,000). Both α and β chains each consist of four DOMAINS. Two domains, α_1 and α_2 and β_1 and β_2 (~90 amino acid residues each) are external to the cell surface, the α_1 and β_1 being amino-terminal. In each chain, there is also a transmembrane segment of approximately 25 residues and a short intracytoplasmic domain of 10–15 residues. The α_2 and β_2 domains, have intrachain disulfide bonds spanning approximately 60 amino acid residues, and these domains resemble constant region-like domains (*see* IMMUNOGLOBULIN SUPERFAMILY). The α chain has two N-LINKED OLIGOSACCHARIDES, one in the α_1 domain and the other in the α_2 domain; the β chain has one N-linked oligosaccharide in the β_1 domain. The α genes contain five exons: one exon encodes the SIGNAL SEQUENCE and two encode the two extracellular domains. The fourth exon encodes the transmembrane domain, the short cytoplasmic domain, and part of the 3′ untranslated region; the fifth exon encodes the rest of the 3′ untranslated region. In the case of the β genes, there are six exons: these are similar to the first three exons of the α genes, the fourth encodes the transmembrane domain and a part of the cytoplasmic domain, the fifth the rest of the cytoplasmic domain, and the sixth the 3′ untranslated region. Most of the sequence diversity in class II molecules lies in the β_1 domain. In mice, the α_1 domain of I–A molecules, but not of I–E molecules, also has considerable sequence diversity.

In mice and humans, class II molecules are associated with a third polypeptide chain that exhibits little or no polymorphism. It is designated the I INVARIANT CHAIN (Ii).

class III molecules. Molecules, encoded by genes in the S REGION of the MAJOR HISTOCOMPATIBILITY COMPLEX (MHC). They are not determinants of histocompatibility. Originally, COMPLEMENT components (FACTOR B, C2 and C4) were found to be linked to genes encoding HLA on the short arm of chromosome 6 in humans and to *H-2* on chromosome 17 in mice; they were called CLASS III MOLECULES to distinguish them from CLASS I and CLASS II HISTOCOMPATIBILITY MOLECULES. The genes encoding class III molecules occupy a segment of approximately 100 kilobases in the MHC between the HLA-B locus and the HLA-D REGION in humans and the I-REGION and H-2D in mice. Subsequently, genes encoding P-450 21-hydroxylase were found to be closely linked to the genes encoding C4.

class switching (isotype switching). Change in IMMUNOGLOBULIN CLASS (ISOTYPE) synthesis that occurs during the differentiation of B LYMPHOCYTES. The switch involves only the CONSTANT REGION of the heavy chain; there is no change in the type of light chain produced nor in the heavy-chain VARIABLE REGION (i.e., the antigen-binding specificity remains the same). Two molecular mechanisms appear to be involved in class switching at different stages in B cell differentiation: (1) produc-

tion of transcripts that are processed to different mRNAs, and (2) IMMUNOGLOBULIN GENE REARRANGEMENTS resulting in transposition of constant-region gene segments.

Immature B lymphocytes express membrane IgM (*see* MEMBRANE IMMUNOGLOBULIN, IMMUNOGLOBULIN MU CHAIN). As the B cells mature, membrane IgD is also expressed. Differential splicing of a long (at least 23 kilobases) transcript is thought to be responsible for the co-expression of the two isotypes. A primary transcript containing sequences corresponding to a heavy chain variable region and both mu and delta constant regions is presumably spliced to yield mRNA encoding each heavy chain (i.e., V_H–D_H–J_H–C_μ and V_H–D_H–J_H–C_δ). It has also been proposed that processing of extremely long transcripts (e.g., containing C_μ and C_α sequences) may be responsible for class switching in memory B lymphocytes.

Immunoglobulin gene rearrangements are thought to account for most cases of switching after B cells have been stimulated by interactions with antigen and T LYMPHOCYTES. These class switches usually occur with 5′ to 3′ polarity with respect to the order of the *C* GENE SEGMENTS encoding the heavy chains of different classes (*see* IMMUNOGLOBULIN GENES). Thus, synthesis of IgM is replaced by synthesis of IgG1, but the reverse does not usually occur. This process appears to be mediated by reiterated sequences within SWITCH (S) REGIONS located within or 5′ to each functional C_H gene (except C_δ). The 5′ rearrangement breakpoint usually lies 5′ to S_μ, the 3′ break-point is within S_γ, S_ϵ or S_α. A V_H–D_H–J_H gene segment is translocated, in the 3′ direction, from the region 5′ to one C_H to the region 5′ to another C_H. B lymphocytes that are in the process of switching may transiently express two or even three different immunoglobulin classes. Several mechanisms for switch recombination have been proposed: (1) looping out of intervening C_H gene segments followed by deletion; most switch–recombination events appear to be consistent with this mechanism; (2) unequal homologous chromosome exchange; and (3) sister chromatid exchange. Recent studies indicate that class switching is preceded by transcriptional activation of those downstream C_H gene segments that will undergo rearrangement.

classical pathway of complement. One of the two known mechanisms (the other being the ALTERNATIVE PATHWAY OF COMPLEMENT) for the activation of C3. The proteins of the classical pathway are C1, C4 and C2. The classical pathway is activated when the C1 subcomponent, C1q, binds to IgG or IgM. The sequential activation of C1 subcomponents C1r and C1s results in cleavage of the two substrates of C1s, C4 and C2. Their active fragments, C4b and C2a, form a bimolecular enzyme (C4b2a) which is the classical pathway C3 CONVERTASE; the catalytic site of the enzyme lies in the C2a fragment. The classical pathway is inhibited by C1 INHIBITOR, which dissociates C1r and C1s from C1q, and by C4 BINDING PROTEIN, which binds to C4b, dissociates it from C2a and allows FACTOR I to cleave the heavy chain of C4b, producing C4bi; C4bi cannot bind C2a and is, therefore, inactive in the classical pathway.

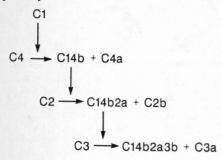

C1

C4 → C14b + C4a

C2 → C14b2a + C2b

C3 → C14b2a3b + C3a

classical pathway

clathrin. Major protein in the coat of many COATED VESICLES. Clathrin molecules are composed of three heavy chains (each M_r 180,000) and three light chains (each M_r 30,000–35,000) assembled into characteristic pentagonal or hexagonal lattices, which can form cage-like structures around the vesicles.

Cleveland procedure. Type of peptide map in which a protein is partially digested with a protease in the presence of sodium dodecyl sulfate (SDS), and the cleavage products are analysed by POLYACRYLAMIDE GEL ELECTROPHORESIS IN SDS. The pattern of peptide fragments produced is characteristic of the protein substrate and the proteolytic enzyme and is highly reproducible. *See* FINGERPRINTING.

clonal selection theory. Theory of antibody formation based on the assumption that each LYMPHOCYTE bears MEMBRANE IMMUNOGLOBULIN receptors of a single specificity and that the binding of a LIGAND (i.e., an ANTIGENIC DETERMINANT) to these receptors stimulates (i.e., 'selects') that lymphocyte to proliferate into a CLONE of antibody-secreting cells. The secreted antibody has the same specificity as that of the membrane receptors. The clonal selection theory is now widely accepted as being correct and has superseded all other SELECTIVE THEORIES.

clone. Population of cells or organisms all derived from a single individual by asexual multiplication. The members of a clone are genetically identical.

cloned DNA. Fragment of DNA (e.g., a gene) that has been inserted into a VECTOR and replicated in a bacterial or eukaryotic cell line.

clonotypic. Characteristic of a clone. The term was introduced to describe the properties of the antigen-specific receptors of a population of B LYMPHOCYTES that would be expected from a CLONE of such cells. Thus, the SPECTROTYPE of secreted antibodies should be restricted, the reactivity with antigens should be highly specific (e.g, as measured by cross-reactivity with a panel of antigens) and the antibodies should have one or more distinct PRIVATE IDIOTYPIC DETERMINANTS. The term has been extended to refer to the characteristic properties of the antigen-specific receptor on a clone of T LYMPHOCYTES, i.e., the uniformity and individuality of antigen recognition and idiotypic expression.

cluster of differentiation (CD). Group of antigenic determinants on a molecule in the membrane of human blood cells that define stages of differentiation of these cells and that are detected by monoclonal antibodies. By extension, CD designations are assigned to equivalent molecules in blood cells of animals (e.g., L3T4 in mice is called CD4). The clusters are designated CD1, CD2, CD3...CD*n*.

c–myc. *See* MYC ONCOGENE.

coated pit. Invagination of the plasma membrane having a CLATHRIN coat on the cytoplasmic side. Many extracellular ligands, such as peptide hormones and growth factors, bind to their specific receptors and cluster in coated pits, which invaginate and pinch off to form COATED VESICLES. Plasma membrane receptor proteins may associate spontaneously with coated pits or may be induced to migrate to the coated pits by the binding of ligand. Coated pits constitute about 2 percent of the cell surface of a cultured fibroblast.

coated vesicle. Cytoplasmic vesicle (about 70–200 nm in diameter) surrounded by a distinct protein coat, often consisting of CLATHRIN molecules. Clathrin-coated vesicles play an important role in receptor-mediated ENDOCYTOSIS and in protein secretion. In receptor-mediated endocytosis, clathrin-coated vesicles, which are derived from COATED PITS, transport macromolecules together with their specific receptors from the extracellular fluid to the interior of the cell. Coated vesicles also transport proteins between intracellular organelles (e.g., ENDOPLASMIC RETICULUM and GOLGI COMPLEX). Intracellular vesicles, coated by proteins other than clathrin, have been described. *See* ENDOCYTOSIS, EXOCYTOSIS.

cobra venom factor (CVF). Protein in venom of the hooded Indian cobra (*Naja naja*) that can be substituted for mammalian C3b in the activation of the ALTERNATIVE PATHWAY OF COMPLEMENT. Since CVF, in contrast to C3b, cannot be inactivated by mammalian FACTOR I, the addition of cobra venom to mammalian serum, results in formation of a stable alternative pathway C3 CONVERTASE (i.e., between CVF and mammalian FACTOR B). Thus, when cobra venom factor is given to a mammal intravenously, the COMPLEMENT activity is destroyed. CVF is derived from cobra C3 and structurally resembles mammalian C3c.

co-capping. Capping of one membrane molecule as the result of the ligand-induced capping of another membrane molecule. Co-capping may occur when two molecules are associated in the membrane. For example, if molecules A and B are associated, then antibodies to A, which cap A, may also cap B; the capping of B is co-capping. If A and B are not associated, then the capping of A will not change the distribution of B in the membrane. For example, the association of BETA-2 MICROGLOBULIN with the heavy chain of CLASS I MAJOR HISTOCOMPATIBILITY MOLECULES and that of CD3 and the T CELL RECEPTOR were demonstrated by co-capping.

coccidioidin. Crude extract of *Coccidioides immitis* used to test CELL-MEDIATED IMMUNITY to the fungus.

co-dominance. Expression of two traits corresponding to a pair of different alleles (i.e., the heterozygote has the phenotype of both homozygotes). An example of co-dominance is the expression of both A and B blood group antigenic determinants in AB individuals. *See* ABO BLOOD GROUP.

codon. Triplet of contiguous nucleotides in mRNA (e.g., UUU) that encodes a particular amino acid residues (phenylalanine) or that specifies termination of translation. The codon pairs with a triplet of three complementary nucleotides (AAA) in the ANTICODON loop of a tRNA molecule. The sequence of triplet codons in mRNA determines (encodes) the linear sequence of amino acid residues in a protein. Sometimes, the corresponding triplet of bases in DNA (TTT) is also referred to as a codon.

Table of codons

First position (5' end)	Second position				Third position (3' end)
	U	C	A	G	
U	Phe	Ser	Tyr	Cys	U
	Phe	Ser	Tyr	Cys	C
	Leu	Ser	Stop	Stop	A
	Leu	Ser	Stop	Trp	G
C	Leu	Pro	His	Arg	U
	Leu	Pro	His	Arg	C
	Leu	Pro	Gln	Arg	A
	Leu	Pro	Gln	Arg	G
A	Ile	Thr	Asn	Ser	U
	Ile	Thr	Asn	Ser	C
	Ile	Thr	Lys	Arg	A
	Met	Thr	Lys	Arg	G
G	Val	Ala	Asp	Gly	U
	Val	Ala	Asp	Gly	C
	Val	Ala	Glu	Gly	A
	Val	Ala	Glu	Gly	G

cognate interaction. Direct interaction between a processed antigen on the surface of a B LYMPHOCYTE and a T LYMPHOCYTE receptor, leading to terminal differentiation of the B lymphocyte and antibody production. In cell culture, B cells can also be activated by antibodies to IMMUNOGLOBULIN MU CHAINS and by LYMPHOKINES without the need for cognate interaction. *See* T–B CELL COLLABORATION.

cognate recognition. *See* COGNATE INTERACTION.

cohesive end. Single-stranded overhanging segment of DNA produced in a DNA duplex. Cohesive ends can be produced by cleavage with certain RESTRICTION ENDONUCLEASES (e.g., *Eco* RI). A cohesive or sticky end can associate by base pairing with a segment containing the complementary sequence (generally generated by cleavage of another DNA duplex using the same restriction enzyme). Two segments of DNA, which are non-covalently associated through their cohesive ends, can be covalently joined by DNA ligase.

coisogenic strains. INBRED STRAINS of mice that differ at a single genetic locus. True coisogenic strains can be produced when a point mutation occurs in an inbred strain. If the individual carrying the mutation is inbred, the new line will be coisogenic with the original line. Since mutations in particular loci cannot be produced at will (unless methods of site-directed mutagenesis are used), it is difficult to obtain lines that are coisogenic at a specified locus. Therefore, CONGENIC STRAINS, which differ in a short chromosomal region, have been developed.

cold agglutinin. Antibody that agglutinates more effectively at temperatures below 37°C than at 37°C. *See* AGGLUTINATION, COLD AGGLUTININ SYNDROME.

cold agglutinin syndrome. Form of HEMOLYTIC ANEMIA caused by monoclonal IgM AUTOANTIBODIES to the I and/or i antigen of red blood cells (*see* Ii ANTIGEN). These IgM anti-I antibodies agglutinate red blood cells optimally at 20–25°C and fix COMPLEMENT efficiently when warmed to 37°C (*see* AGGLUTINATION). They are found in patients with LYMPHOMA or who have recovered from mycoplasma pneumonia. *In vivo*, HEMOLYSIS occurs in the blood through COMPLEMENT FIXATION or by attachment of affected red blood cells to COMPLEMENT RECEPTORS 1 and 3 on the MACROPHAGES of liver and SPLEEN.

colony-forming unit–spleen (CFU-S). Hematopoietic progenitor cell that, upon inoculation into a lethally irradiated mouse, forms a small nodule in the spleen. The nodules, visible to the naked eye, represent foci of cell proliferation. Each nodule is derived from a single cell called a colony-forming unit. There are three types of progenitor cells: (1) those that give rise to red blood cells; (2) those that give rise to MEGAKARYOCYTES and PLATELETS; (3) those that give rise to POLYMORPHONUCLEAR LEUKOCYTES and MONOCYTES.

colony stimulating factors (CSF). Factors that promote the growth and differentiation of HEMATOPOIETIC STEM CELLS and stimulate end-cell functional activity. The target cells of each CSF express a cell surface receptor for the appropriate CSF. These factors are synthesized by T LYMPHOCYTES, endothelial cells, fibroblasts and other cells. Four of these factors have been identified in mouse and humans, and cDNA clones have been obtained; they are all glycoproteins.

colostrum. First fluid produced by the mammalian breast after childbirth. It contains large amounts of immunoglobulins, principally IgA and is a source of PASSIVE IMMUNITY for the newborn of most species.

combined immunodeficiency. Any PRIMARY IMMUNODEFICIENCY that affects both T and B LYMPHOCYTES. SEVERE COMBINED IMMUNODEFICIENCY, in contrast to combined immunodeficiency, is a term restricted to infants with potentially fatal defects of both T and B lymphocytes. Combined immunodeficiency is a term that describes less severe forms of immunodeficiency in children and adults. *See* COMMON VARIABLE IMMUNODEFICIENCY.

commensal mouse. WILD MOUSE that lives in close association with humans. *See* FERAL MOUSE.

common acute lymphocytic leukemia antigen (CALLA). Surface glycoprotein (M_r 100,000) that is expressed in 80 percent of non–T cell leukemias, on poorly differen-

Colony stimulating factor (CSF)	Alternative name	Target cells	Approx. M_r Mouse	Human	No. of amino acids/chain* Mouse	Human
1. Granulocyte-macrophage (GM-CSF)	CSF-2 CSF-α	pluripotential stem stells; promyelocytes, neutrophils, eosinophils; promonocytes, monocytes	23,000	22,000	118	144
2. Macrophage (M-CSF)	CSF-1	pluripotential stem cells; promonocytes, monocytes	70,000 (homo-dimer)	45,000 (homo-dimer)	–	256
3. Granulocyte (G-CSF)	CSF-β	pluripotential stem cells; myelocytes, neutrophils	25,000	30,000	–	207
4. Multi-potential (Multi-CSF)	Interleukin-3 (IL-3)	pluripotential stem cells; promyelocytes, myelocytes, neutrophils, eosinophils; promonocytes, monocytes; megakaryocytes; mast cells	25,000	18,000	167	152

* including signal sequence and in the case of M-CSF a putative transmembrane segment and cytoplasmic domain.

tiated LYMPHOMAS, as well as normal tissue, especially kidney. CALLA is detected by mouse MONOCLONAL ANTIBODIES. One percent of normal bone marrow cells express CALLA. Anti-CALLA and COMPLEMENT have been used to eliminate acute lymphocytic leukemia cells from bone marrow before AUTOLOGOUS bone marrow transplants. CALLA is identical to neutral endopeptidase (EC 3.4.24.11).

common variable immunodeficiency (CVI). Group of disorders characterized predominantly by antibody deficiency and by variable defects in CELL-MEDIATED IMMUNITY. It is the most common primary immunodeficiency in adults. Patients whose immunodeficiency cannot be readily classified as one of the known heritable or acquired immunodeficiency syndromes are grouped under the term CVI. These patients may have intrinsic defects in B LYMPHOCYTES, which do not differentiate normally; there may be defects in the regulatory functions of T LYMPHOCYTES (eg., too few HELPER T LYMPHOCYTES); in rare cases, there are AUTOANTIBODIES to B lymphocytes. Patients frequently have PYOGENIC INFECTIONS. This ill-defined immunodeficiency, which was formerly called 'acquired agammaglobulinemia', may have its onset at any age and occurs with equal frequency in males and females.

complement (C). Group of serum proteins, sequentially activated by limited proteolysis,

that are important effectors of HUMORAL IMMUNITY. Typically the activation of C is triggered by ANTIGEN–ANTIBODY COMPLEXES. It may also be triggered by proteolytic enzymes (e.g., plasmin) or by complex carbohydrates (e.g., INULIN). Many biological activities are mediated by the components of the complement system, e.g., immune cytolysis, ANAPHYLATOXIN production, BACTERIOLYSIS, CHEMOTAXIS, HEMOLYSIS, OPSONIZATION, PHAGOCYTOSIS. The components of the complement system are C1, C4, C2, C3, C5, C6, C7, C8, C9, FACTOR B, FACTOR D, FACTOR H, FACTOR I, PROPERDIN, C1 INHIBITOR and C4 BINDING PROTEIN.

complement deficiency. Decrease in serum concentration of one or more complement components of sufficient magnitude to lower the total hemolytic activity (CH_{50}). Genetic deficiencies of C1q, C1r/C1s, C1 INHIBITOR, C2, C3, C4, C5, C6, C7, C8, C9, FACTOR H, FACTOR I, FACTOR D or PROPERDIN have been found in humans, rabbits, guinea-pigs and mice. The genetic deficiencies in humans are listed and are grouped according to the main symptoms. Complement deficiency may be acquired due to (1) increased consumption of complement components in immune complex disease (e.g., SYSTEMIC LUPUS ERYTHEMATOSUS) or (2) decreased synthesis of complement components (e.g., acute hepatic necrosis). Synonym for hypocomplementemia. See C1 DEFICIENCY, C2 DEFICIENCY, C3 DEFICIENCY, C4 DEFICIENCY, C5 DEFICIENCY,

Complement components

Component	Serum conc. (mg/ml)	No. of polypeptide chains	No. of amino acid residues/chain	M, of polypeptide chains	Human chromosome map location
C1q	0.1	18	A chain 224 B chain 226 C chain 222	each ~ 23,000	B chain:1p
C1r	0.1	2	α463;β243	α56,000;β27,000	12p
C1s	0.05	2	α431;β242	α58,000;β27,000	12p
C2	0.01	1	732	100,000	6p
C3	1.5	2	α992;β645	α117,000;β75,000	19q
C4	0.6	3	α772;β660;γ288	α93,000;β75,000;γ30,000	6p
C5	0.1	2	α1002;β643	α115,000;β75,000	
C6	0.2	1		124,000	
C7	0.1	1	843	104,000	
C8	0.1	3	α583;β590;γ?	α64,000;β64,000;γ22,000	
C9	0.2	1	537	71,000	
C1 inhibitor	0.2	1	478	105,000	11q
C4 binding protein	0.2	7 identical	549 each	107,000 each	1q
Factor B	0.2	1	739	100,000	6p
Factor D	0.003	1	222	24,000	
Factor H	0.5	1	1216	150,000	1q
Factor I	0.03	2	α321;β244	α50,000;β38,000	4q
Properdin	0.02	4 identical	441	56,000 each	X

C6 DEFICIENCY, C7 DEFICIENCY, C8 DEFICIENCY, C9 DEFICIENCY, FACTOR D DEFICIENCY, FACTOR H DEFICIENCY, FACTOR I DEFICIENCY, HEREDITARY ANGIONEUROTIC EDEMA, PROPERDIN DEFICIENCY.

Genetic deficiencies of human complement components

Group I: immune complex disease
  1. C1q　　　　　　　　　　　AR
  2. C1r or C1r/C1s　　　　　　AR
  3. C2　　　　　　　　　　　　AR
  4. C4　　　　　　　　　　　　AR
Group II: angioedema
  1. C1 inhibitor (*see* HEREDITARY ANGIONEUROTIC EDEMA)　AD
Group III: recurrent pyogenic infections
  1. C3　　　　　　　　　　　　AR
  2. Factor I　　　　　　　　　　AR
  3. Factor H　　　　　　　　　　AR
Group IV: recurrent neisserial infections
  1. C5　　　　　　　　　　　　AR
  2. C6　　　　　　　　　　　　AR
  3. C7　　　　　　　　　　　　AR
  4. C8　　　　　　　　　　　　AR

  5. properdin　　　　　　　　　XL
  6. Factor D　　　　　　　　　XL(?)
Group V: asymptomatic
  1. C9　　　　　　　　　　　　AR

AR = autosomal recessive
AD = autosomal dominant
XL = X-linked recessive

complement deviation. Inhibition of COMPLEMENT FIXATION in ANTIBODY EXCESS. *See* PROZONE.

complement fixation. Activation of COMPLEMENT with the result that complement activity disappears. *See* COMPLEMENT FIXATION TEST.

complement fixation test. Test for COMPLEMENT FIXATION, typically by ANTIGEN–ANTIBODY COMPLEXES or non-specifically by aggregated immunoglobulins. To determine whether complement has been fixed (step I) an indicator system, consisting of sheep red blood cells sensitized (coated) with rabbit antibodies, is added (step II). Diminished (or absent) lysis indicates that complement has been fixed. This is a sensitive test for the detection of antibodies or antigens.

STEP I

1. Ab + Ag + C → Ab–Ag–C
2. Ab + C → Ab + C
3. Ag + C → Ag + C

STEP II

+ EA → no lysis
+ EA → lysis
+ EA → lysis

Ab = antibody

Ag = antigen

C = complement

EA = sensitized sheep red blood cells

complement fixation test

complement receptors.   Receptors for complement components or fragments derived from these components. There are four such receptors: COMPLEMENT RECEPTOR 1 (CR1), COMPLEMENT RECEPTOR 2 (CR2), COMPLEMENT RECEPTOR 3 (CR3) and COMPLEMENT RECEPTOR 4 (CR4). Their cell distribution, ligands, molecular properties and functions are shown in the table.

complement receptor 1 (CR1) (CD35). Receptor for C3b and C4b. CR1 is a membrane glycoprotein of PHAGOCYTIC CELLS, MAST CELLS, B LYMPHOCYTES, some T LYMPHOCYTES, red blood cells (in primates), renal glomerular epithelial cells (in primates) and platelets (in sub-primate mammals). CR1 interacts with its ligands more efficiently when they are aggregated. CR1 mediates IMMUNE ADHERENCE, which is thought to be important in the clearance of immune complexes from the blood. CR1 is also a cofactor for the cleavage of C3b and C4b by FACTOR I. Human CR1 is a single polypeptide chain; it is composed of 21 short consensus sequence repeats (*see* CONSENSUS SEQUENCE OF C3/C4 BINDING PROTEINS) arranged in three long homologous repeating sequences, each of which consists of seven short consensus repeats (a b c d e f g a′ b′ c′ d′ e′ f′ g′ a″ b″ d″ e″ f″ g″). The corresponding short consensus repeats (e.g., a, a′, a″) of approximately 60 amino acid residues have 60–100 percent amino acid sequence identity, whereas the long repeats generally have approximately 50 percent identity. CR1 is polymorphic; in 70 percent of humans, CR1 has an M_r of 250,000 and in 3 percent, it has an M_r of 290,000. The remainder of the population is heterozygous. The gene encoding CR1 has been mapped to chromosome 1q3.2 It is closely linked to the genes for COMPLEMENT RECEPTOR 2, C4 BINDING PROTEIN, FACTOR H and DECAY ACCELERATING FACTOR. *See* RCA LOCUS.

complement receptor 2 (CR2) (CD21). Receptor for C3dg or C3d. CR2 is a membrane glycoprotein of B LYMPHOCYTES, the growth of which is stimulated by C3d. CR2 is also the receptor for EPSTEIN–BARR VIRUS. CR2 consists of a single polypeptide chain (M_r 145,000). It contains 13 consensus sequence repeats (*see* CONSENSUS SEQUENCE OF C3/C4 BINDING PROTEINS). The gene encoding CR2 has been mapped to chromosome 1q3.2. It is closely linked to the genes for COMPLEMENT RECEPTOR 1, C4 BINDING PROTEIN, FACTOR H and DECAY ACCELERATING FACTOR. *See* RCA LOCUS.

Receptors	Cell distribution	Ligand	M_r of chains	Function
CR1	erythrocytes, granulocytes, mast cells, macrophages, renal epithelial cells	C3b C4b	190,000–290,000*	IMMUNE ADHERENCE
CR2	B lymphocytes	C3d	140,000	B cell growth and differentiation
CR3	phagocytes, natural killer cells	C3bi	α155,000 (CD11b) β95,000 (CD18)	PHAGOCYTOSIS
CR4	neutrophils	C3dg	α150,000 (CD11c) β95,000 (CD18)	phagocytosis

*Range of M_r includes all genetic forms of CR1.

complement receptor 3 (CR3) (CD11b, 18). Receptor for C3bi (iC3b). CR3 is a membrane glycoprotein of NEUTROPHILS, MONONUCLEAR PHAGOCYTES and NATURAL KILLER CELLS. CR3 mediates PHAGOCYTOSIS of particles coated with C3bi. CR3 consists of an alpha chain (M_r 170,000) and a beta chain (M_r 95,000), which is identical to the beta chain of LYMPHOCYTE FUNCTION ASSOCIATED ANTIGEN-1 (LFA-1) and of p150,95. Human CR3 is also known as Mo1 and mouse CR3 as Mac1. CR3 expression is greatly increased when phagocytic cells are stimulated (e.g., with C5a or FORMYL-METHIONYL–LEUCYL–PHENYLALANINE). Genetic deficiency of CR3 in humans results in recurrent PYOGENIC INFECTIONS. *See* LEUKOCYTE ADHESION DEFICIENCY.

complement receptor 4 (CR4). Membrane glycoprotein of NEUTROPHILS that is a receptor for C3dg. CR4 mediates PHAGOCYTOSIS. One form of CR4 is identical to p150,95 (CD11c, 18).

complementarity-determining region (CDR). Segment of a VARIABLE REGION containing amino acid residues that determine antigen-binding specificity. Residues in CDRs often make contact with antigen. *See* HYPERVARIABLE REGION, ANTIBODY COMBINING SITE.

complete Freund's adjuvant. ADJUVANT containing a suspension of killed, dried Mycobacteria in a water-in-oil emulsion. *See* FREUND'S ADJUVANT.

complex allotype. ALLOTYPE that differs at a considerable number of amino acid residue positions from another allotype at the same locus (e.g., the a ALLOTYPES of rabbit heavy chains or the b ALLOTYPES of rabbit light kappa chains).

complotype. A specific combination of linked alleles of genes encoding CLASS III MOLECULES of the human MAJOR HISTOCOMPATIBILITY COMPLEX (C2, FACTOR B, C4A and C4B). A complotype is a HAPLOTYPE of the class III region. There are 12 common (more than 1 percent in the population) complotypes in Caucasians. The complotype SCO1, for example, indicates an individual with alleles for 'slow' Factor B, the 'common' variant of C2, no C4A and type 1 C4B. These complotypes are in positive LINKAGE DISEQUILIBRIUM. *See* EXTENDED HAPLOTYPE.

concanavalin A (Con A). Plant LECTIN that is mitogenic for T LYMPHOCYTES and induces the selective proliferation of these cells in culture. Con A, a globular protein (M_r 102,000), extracted from the jack bean (*Canavalia ensiformis*) is composed of four identical subunits, each consisting of 237 amino acid residues. Each subunit has a binding site for Ca^{2+}, for a transition metal ion (usually Mn^{2+}) and for one saccharide. Con A has particularly high affinity for high-mannose sugars and has been used to fractionate glycoproteins and as a ligand to cell surface carbohydrates. It binds to a wide variety of mammalian cells and also microorganisms. The molecular events in the proliferative response of T lymphocytes to Con A are complex and require the presence of macrophages in the culture. Resting T lymphocytes undergo early changes in Ca^{2+} flux, in membrane transport sites, and in phospholipid biosynthesis; after 24 to 48 hours DNA and RNA are synthesized. Con A induces release of INTERLEUKIN-2, which stimulates the growth of T lymphocytes. Con A also promotes the ability of CYTOTOXIC T LYMPHOCYTES to lyse inappropriate TARGET CELLS, regardless of the antigen specificity of the cytotoxic T cell or the antigens on the target cells. It is thought that this antigen non-specific cytotoxicity is brought about by lectin-induced cross-linking of the cytotoxic and target cells. Con A simultaneously binds to high-mannose oligosaccharides (*see* N-LINKED OLIGOSACCHARIDE) on the surface of the target cell and also to sugars (probably of the high-mannose type) on the antigen-specific T CELL RECEPTOR or the cytotoxic T lymphocyte.

conformation. Spatial configuration of a macromolecule.

conformational determinant. ANTIGENIC DETERMINANT that is dependent on conformation (i.e., three-dimensional structure). The amino acid residues comprising a conformational determinant of a protein are not all contiguous in the amino acid sequence, but are brought together on the surface by the folding of the protein. Such a determinant is usually disrupted by denaturation of the protein. Usually, the binding of antibodies to a conformational determinant is not expected to be inhibited by small peptides derived from the protein. *See* SEQUENTIAL DETERMINANT.

congenic strains. Two INBRED STRAINS of mice that are presumed to be identical except for a short chromosomal segment that has been introduced by appropriate crosses with an unrelated stock. The introduced segment need not be from an inbred strain. If the introduced chromosomal segment bears a foreign histocompatibility gene, the strain is called 'congenic resistant' because tumor grafts exchanged between it and the inbred partner will be rejected. The production of a congenic line begins with the crossing of two strains – donor and background. The F_1 offspring are repeatedly back-crossed to the background strain with selection in each generation for the desired trait. After the procedure has been repeated at least 12 times, the offspring are inbred by brother–sister mating to produce a homozygous inbred strain. As the number of back-crosses increases, congenic strains become more nearly coisogenic. Congenic strains are usually designated by a compound symbol consisting of two parts separated by a period, the first of which denotes the background strain and second of which denotes the donor strain or a genetic symbol of the donor locus. For example B10.A is a congenic line carrying a gene (*H-2a*) of the donor A strain on the C57BL/10 (abbreviated B10) background strain. *See* COISOGENIC STRAINS.

congenital agammaglobulinemia. *Synonym for* X-LINKED AGAMMAGLOBULINEMIA.

conglutination. AGGLUTINATION by CONGLUTININ of bacteria or red blood cells sensitized with antibody and sublytic amounts of complement.

conglutinin (K). Serum protein of ruminants (e.g., cows, antelopes) that binds to complexes of antigen, antibody and complement in the presence of Ca^{2+}. The ligand for K is the N-LINKED OLIGOSACCHARIDE in the alpha chain of C3bi. The binding of K to immune complexes containing C3bi enhances their PHAGOCYTOSIS; a receptor for K has not yet been defined on membranes of phagocytic cells.

K is composed of 12 identical polypeptide chains (M_r 33,000), arranged into four subunits. Following an amino-terminal sequence of 25 residues, each chain has a collagen-like sequence (M_r 13,000), which forms a triple helical structure; the carboxy-terminal segments (M_r 20,000) form 'globular heads', in which there are disulfide bridges between the chains.

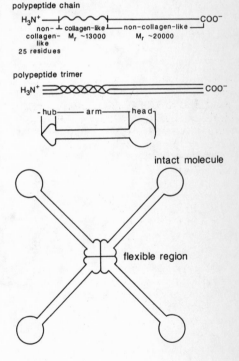

conglutinin

connective tissue disease. Disease characterized by inflammation affecting mainly blood vessels and connective tissue. Included in this generic term are SYSTEMIC LUPUS ERYTHEMATOSUS, SYSTEMIC SCLEROSIS, RHEUMATOID ARTHRITIS, SJÖGREN'S SYNDROME,

POLYMYOSITIS, DERMATOMYOSITIS, POLY-ARTERITIS NODOSA and ANKYLOSING SPONDYLITIS. All these diseases are thought to have an immunological cause.

consensus sequence. Idealized or 'typical' sequence (nucleic acid or protein) in which each position is the nucleotide or amino acid residue found most frequently when many actual sequences are compared.

consensus sequence of C3/C4 binding proteins. Segment of 60 amino acid residues that occurs repeatedly (2 to 21 times) in proteins that interact with C3 and/or C4 or once in Factor I (see table). In addition, the same consensus sequence has been found in beta₂-glycoprotein I, the INTERLEUKIN-2 RECEPTOR, Factor XIII of the clotting system and haptoglobin. In this consensus sequence, 12 of the positions are always or almost always occupied by the same amino acid residues: cysteine at positions 4, 32, 46 and 59; proline at 7 and 57; glycine at 35, 40 and 50; tryptophan at 52; and phenylalanine or tyrosine at 30 and 36.

Repeats of the 60 amino acid residue segments are frequently referred to as 'short' consensus repeats. When a series of 'short' consensus repeats are repeated, they are referred to as 'long' consensus repeats (as in COMPLEMENT RECEPTOR 1).

Protein	No. of consensus regions
FACTOR H	20
FACTOR I	1
C4 BINDING PROTEIN	8/subunit
FACTOR B (Ba fragment)	3
C2 (C2b fragment)	3
CR1 (COMPLEMENT RECEPTOR 1)	21
CR2 (COMPLEMENT RECEPTOR 2)	13
C1r	2
C1s	2
DAF (DECAY ACCELERATING FACTOR)	4

constant region (C region). In a set of equivalent proteins, that portion of each protein (or constituent polypeptide chain) that does not vary in sequence from one molecule to the next. In the IMMUNOGLOBULINS, the constant region is the segment of a heavy or light chain that is identical in sequence in chains of the same ISOTYPE and ALLOTYPE. In IMMUNOGLOBULIN LIGHT CHAINS, the constant region is a single DOMAIN. In IMMUNOGLOBULIN HEAVY CHAINS, the constant region consists of at least two domains (usually three or four), and in some IMMUNOGLOBULIN CLASSES a HINGE REGION and a carboxy-terminal segment (a 'tail piece'). The constant region of a light chain is encoded by a single EXON and that of a heavy chain by several exons (see IMMUNOGLOBULIN GENES). The constant regions of immunoglobulin heavy chains mediate EFFECTOR FUNCTIONS of antibodies. Most ISOTYPIC and ALLOTYPE DETERMINANTS are in the constant region. Constant regions (encoded by three or four exons) are also found in the alpha, beta, gamma and delta chains of T CELL RECEPTORS. The term 'constant region' is also used to refer to segments of major histocompatibility molecules (class I or class II) that hardly vary in sequence when different alleles are compared. See VARIABLE REGION.

contact system. Group of sequentially interacting plasma proteins that are activated upon contact with negatively charged particles or surfaces such as glass, kaolin or asbestos, or with negatively charged organic substances such as LIPOPOLYSACCHARIDES, collagen, ellagic acid, HERPARIN or dextran sulfate. Their sequential interaction results in the release of BRADYKININ. The contact system plays a major role in generating INFLAMMATION as well as in anaphylactic shock and ENDOTOXIC SHOCK. The contact system is inhibited by C1 INHIBITOR. See KALLIKREIN, KININOGEN.

convalescent serum. Serum sample taken from a patient two or more weeks after the onset of a disease. If the TITER or antibody to a pathogenic organism has risen significantly relative to serum taken in the early phase of the disease, it is considered to be presumptive evidence of infection caused by that organism.

conventional mouse. Mouse raised under usual housing conditions and fed water and food freely.

Coombs test. See ANTIGLOBULIN TEST OF COOMBS.

negatively charged
surfaces e.g. glass

Hageman factor ⟶ activated Hageman factor

prekallikrein ⟶ kallikrein

kininogen ⟶ bradykinin

contact system

coproantibody. Antibody, usually of the IgA class, found in the intestinal lumen or feces.

corticosteroids. Steroid hormones (e.g., cortisone) of the adrenal cortex or their analogs, which have important effects on carbohydrate metabolism (glucocorticoids) and on electrolyte balance (mineralocorticoids). Corticosteroids all have 21 carbon atoms, a double bond at C4 and keto groups at C3 and C20. Many corticosteroids have powerful anti-inflammatory activity and also suppress the IMMUNE RESPONSE. Corticosteroids inhibit accumulation of POLYMORPHONUCLEAR LEUKOCYTES at sites of INFLAMMATION and deplete the number of circulating LYMPHOCYTES. Corticosteroids are used in the treatment of severe ASTHMA, RHEUMATOID ARTHRITIS, INFLAMMATORY BOWEL DISEASE, SYSTEMIC LUPUS ERYTHEMATOSUS, etc.

cosmid. Hybrid cloning VECTOR in which the COHESIVE END (cos) sites of LAMBDA BACTERIOPHAGE have been cloned into a PLASMID (hence the name cosmid). Cosmids have been specifically designed to accommodate large fragments of eukaryotic DNA. The essential components of a cosmid are: (1) a plasmid origin of replication; (2) a DNA fragment carrying the cos site of phage lambda; (3) a drug-resistance marker that can be used for selection; (4) unique restriction sites for inserting foreign DNA; (5) small size so that DNA fragments up to

betamethasone

cortisone

corticosterone

hydroxycortisone

45 kilobases can be accommodated. The cosmid, which has been cleaved to linear form with a RESTRICTION ENDONUCLEASE, and the foreign DNA, which has been partially cleaved to generate large (35–45 kilobases) fragments, are mixed and ligated. The foreign DNA will be linked to two cosmids, such that both cos sites are in the same orientation. When such molecules are incubated with 'packaging mix', the cos sites flanking the foreign DNA are cleaved by a site-specific nuclease and the intervening DNA is packaged into mature phage particles, which are used to infect E. coli. After injection into the bacterial cell, the recombinant DNA circularlized via the cos sites, replicates as a plasmid, and expresses the drug-resistance marker. The packaging step requires recombinants of total size 40–50 kilobases; the plasmid can be as small as four to six kilobases so up to 45 kilobases of foreign DNA can be accommodated.

Cot. The product of DNA concentration (C_0) and incubation time (t) in a DNA annealing reaction. The Cot is a measure of the annealing (reassociation) rate of single-stranded DNA into duplex DNA and can be used to determine the relative concentration of a specific DNA sequence in a mixture. The annealing rate is a function of the complexity and frequency of a particular sequence in the total DNA. Short, simple, highly repetitive sequences renature quickly; long, complex scarce sequences renature slowly. The $Cot_{1/2}$ is the Cot value at 50 percent reassociation. In addition, hybridization of labeled trace amounts of RNA with excess DNA (i.e., a DNA-driven reaction) can be used to determine the amount of DNA complementary to the RNA probe. *See* Rot.

C-reactive protein (CRP). Serum GLOBULIN that increases dramatically in concentration during INFLAMMATION. CRP is normally present at a level of only 1–2 μg/ml and may increase to as much as 1 mg/ml. It is a pentamer of identical subunits, each composed of 206 amino acid residues. CRP is so named because it binds to phosphoryl choline in the C carbohydrate of the pneumococcus (*Streptococcus pneumoniae*) in the presence of Ca^{2+}. CRP binds to

chromatin and also to C1q thereby activating COMPLEMENT. The gene encoding CRP has been mapped to chromosome 1q2.1; SERUM AMYLOID P COMPONENT maps to the same chromosome band.

CREST syndrome. Acronym for a mild variant of SYSTEMIC SCLEROSIS, characterized by *c*alcinosis, *R*aynaud's phenomenon, *e*sophageal dysfunction, *s*clerodactyly and *t*elangiectasia. Serum contains anti-nucleolar autoantibodies, which react with antigens of the inner and outer plates of the kinetochore.

cromolyn   (1,3-bis[2-carboxychromon-5-yloxy-2-hydroxypropane]).   Drug that inhibits degranulation of MAST CELLS. It is useful in the treatment of ASTHMA, ALLERGIC RHINITIS and other forms of ALLERGY.

cromolyn sodium

cross-reacting antibody. Antibody that reacts with an antigen that was not used in stimulating the production of that antibody.

cross-reacting antigen. Antigen that reacts with an antibody (antiserum) that was induced by a different antigen. In addition, two antigens that are not identical but react with the same antiserum, are said to be cross-reacting. Some, but not all, of the ANTIGENIC DETERMINANTS of cross-reacting antigens must be similar or identical.

cross reaction. Reaction of an antibody with an antigen that was not used to induce that antibody. *See* CROSS-REACTING ANTIBODY.

crossed immunoelectrophoresis. Two-dimensional IMMUNOELECTROPHORESIS. In the first step, antigens are separated by ELECTROPHORESIS in a gel. Then, the gel containing the separated antigens is inserted into another gel that contains antiserum, and a second step of electrophoresis is carried out at right angles to the first. Rocket-shaped zones of precipitation, which are proportional in height to antigen concentration, are formed. The method combines the resolution of immuno-electrophoresis with the quantitation of ROCKET IMMUNOELECTROPHORESIS.

cryoglobulin. IMMUNOGLOBULIN that pre-cipitates when it is cooled below 37°C. Cryoglobulins are not found in normal serum but occur in certain diseases. *See* CRYOGLOBULINEMIA.

cryoglobulinemia. Presence of CRYO-GLOBULIN in blood. Cryoglobulins are almost always MONOCLONAL IgG or IgM and are found in MULTIPLE MYELOMA, MACROGLO-BULINEMIA OF WALDENSTRÖM and SYSTEMIC LUPUS ERYTHEMATOSUS. Patients with cryoglobulinemia may develop occlusion of peripheral blood vessels which can lead to skin ulcers and gangrene or RAYNAUD'S PHENOMENON when extremities are exposed to cold. Some cryoglobulins cause cold URTICARIA. *See* ESSENTIAL MIXED CRYOGLOBULINEMIA.

cutaneous basophil hypersensitivity *Synonym for* JONES–MOTE REACTION.

cyclophosphamide (*N,N*-bis[2-chloroethyl]-tetrahydro-2*H*-1,3,2-oxazaphosphorine-2-amine-2-oxide). Nitrogen mustard deriva-tive frequently used in cancer chemotherapy or to achieve IMMUNOSUPPRESSION. Cyclophosphamide acts mainly during the S phase of the cell cycle. It can damage both proliferating and resting lymphocytes.

cyclophosphamide

cyclosporin A. Cyclic peptide of 11 amino acid residues produced by two strains of fungus (*Cylindrocapon lucidum* Booth and *Tolypocaldium inflatum* Gams), which has immunosuppressive activity. Cyclo-sporin A is frequently used in clinical transplantation to prevent GRAFT REJECTION. It has a direct effect on both T and B LYMPHOCYTES, but the exact mode of action is not known. In T lymphocytes, no mRNA for INTERLEUKIN-2 is found after treatment with cyclosporin A. Secretion of INTERFERON-GAMMA by T lymphocytes is also suppressed.

cytochalasin. Fungal metabolite, char-acterized by highly substituted isoindole rings. Cytochalasins perturb microfilaments (*see* CYTOSKELETON) by blocking the polymerization of actin filaments. Cytochalasins thereby interfere with cell functions such as locomotion, CAPPING and PHAGOCYTOSIS.

cytochrome b deficiency. *See* CHRONIC GRANULOMATOUS DISEASE.

cytokine. Secreted polypeptide that affects the functions of other cells. Cytokines are important for the interactions between cells in the IMMUNE RESPONSE. Cytokines produced by MONONUCLEAR PHAGOCYTES are called MONOKINES; those produced by LYMPHOCYTES are called LYMPHOKINES. Other cell types (e.g., endothelial cells, fibroblasts) also produce cytokines.

cytolysin. *Synonym for* PERFORIN.

cytolytic. Having the property of cytotoxicity. *Synonym for* CYTOTOXIC.

cytophilic antibody. Antibody that binds to high affinity Fc RECEPTORS of cells. In humans, IgG1 and IgG3 and in mice, IgG1, IgG2a and IgG3 are cytophilic for MONO-NUCLEAR PHAGOCYTES. In all species, IgE is cytophilic for MAST CELLS and BASOPHILS. *See* Fcγ RECEPTOR, Fcε RECEPTOR.

cytosine arabinoside. (ARA-C). Synthetic nucleoside that differs from cytidine and deoxycytidine in that the ribose or deoxyribose is replaced by arabinose. ARA-C kills cells in S phase by inhibiting DNA polymerase. It is used in cancer chemotherapy and occasionally in bone marrow transplantation. ARA-C suppresses both the primary and the secondary antibody response, as well as the development of CELL-MEDIATED IMMUNITY, but it has no effect on established cell-mediated immunity.

cyclosporin A

cytosine arabinoside

cytoskeleton. Network of different types of protein filaments present throughout the cytoplasm of eukaryotic cells. These filaments serve as a scaffold or framework for other cell constituents and are essential for maintaining the shape, internal organization, and motility of the cell. The cytoskeleton interacts with the cell membrane and with cytoplasmic organelles. Three types of cytoskeletal filaments are recognized: microtubules, microfilaments, and intermediate filaments. Microtubules are long hollow cylinders about 24 nm in diameter. The walls of the cylinders are made up of 13 protofilaments, each of which is composed of dimers of alpha and beta tubulin, proteins of M_r approximately 55,000. Microtubules polymerize and depolymerize, affecting the shape of cells; they form the mitotic spindle and are the main structural elements of flagella and cilia. Drugs, such as colchicine and vinblastine, bind to alpha–beta dimers of tubulin, preventing polymerization into microtubules and the formation of the mitotic spindle, thereby blocking cell division.

Microfilaments (~7.5 nm in diameter) are polymers of actin (M_r of subunit ~42,000). In muscle cells, stable actin filaments interact with thick filaments of myosin to produce muscle contraction. In non-muscle cells, actin filaments exist transiently, polymerizing and depolymerizing in controlled ways that create movement or determine cell shape. These filaments are involved in a variety of cell functions, such as PHAGOCYTOSIS, membrane ruffling and cytoplasmic streaming. Actin filaments occur as networks or bundles just beneath the cell membrane and may restrict the movement of membrane proteins. In some cells, actin filaments form the core of microvilli, stable evaginations of the plasma membrane. A variety of actin-binding proteins regulate the polymerization of actin filaments. Drugs such as the cytochalasins inhibit cell movement by blocking polymerization of these filaments.

Intermediate filaments (~10 nm in diameter) are composed of different proteins in different cell types (e.g., keratin in epithelial cells, desmin in muscle and vimentin in lymphocytes, macrophages and endothelial cells). These filaments have important roles in maintaining the structure of differentiated cells.

cytotoxic. Having the property of CYTOTOXICITY. *Synonym for* cytolytic.

cytotoxic T lymphocyte (CTL or T_C). T LYMPHOCYTE that kills other cells. Most CTL are CD8+; these CTL recognize class I alloantigens or conventional antigens (e.g., viruses) associated with self CLASS I HISTOCOMPATIBILITY MOLECULES. Some CTL are CD4+; these CTL recognize antigen associated with class II alloantigens or self CLASS II HISTOCOMPATIBILITY MOLECULES. The mechanisms of killing have been studied in detail with CD8+ T lymphocytes. Once a cytoxic T lymphocyte has recognized antigen, it binds to the target cell and kills it within a few hours. The mechanism of target killing is not well understood and appears to include release of trypsin-like serine proteases and cytotoxic LYMPHOKINES (e.g., PERFORIN). Activated cytotoxic T lymphocytes are derived from inactive CYTOTOXIC T LYMPHOCYTE PRECURSORS whose proliferation and activation requires lymphokines derived from INDUCER T LYMPHOCYTES (e.g., INTERLEUKIN-2). CTL produce INTERFERON-GAMMA which activates MACROPHAGES. CTL are important in the immunological response to tumors and in GRAFT REJECTION.

cytotoxic T lymphocyte precursor (CTLp). Resting T lymphocyte that will become a CYTOTOXIC T LYMPHOCYTE following encounter with antigen and INDUCER T LYMPHOCYTES. CTLp are usually defined operationally by LIMITING DILUTION ANALYSIS.

cytotoxicity. Killing of TARGET CELLS. Cytotoxicity can be effected by CYTOTOXIC T LYMPHOCYTES, NATURAL KILLER CELLS or ACTIVATED MACROPHAGES. These cells release cytotoxic substances (e.g., PERFORIN, LYMPHOTOXIN). Cytotoxicity can also be mediated by COMPLEMENT-fixing antibodies. Tests for cytotoxicity include: (1) estimation of cell death by the release of constituents of target cells (e.g., hemoglobin from red blood cells, chromium-labeled proteins from nucleated cells); (2) enumeration of viable cells by exclusion of vital dyes such as trypan blue or eosin Y.

D

d allotype. Allotype associated with the heavy (γ) chain of rabbit IgG. The d allotypes are SIMPLE ALLOTYPES, the result of an amino acid substitution at position 225 in the hinge region. Heavy chains of allotype d11 have methionine at this position and chains of allotype d12 have threonine at this position. d allotypes and the e ALLOTYPES are products of allelic genes at a single locus, called *de*, which encodes the constant region of rabbit γ chains.

D gene segment. Segment of DNA that encodes the 'diversity' or D region of an IMMUNOGLOBULIN HEAVY CHAIN or a T CELL RECEPTOR beta or delta chain gene, i.e., that portion of the VARIABLE REGION (part of the third HYPERVARIABLE REGION) that lies between the segments of chain encoded by the V GENE SEGMENT and the J GENE SEGMENT. In many antibodies this portion of the heavy chain variable region is important in determining specificity. As a consequence of gene rearrangement, a *D* gene segment joins a *V* gene segment to a *J* gene segment. The number and location of *D* gene segments is discussed in the definitions of IMMUNOGLOBULIN GENES and T CELL RECEPTOR GENES. *See* IMMUNOGLOBULIN GENE REARRANGEMENTS and J REGION.

D region. Portion of the VARIABLE REGION of an IMMOUNOGLOBULIN HEAVY CHAIN or a T CELL RECEPTOR beta or delta chain that is encoded by a *D* GENE SEGMENT. In most immunoglobulin heavy chains, the D region consists of a few residues in the third HYPERVARIABLE REGION; the remaining (carboxy-terminal) residues of this hypervariable region are part of the J REGION. The D region is important in determining the specificity of antibodies (D denotes diversity) and, presumably, also of T cell receptors.

Danysz phenomenon. Variation in the ability of ANTITOXIN to neutralize a set amount of TOXIN, depending on the way the antitoxin is added, i.e., all at once or in stages. If an equivalent amount (*see* PRECIPITIN CURVE) of toxin is added all at once to the antitoxin, the mixture is not toxic. However, if the same total amount of toxin is added in stages, with intervals of about 30 minutes between additions, the mixture is toxic. The reason for this apparent discrepancy is that relatively more antibody is bound in ANTIBODY EXCESS, as after the first addition of a portion of the toxin. There is, therefore, not enough antitoxin left to neutralize all the remaining toxin. This phenomenon led to the early (but mistaken) belief that the formation of ANTIGEN–ANTIBODY COMPLEXES is irreversible. In sufficient (but possibly very long) time, the mixture should re-equilibrate and become nontoxic.

decay accelerating factor (DAF). Membrane glycoprotein of erythrocytes, leukocytes and platelets that accelerates the dissociation of the C3 CONVERTASE of the CLASSICAL PATHWAY OF COMPLEMENT (C4b2a) to C4b and C2a or of the ALTERNATIVE PATHWAY OF COMPLEMENT (C3bBb) to C3b and Bb. DAF inhibits amplification of the complement cascade on cell surfaces and, thereby, protects hosts cells from damage by autologous complement.

DAF is a single chain of M_r 70,000 that is anchored in the membrane by phosphatidylinositol, similar to the anchoring of Thy-1. Analysis of cDNA clones and cellular RNA has shown that there are two forms of mRNA that could encode DAF. The shorter and major (90 percent) form appears to be derived from the longer minor form by the removal of an intron located near the 3′ end of the coding region. This intron contains no stop codons and so could encode part of a protein. The splicing results in a frame shift so that the two predicted proteins also differ at their carboxy-terminal ends. The shorter protein (381 residues including a signal sequence) is probably the membrane form; it has a hydrophobic carboxy-terminus that may be cleaved off and replaced with the glycophospholipid that anchors it in the membrane. The longer predicted protein (440 residues including a signal sequence) has a hydrophilic carboxy-terminus and may be a soluble form of DAF. In the amino-terminal section shared by both forms of DAF, there are four contiguous SHORT HOMOLOGOUS REPEATS (~63 residues each) of C3 and/or C4 binding proteins see CONSENSUS SEQUENCE of C3/C4 BINDING PROTEINS, followed by a 77-residue region that is rich in threonine and serine residues, which may be sites for attachment of O-LINKED SACCHARIDES. There is a single site for an N-LINKED OLIGOSACCHARIDE.

DAF is deficient or absent in cells from patients with PAROXYSMAL NOCTURNAL HEMO-GLOBINURIA. The red blood cells in patients with this disease have enhanced sensitivity to complement-mediated lysis. The gene encoding DAF has been mapped to human chromosome 1q3.2. See RCA LOCUS.

deficiency of secondary granules. Rare defect of NEUTROPHILS characterized by the absence of SECONDARY GRANULES. It results in increased susceptibility to PYOGENIC INFECTIONS and is inherited as an autosomal recessive.

delayed-type   hypersensitivity (DTH). Inflammatory reaction that occurs 24 – 48 hours after challenge with antigen and is a result of CELL-MEDIATED IMMUNITY. In contrast, anaphylactic reactions (see ANA-PHYLAXIS) or ARTHUS REACTIONS take place immediately or a few hours after antigen administration and are results of antibody-mediated immunity. DTH reactions in the skin are characterized grossly by induration (hardening) and ERYTHEMA and microscopically by heavy infiltration with macrophages. DTH reactions are induced when T LYMPHOCYTES recognize antigen on Ia-positive (see Ia ANTIGENS) macrophages and elaborate LYMPHOKINES. The lymphokines attract more macrophages and activate them locally. In clinical medicine, skin tests are used to measure DTH to infectious agents

suspected of causing disease. For example, in tuberculosis, one can test with extracts of the tubercle bacillus (TUBERCULIN or PURI-FIED PROTEIN DERIVATIVE). The term DTH has replaced the older designation 'delayed hypersensitivity' in order to deemphasize the element of time, thereby emphasizing the cellular mechanism of the reaction.

dendritic cell. *Synonym for* LANGERHANS CELL.

dendritic epidermal cell (DEC). A cell in mouse epidermis that is of bone marrow origin and is thought to be a type of T LYMPHOCYTE. DEC are THY-1+ and express the γδ T CELL RECEPTOR in association with CD3. DEC do not contain CLASS II HISTO-COMPATIBILITY MOLECULES and are distinct from LANGERHAN CELLS, which are also found in the epidermis.

dense-deposit disease. Form of MEMBRA-NOPROLIFERATIVE GLOMERULONEPHRITIS.

deoxyribonuclease I (DNase I; pancreatic DNase: EC 3.1.21.1). Endonuclease, from bovine pancreas, which hydrolyses double-stranded (preferentially) or single-stranded DNA to a mixture of mono- and oligo-nucleotides with 5′-phosphoryl termini. In the presence of Mg^{2+}, DNase I attacks each strand of DNA at random sites; in the presence of Mn^{2+}, DNase I cleaves both strands of DNA at approximately the same site, yielding fragments that are blunt-ended or that have protruding termini one or two nucleotides in length.

There are four chromatographically separable forms of the enzyme: A, B, C and D. All consist of 257 amino acid residues and have a single N-LINKED OLIGOSACCHARIDE at position 18. The C and D forms differ from the A and B forms in having proline instead of histidine at position 118. The only difference between the A and B forms and the C and D forms is in the composition of the N-linked oligosaccharide.

DNase I is used in 'NICK TRANSLATION' and in nicking DNA for subsequent muta-genesis. Another important application is in mapping regions of transcriptional activity in chromosomes. Regions (up to 100 kilobases) containing active genes are an order of magnitude more sensitive to digestion by this enzyme than are regions containing inactive genes. In addition, within these sensitive chromosomal regions there are specific hypersensitive sites (approximately 200 base pairs), near the PROMOTER and ENHANCER, that are yet another order of magnitude more sensitive to the enzyme.

dermatitis herpetiformis. Itchy skin disease, characterized by crops of vesicles on a red base. Granular deposits of IgA at the dermal–epidermal junction are seen by IMMUNOFLUORESCENCE; 90 percent of Caucasian patients have the EXTENDED HAPLOTYPE HLA-B8, HLA-DR3, COMPLOTYPE SCO1 and/or HLA-B44, HLA-DR7, complotype FC31. *See* GLUTEN-SENSITIVE ENTEROPATHY.

dermatomyositis. Form of POLYMYOSITIS, accompanied by a distinctive rash of purplish hue, that is described as being heliotrope in color. The rash appears most prominently on the upper eyelids, over the extensor surfaces of joints and at the base of the neck. Patients have muscle pain, weakness and edema; subcutaneous calcium deposits occur late in the course of the disease. Microscopically there are heavy infiltrates of lymphocytes surrounding blood vessels. Serum of patients contains autoantibodies to tRNA synthetases. CORTICOSTEROIDS and METHOTREXATE are used in the treatment of dermatomyositis.

dermatophagoides. Genus of house mite. These mites contain the principal ALLERGEN of house dust.

desensitization. Attempt, by repeated injections of ALLERGENS, to decrease the symptoms of ATOPY (e.g., ASTHMA or ALLERGIC RHINITIS) or to prevent anaphylactic reactions (e.g. to bee venom) (*see* ANAPHYLAXIS). The immunological basis for the success of desensitization is not understood, but is thought to result from the production of IgG antibodies that bind to the antigen and thereby block interactions of antigens with cell-bound IgE.

desetope. In antigen presentation, the part of a CLASS II HISTOCOMPATIBILITY MOLECULES that interacts with antigen. It is believed that the contact residues vary depending on the allelic form of the histocompatibility molecule and that this variation is one factor that selects for the antigenic determinant being presented. Desetope is derived from *de*terminant *se*lection. *See* AGRETOPE, HISTOTOPE, RESTITOPE.

dextran. Polydisperse very high molecular weight polysaccharide synthesized by certain microorganisms. Dextrans are homopolymers of D-glucose linked alpha-glycosidically with predominant α-1,6 bonds; some α-1,2 α-1,3 and α-1,4 linkages also occur and are responsible for branching of the dextran chains. Lower molecular weight dextrans (M_r ~75,000), produced by partial hydrolysis of the high molecular weight form, have been used as blood volume expanders. Dextrans are THYMUS-INDEPENDENT ANTIGENS.

diazotization. Introduction of a diazo group ($N≡N^+$) into a molecule. The coupling, *via* diazo linkage, of derivatives of aromatic amines to the side chains of certain amino acid residues has been used extensively to introduce small molecules ('HAPTENS') into proteins. Immunization with such protein–hapten conjugates usually elicits some antibodies whose specificity is directed entirely to the hapten. The first step in the reaction is the formation of a diazonium salt by reacting an aromatic amine with nitrous acid. At slightly alkaline pH, the diazonium salt is then reacted with the protein. The main products of the reaction are monosubstituted tyrosine and histidine, and disubstituted lysine residues.

p-aminobenzenearsenate

p-azobenzenearsenate-diazonium salt

p-azobenzenearsenate tyrosine residue

tyrosine residue

diazotization

Dick test. SKIN TEST for circulating antibodies to erythrogenic toxin of strains of *Streptococcus pyogenes* that cause scarlet fever. A culture filtrate containing TOXIN is diluted 1/1,000, and 0.2 ml of the diluted filtrate is injected into the skin. A bright red flush at the site of injection, appearing in 6 to 12 hours, indicates a lack of antibodies to the erythrogenic toxin (i.e., susceptibility to scarlet fever). As a control, 0.2 ml of the diluted filtrate is used after it has been heated to 96°C for 45 minutes.

differentiation antigen. Antigen that is found at different developmental stages or in different tissues. *See* CLUSTER OF DIFFERENTIATION, ONCOFETAL ANTIGENS.

DiGeorge's syndrome (third and fourth arch/pouch syndrome). Congenital malformation of organs – the parathyroid glands and THYMUS – derived from the third and fourth pharyngeal pouches. Affected infants also have congenital anomalies of the heart, aortic arch and facial features. Neonatal hypocalcemia and tetany are almost invariably present due to aplasia of the parathyroid glands. The extent of the malformations is variable. Affected infants may have a deficiency of T LYMPHOCYTES and of CELL-MEDIATED IMMUNITY, depending on the severity of the thymic hypoplasia. Deficient cell-mediated immunity may lead to OPPORTUNISTIC INFECTIONS and to GRAFT-*VERSUS*-HOST DISEASE following blood transfusions. As these infants get older their T lymphocyte function improves.

dinitrophenyl (DNP). Usually refers to the 2,4-dinitrophenyl group. Proteins substituted with DNP groups have been used as model antigens. Many of the induced antibodies react with low molecular weight ligands containing the DNP group (e.g., epsilon-amino-DNP-lysine). Studies of the reactions of anti-DNP antibodies with DNP-ligands have shown that: (1) antibodies are heterogeneous with respect to association constant for ligand; and (2) the average association constant for ligand increases with time after immunization. *See* DNBS, DNCB, DNFB, MATURATION OF AFFINITY.

dinitrophenyl group

diploid. Descriptive of a nucleus, cell, or organism having twice the HAPLOID number of chromosomes (i.e., two copies of each autosome and two sex chromosomes). The diploid number of chromosomes in humans is 46.

discoid lupus. *See* SYSTEMIC LUPUS ERYTHEMATOSUS.

dissociation constant (K_D). Reciprocal of ASSOCIATION CONSTANT. It is the usual practice to describe the interactions of enzymes and substrates in terms of dissociation constants, and the interactions of antibodies and antigens in terms of association constants. In describing the reaction between an enzyme and a substrate, it is sometimes stated that the Michaelis constant K_M (which is equal to the substrate concentration when the velocity of the reaction is half-maximal) is the dissocation constant. This is true *only* when the binding of enzyme to substrate reaches equilibrium before catalysis occurs. In general, however, K_M is *not* equal to K_D.

DNA library. Collection of recombinant DNA clones corresponding to DNA sequences in a genome or in a population of cDNA. It is sometimes called a gene bank. The DNA fragments are cloned into PLASMIDS (*see* pBR322) bacteriophage VECTORS (*see* LAMBDA BACTERIOPHAGE) or COSMID vectors. (Phage vectors are convenient for storing and screening large numbers of recombinant clones; cosmids are specifically designed to accept large inserts.) In constructing genomic libraries, it is useful to clone random and relatively large (~20 kilobases) DNA fragments. The advantage of cloning *random* fragments is that there will be no systematic exclusion of any particular sequence. In addition, clones will overlap one another, providing the possibility of 'walking' from one clone to an adjacent one (*see* CHROMOSOME WALKING). Cloning large (rather than small) fragments is advantageous because fewer recombinants are required to achieve a particular level of probability that all sequences will be represented in the library; moreover, the chance of cloning a single fragment containing all of a relatively large gene will be increased.

Suppose a population of DNA has been fragmented to a size such that each fragment represents a fraction (f) of the total genome.

The probability (p) that a unique DNA segment is present in a collection of n transformants is:

$$p = 1 - (1-f)^n$$

For the human genome (2.8×10^9 base pairs) and for a cloned fragment size of 20 kilobases, 650,000 recombinants are required to achieve a 99 percent probability of including any particular sequence in a random genomic library. The usual method for preparing such a library is partial digestion of the genomic DNA with one or two RESTRICTION ENDONUCLEASES having tetranucleotide recognition sites, followed by size fractionation to give a random population of ~20 kilobase fragments that can then be cloned into a lambda bacteriophage vector. Packaging the phage *in vitro* ensures that an appropriately large number of independent recombinants can be recovered, which should be an almost completely representative library.

To prepare libraries of cDNA, cloning into plasmid vectors is frequently sufficient. However, to isolate cDNA corresponding to a rare message, a large number of recombinants may be required and cloning into lambda phage vectors may be advantageous.

DNA ligase. *See* POLYDEOXYRIBONUCLEOTIDE SYNTHASE (ATP) and POLYDEOXYRIBONUCLEOTIDE SYNTHASE (NAD$^+$).

DNA nucleotidylexotransferase (terminal deoxyribonucleotidyltransferase; terminal addition enzyme; terminal transferase (TdT); EC 2.7.7.31). Template-independent DNA polymerase that catalyses the random addition of deoxynucleotides to the 3'-hydroxyl ends of single-stranded DNA. Mouse TdT is a single chain consisting of 508 amino acid residues. TdT is found in immature T and B LYMPHOCYTES; therefore its concentration in the THYMUS is high, but it can also be detected in bone marrow. It appears to be responsible for the insertion of a few nucleotides at the *V–D, D–J or V–J* junctions of IMMUNOGLOBULIN GENE and T CELL RECEPTOR GENE segments, thereby increasing sequence diversity. In recombinant DNA experiments, TdT is used to add homopolymer tails to VECTOR DNA and to cDNA.

DNA polymerase. *See* DNA-DIRECTED DNA POLYMERASE.

DNA-directed DNA polymerase (DNA nucleotidyltransferase (DNA-directed)). Enzyme that catalyses the formation of phosphodiester bonds resulting in the elongation of DNA strands in the 5'→3' direction. It requires DNA as a template, as well as a primer with a free 3'-hydroxyl end. Both prokaryotic and eukaryotic cells contain more than one DNA polymerase, but only one of these enzymes provides most of the replicase activity *in vivo*. The others may have a subsidiary role in replication and/or they participate in DNA repair. Three DNA polymerases (Pol I, Pol II and Pol III) have been isolated from *E. coli* and are active in the elongation of DNA chains *in vitro*.

In addition to 5'→3' polymerization, the *E. coli* enzymes all have a 3'→5' exonuclease activity. This degradative activity acts preferentially on incorrectly paired bases and so has a 'proofreading' function, i.e., removal of mismatched bases before polymerization continues. The proofreading step greatly increases the fidelity of DNA replication. However, ordinarily, in the presence of even moderate levels of deoxynucleoside triphosphates, synthesis is favored over degradation so the enzyme is a *net* polymerase. Pol I and Pol III (but not Pol II) also have a 5'→3' exonuclease activity. *See* DNA-DIRECTED DNA POLYMERASE I (*E. coli*), KLENOW FRAGMENT.

DNA-directed DNA polymerase (T4) (DNA nucleotidyltransferase (DNA-directed); EC 2.7.7.7). DNA polymerase that, like the KLENOW FRAGMENT of DNA-DIRECTED DNA POLYMERASE I (*E. coli*), has two activities: 5'→3' polymerase and 3'→5' exonuclease. The exonuclease activity on single-stranded DNA is much greater than that on double-stranded DNA. Therefore, the enzyme is frequently used to 'blunt-end' a DNA molecule, i.e., to remove a 3' 'overhang' (a few single-stranded nucleotides at the 3'-end of a DNA duplex). It can also be used to fill in 5' overhangs.

DNA-directed DNA polymerase I (*E. coli*) (Pol I; EC 2.7.7.7). DNA polymerase having three separate enzymatic activities: (1) polymerase activity (5'→3' elongation of DNA strands), which requires the presence of a single-stranded DNA template, a primer with a free 3'-hydroxyl end, and deoxynucleotide triphosphates; (2) 5'→3' exonuclease activity that degrades double-stranded DNA from a free 5'-end; (3) 3'→5' exonuclease activity that degrades double-stranded or single-stranded DNA from a free 3'-hydroxyl end; this activity removes mismatched nucleotides during DNA synthesis (proofreading). *In vivo,* Pol I is used for filling in short single-stranded regions in double-stranded DNA during replication and in DNA excision repair.

Pol I is a single polypeptide chain of 928 amino acid residues (M_r 103,000). Limited proteolysis cleaves the molecule into two fragments. The larger fragment (known as KLENOW FRAGMENT), consisting of residues 324–928, has both the DNA polymerase and 3'→5' exonuclease activity; the smaller fragment, consisting of residues 1– 323, retains the 5'→3' exonuclease activity. The intact enzyme is used in 'NICK TRANSLATION' of DNA; this reaction resembles the enzyme's role *in vivo.* Pol I was originally used for second-strand synthesis of cDNA, but now the Klenow fragment is used more frequently for this purpose.

DNA-directed RNA polymerase (RNA nucleotidyltransferase (DNA-directed); EC 2.7.7.6). Enzyme that catalyses the synthesis of RNA from a DNA template. In bacteria, a single type of RNA polymerase is responsible for the synthesis of all types of RNA (messenger RNA (mRNA); ribosomal RNA (rRNA); transfer RNA (tRNA)). *E. coli* RNA polymerase is a large (M_r ~450,000) enzyme consisting of five subunits (two alpha, one beta, one beta' and one sigma) that are associated noncovalently. The sigma chain is an initiation factor that facilitates the attachment of the enzyme to specific initiation (PROMOTER) sites on the DNA and is then released. The remaining four subunits, which carry out the elongation, are known as the core enzyme. It is thought that the alpha subunits are involved in promoter recognition, the beta subunit in binding the nucleotide substrates, and the beta' subunit in binding of the core enzyme to the DNA template.

In eukaryotes, there are three nuclear RNA polymerases. RNA polymerase I is in the nucleolus and synthesizes only rRNA (except 5S rRNA). RNA polymerase II is in the nucleoplasm (i.e., the nucleus outside the nucleolus) and synthesizes the precursors of all mRNA (i.e., it is responsible for the transcription of genes encoding proteins) as well as the synthesis of certain small nuclear RNAs. RNA polymerase III is also in the nucleoplasm and synthesizes tRNA, 5S rRNA and certain other small RNAs.

These RNA polymerases are large (M_r at least 500,000) proteins with two large subunits and, depending on the organism, up to ten small subunits. In addition, mitochondria and chloroplasts contain RNA polymerases (encoded in the nuclear genome) that are different from those in the nucleus.

DNBS (2, 4-dinitrobenzene sulfonate). Reagent used to prepare dinitrophenylated proteins for use as model antigens. At alkaline pH, DNBS reacts almost exclusively with free ε-amino groups of lysine residues. *See* DNCB, DNFB, DINITROPHENYL.

DNCB (2,4-dinitrobenzene-1-chlorobenzene). Reagent that reacts with free alpha-amino-terminal groups in polypeptide chains and also with the side chains of certain amino acid residues (e.g., lysine, tyrosine, histidine, cysteine). It is less reactive than DNFB. DNCB has been used to identify the amino-terminal amino acid residue in polypeptide chains and also to introduce DINITROPHENYL groups into proteins, which are then used as model antigens. DNCB, when applied to the skin, induces ALLERGIC CONTACT DERMATITIS, a form of DELAYED-TYPE HYPERSENSITIVITY, by virtue of its reaction with proteins in the skin. *See* DNFB.

DNFB (2, 4-dinitro-1-fluorobenzene). Reagent that reacts with free alpha-amino-terminal groups in polypeptide chains and also with the side chains of certain amino acid residues (e.g., lysine, tyrosine, histidine, cysteine). It is more reactive than DNCB. DNFB has been used to identify the amino-terminal amino acid residue in polypeptide chains and also to introduce DINITROPHENYL groups into proteins, which are then used as model antigens. DNFB, when applied to the skin, induces ALLERGIC CONTACT DERMATITIS, a form of DELAYED-TYPE HYPERSENSITIVITY, by virtue of its reaction with proteins in the skin.

domain. Segment of a protein that assumes a discrete structure or has a functional role independent of the rest of the protein. Domains are often encoded by discrete EXONS. *See* IMMUNOGLOBULIN DOMAIN.

domesticated mouse. Mouse that has been deliberately adapted to life in captivity.

dominant phenotype (trait). Phenotype that is expressed when the individual is heterozygous at the relevant gene locus, e.g. HEREDITARY ANGIONEUROTIC EDEMA.

Donath–Landsteiner antibody. *See* PAROXYSMAL COLD HEMOGLOBINURIA.

double immunodiffusion. Type of IMMUNODIFFUSION in which both reactants (e.g. antiserum and antigen), typically separated by a gel, diffuse toward each other and, when equivalence is reached, form precipitin lines (*see* PRECIPITIN CURVE). Double immunodiffusion may be carried out in a tube (one-dimensional, method of Preer or Oakley–Fulthorpe) or on a plate (two-dimensional, method of Ouchterlony), and is usually used to analyse the specificity of antigens and antibodies and to determine antigenic relationships. *See* REACTION OF IDENTITY, REACTION OF NON-IDENTITY, REACTION OF PARTIAL IDENTITY.

drug allergy. Adverse immunological reaction to a drug. Drugs may bind to CARRIER proteins and act as HAPTENS. Drug allergies may involve antibodies (IMMEDIATE HYPERSENSITIVITY) or T lymphocytes (DELAYED-TYPE HYPERSENSITIVITY). Examples of antibody-mediated drug allergy are generalized ANAPHYLAXIS, SERUM SICKNESS, URTICARIA, THROMBOCYTOPENIA and HEMOLYTIC ANEMIA. Drug reactions mediated by T lymphocytes are usually manifested as skin rashes. Fever is a common manifestation of drug allergy.

Duffy blood group. Antigenic determinant of human red blood cells detected by ALLOANTIBODIES to the products of two genes: *Fya* and *Fyb*. The Duffy antigens are the receptors for the malaria parasite (*Plasmodium vivax*). The Fy(a−b−) phenotype is very common in Blacks and causes resistance to this form of malaria. The Duffy antigens have not been biochemically characterized. The genes for the Duffy blood group have been mapped to chromosome 1. ALLOIMMUNIZATION of mothers with Duffy antigens in fetal blood can cause HEMOLYTIC DISEASE OF THE NEWBORN.

Duncan's syndrome. *See* IMMUNODEFICIENCY FOLLOWING HEREDITARY DEFECTIVE RESPONSE TO EPSTEIN–BARR VIRUS.

E

e allotype. Allotype associated with the heavy (γ) chain of rabbit IgG. The e allotypes are SIMPLE ALLOTYPES, the result of an amino acid substitution at position 309 in C_H2. Heavy chains of allotype e14 have threonine at this position and chains of allotype e15 have alanine. The e allotypes and the D ALLOTYPES are products of allelic genes at a single locus, called *de*, which encodes the constant region of rabbit γ chains.

E rosette. Attachment of erythrocytes (E) to cells: for example, unsensitized sheep erythrocytes bind to human T LYMPHOCYTES. This phenomenon is used to enumerate and separate T lymphocytes. The E-receptor of human T lymphocytes has been designated CD2 and is recognized by monoclonal antibodies named anti–T11 or anti–Leu5.

EA. Erythrocytes (E) coated with specific antibodies (A). EA made with IgG antibodies are used as indicator cells to test for Fcγ RECEPTORS. Erythrocytes, usually from sheep, are reacted with subagglutinating amounts of IgG antibodies and are layered on test cells at room temperature. Cells with Fc receptors for IgG will bind the EA and be detected as ROSETTES. EA made with antibodies of the IgM class (*see* AMBOCEPTOR) are used to bind COMPLEMENT components. *See* EAC.

EA rosette. *See* EA.

EAC. Erythrocytes (E) coated with antibodies (A) and COMPLEMENT (C). EAC are used as indicator cells to test for complement receptors (*see* COMPLEMENT RECEPTOR 1, COMPLEMENT RECEPTOR 2, COMPLEMENT RECEPTOR 3, COMPLEMENT RECEPTOR 4). Erythrocytes, usually from sheep, are incubated with IgM antibodies, followed by a non-lytic dilution of fresh serum as a source of complement. EAC are layered on test cells at room temperature. Cells with complement receptors will bind EAC and form rosettes.

EAC rosette. *See* EAC.

EAC1. *See* C1.

EAC14b. *See* C4.

EAC14b2a. *See* C2.

EAC14b2a3b. *See* C3.

eczema vaccinatum. Severe, often fatal, GENERALIZED VACCINIA that frequently occurs following a smallpox vaccination in a child with ATOPIC DERMATITIS. It is also called Kaposi's varicelliform eruption.

effector function. Any biological activity of an ANTIBODY molecule other than antigen binding. Effector functions are mediated by the CONSTANT REGION of the heavy chain (e.g., COMPLEMENT FIXATION, binding to Fc RECEPTORS, binding to MAST CELLS). Most effector functions lead to the elimination of antigen from the body (e.g., by complement-dependent lysis, phagocytosis).

Biological properties (effector functions) of subclasses of human IgG

Property	IgG1	IgG2	IgG3	IgG4
Binding to C1q	+	+	+	−
Activation of ALTERNATIVE PATHWAY OF COMPLEMENT	+	+	+	+
Passage through placenta	+	+	+	+
Binding to Fcγ RECEPTOR I	+	−	+	−
Binding to Fcγ RECEPTORS II and III	+	+	+	+
PASSIVE CUTANEOUS ANAPHYLAXIS in guinea-pigs (*see* HETEROCYTOTROPIC ANTIBODY)	+	−	+	+
Binding to PROTEIN A of *Staphylococcus aureus*	+	+	−	+
Binding to PROTEIN G of *Staphylococcus aureus*	+	+	+	+

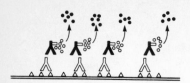

Assay for Antibodies △ in Human
Serum to Antigen △

Add:

1. Antigen △

2. Test serum △

3. Antibody to Human Ig 人
   coupled to enzyme ▫

4. Substrate °°° for enzyme

Measure product ⦂•

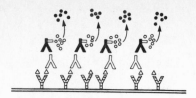

Assay for Antigen △

Add:

1. Excess antibodies Y to △

2. Test antigen △

3. Standard amount of antibodies △
   to △

4. Antibody to Ig 人 coupled to enzyme ▫

5. Substrate °°° for enzyme

Measure product ⦂•

enzyme linked immunosorbent assay (ELISA)

electroimmunodiffusion.   *See* ROCKET IMMU-
NOELECTROPHORESIS.

electrophoresis.   Transport of particles in
an electric field. Various types of electro-
phoresis are used in the characterization and
separation of macromolecules (*see* CROSSED
IMMUNOELECTROPHORESIS,   IMMUNOELECTRO-
PHORESIS, IMMUNOFIXATION, POLYACRYLAMIDE
GEL, PULSED FIELD GRADIENT GEL ELECTRO-
PHORESIS,   RADIOIMMUNOELECTROPHORESIS,
ROCKET IMMUNOELECTROPHORESIS).

electroporation.   Method for introducing a
variety of molecules into cells by subjecting
them to brief high-voltage electric pulses.
Electroporation has been found to be an
effective method for introducing DNA into
animal cells (such as B and T LYMPHOCYTES)
and into plant protoplasts that are difficult to
transfect by other methods. As a result of
the electric discharge (250–1000 volts/cm in
pulses of 10–100 milliseconds), nanometer-
sized pores are formed in the plasma membrane, allowing the penetration of molecules
such as supercoiled or linear DNA. *See*
TRANSFECTION and TRANSFORMATION.

ELISA   (enzyme-linked immunosorbent
assay).   Method for detecting antigens or

antibodies utilizing enzyme–substrate reactions. The enzymes are usually coupled to
antibodies (either to antibodies specific for
the antigen or to anti-immunoglobulin). It is
essential that both the enzymatic activity and
the immunological reactivity of the conjugate be preserved. The amount of enzyme
conjugate is determined from the turnover
of an appropriate substrate. Enzymes having
substrates that yield easily detected colored
or fluorescent products are used. ALKALINE
PHOSPHATASE and *p*-nitrophenyl phosphate
are a useful enzyme–substrate pair; the
product of the reaction, *p*-nitrophenol, has a
strong yellow color and can be detected
easily. The ELISA method is, in principle,
very similar to RADIOIMMUNOASSAY, but it has
several advantages: speed, lower cost, relative simplicity of equipment for detection,
and elimination of the necessity for handling
radioactive   substances.   *See*   IMMUNO-
FLUORESCENCE.

emperipolesis.   Process whereby LYMPHO-
CYTES enter and pass through another cell.

endocytosis.   Uptake by cells of materials
from the extracellular fluid by means of
vesicles formed from the plasma membrane.
There   are   two   types   of   endocytosis:

receptor-mediated endocytosis and fluid phase (pinocytosis).

Receptor-mediated endocytosis is the process by which a cell internalizes extracellular ligands and their receptors subsequent to the binding of the ligands to these receptors; this internalization takes place via COATED PITS and COATED VESICLES. Coated vesicles rapidly (within minutes) lose their CLATHRIN coats and fuse with other such vesicles to form larger vesicles called endosomes; within the endosome, which is acidic (pH~5), the receptor may dissociate from the ligand and be recycled back to the cell surface. The endosomes then fuse with primary lysosomes to form secondary lysosomes in which degradation of the ligand may take place. Examples of receptor-mediated endocytosis are the internalization of low-density lipoproteins by all cells except red blood cells and of asialoglycoproteins (glycoproteins lacking terminal sialic acid, so that galactose residues are exposed) by hepatocytes (liver cells).

Fluid-phase endocytosis (pinocytosis) is the process in which a cell incorporates a sample of extracellular fluid by entrapping it within a vesicle formed from the plasma membrane. MACROPHAGES, particularly if activated, have a high rate of fluid-phase endocytosis. *See* EXOCYTOSIS, PHAGOCYTOSIS, TRANSCYTOSIS.

endogenous pyrogen. Fever-producing substance found in plasma during infection or during cell-mediated immunological reactions. The known endogenous pyrogens are INTERLEUKIN-1, INTERLEUKIN-6, and TUMOR NECROSIS FACTOR.

endoplasmic reticulum (ER). Organelle in a eukaryotic cell that is the site of synthesis of lipids and certain proteins. The ER consists of a highly convoluted, but presumably continuous membrane, which encloses an internal space called the lumen. The ER is continuous with the outer nuclear membrane. Two distinct regions of the ER have been differentiated by electron microscopy: the rough ER, which is studded with ribosomes on its cytoplasmic side, and the smooth ER, which lacks attached ribosomes. The smooth ER is the site of synthesis and metabolism of fatty acids and phospholipids; in liver cells, it contains enzymes that modify (e.g., detoxify,

degrade, activate) endogenous and exogenous small molecules. The rough ER is the site of synthesis of certain membrane and organelle (e.g., lysosome) proteins and of secreted proteins. Ribosomes are directed to the rough ER by the SIGNAL SEQUENCE of the nascent polypeptide chain via a polypeptide–RNA complex known as signal recognition particle and its receptor, known as docking protein, which is an integral membrane protein of the rough ER.

Rough ER is found in great abundance in cells that are specialized for the production of secretory proteins (e.g., PLASMA CELLS, which synthesize antibodies). In these cells, much of the cytosol is filled with rough ER. A few minutes after synthesis, proteins in the rough ER move to the GOLGI COMPLEX, probably within vesicles that bud from the ER, and then fuse with membranes of the Golgi complex. The lumen of the ER is topologically equivalent to the exterior of the cell; once a protein destined for secretion has reached this compartment, it need not cross any additional membranes before it leaves the cell. Membrane proteins are initially inserted into the membrane of the ER and remain membrane-associated as they travel to their final destination.

endosome. Intracellular vesicle (0.1–0.2 μm) formed in the process of ENDOCYTOSIS (receptor-mediated endocytosis or pinocytosis).

endothelial–leukocyte adhesion molecule-1 (E–LAM 1). Protein expressed by cultured endothelial cells following their exposure to INTERLEUKIN–1 or TUMOR NECROSIS FACTOR. E–LAM 1 mediates the attachment of NEUTROPHILS and MONOCYTES to endothelial cells. Such attachment may be required *in vivo* for the margination and migration of LEUKOCYTES to sites of INFLAMMATION. E–LAM 1 consists of two chains of M_r 115,000 and 100,000.

endotoxic shock. Changes that occur after intravenous injection of small amounts (0.1–100 μg) of LIPOPOLYSACCHARIDE (LPS). After a latent period of 10–20 minutes, fever develops and reaches a peak in two to three hours. Hypotension develops in about 30 minutes and may be so severe as to result in death. Intravascular coagulation occurs as a result of activation of the CONTACT SYSTEM. Severe NEUTROPENIA is observed within a few minutes of LPS injection, usually followed within an hour by a rise in neutrophil count. LPS also activates the ALTERNATIVE PATHWAY OF COMPLEMENT and stimulates synthesis and release of INTERFERON -ALPHA, -BETA and -GAMMA.

endotoxin. Originally defined as a toxin released only on lysis of a cell, in contrast to an EXOTOXIN, which is released by living bacteria. The term is presently used as a synonym for heat-stable LIPOPOLYSAC-CHARIDES, associated with the outer membranes of Gram-negative bacteria.

end-piece. Obsolete term for the COMPLE-MENT components found in the PSEUDOGLO-BULIN fraction of serum. It is now known that this fraction contains all of the C2, no C1, and some of the remaining complement components. *See* MID-PIECE.

enhancer. Region of DNA that stimulates initiation of transcription by RNA polymerase II from a eukaryotic PROMOTER. Enhancer elements have the following properties, which distinguish them from promoters: (1) they can act over considerable distances, up to several thousand base pairs; (2) they can be oriented in either direction ($5' \rightarrow 3'$ or $3' \rightarrow 5'$); (3) they may be located either upstream ($5'$) or downstream ($3'$) of the promoter, but they must be on the same DNA molecule as the gene they regulate (i.e., they are *cis*-acting). Enhancers can stimulate transcription from a variety of promotors; if several promoters are nearby, the enhancer usually acts preferentially on the nearest.

The enhancer effect was discovered in the DNA tumor virus, SV40. Enhancers have recently been identified in the *J–C* intron of immunoglobulin μ and κ genes (*see* IMMU-NOGLOBULIN GENES). The μ enhancer is located $5'$ to the μ SWITCH REGION and is therefore retained after CLASS SWITCHING; it contains the octamer sequence ATTTGCAT that is also present in immunoglobulin promoters. The presence of enhancers $3'$ to the *J* GENE SEGMENTS is thought to account for the efficient transcription of rearranged κ and heavy chain genes. Therefore, unrearranged *V* GENE SEGMENTS are not usually transcribed in mature B cells even though they have an upstream promoter sequence. The rearrangement brings the promoter into range for the enhancer. Enhancers are often tissue-specific. Immunoglobulin enhancers function efficiently in B lymphocytes, probably because of the presence of specific regulatory proteins that interact with the enhancer region. The μ enhancer also functions in some T cells. The κ enhancer contains a sequence of 11 base pairs (GGGGACTTTCC); a protein found in the nucleus of B lymphocytes that express κ chains binds to this sequence.

enhancing antibodies. *See* BLOCKING ANTI-BODIES.

enzyme-linked immunosorbent assay. *See* ELISA

eosinophil. Type of POLYMORPHONUCLEAR LEUKOCYTE characterized by SECONDARY GRANULES that are refractile and stain brilliant red–orange with eosin (as in Wright and Giemsa stains). Eosinophils constitute 5 percent of the white cells in blood. When eosinophils contact TARGET CELLS, they degranulate; cationic peptides, released from the secondary granules, can kill some targets (e.g., the schistosomula of *Schistosoma mansoni*). Eosinophils increase in number (EOSINOPHILIA) during allergic reactions and especially during infection with intestinal parasites.

eosinophil chemotactic factor. Peptide from MAST CELL granules that stimulates CHEMOTAXIS OF EOSINOPHILS and that may be responsible for accumulation of eosinophils at sites of inflammatory and allergic reactions. Two tetrapeptides, Val–Gly–Ser–Glu and Ala–Gly–Ser–Glu have been shown to have such activity. These peptides are also capable of inducing the chemotaxis of neutrophils, but to a lesser extent than that of eosinophils. HISTAMINE also has chemotactic activity for eosinophils. There may be other chemotactic factors for eosinophils, but these are only partially characterized.

eosinophilia. Increase in the number of EOSINOPHILS in the blood. Eosinophilia occurs in parasitic infestations, in ATOPY and in ANAPHYLAXIS.

epithelial thymic-activating factor (ETAF). Substance found in cultures of epithelial cells, originally identified by its ability to stimulate growth of thymocytes. It appears to be identical to INTERLEUKIN-1.

epithelioid cell. Flattened MACROPHAGE containing few organelles that is found in large GRANULOMAS (e.g., in tuberculosis).

epitope. *Synonym for* ANTIGENIC DETERMINANT.

Epstein–Barr virus (EBV). Herpes virus that causes INFECTIOUS MONONUCLEOSIS and is associated with BURKITT'S LYMPHOMA and nasopharangeal carcinoma. EBV is LYMPHOCYTOTROPIC for B LYMPHOCYTES and can transform B lymphocytes. This has proved useful in establishing long-term B lymphocyte lines. Patients with EBV infection form several types of antibodies to EBV: (1) antibodies that appear early in infection (EA); (2) antibodies to viral capsid antigens (VCA); and (3) antibodies to nuclear antigens (EBNA). In addition, patients with infectious mononucleosis form HETEROPHILE ANTIBODIES.

equilibrium constant. Constant that describes the equilibrium state of the reversible reaction between two molecular species: $A + B \rightleftharpoons AB$. It can be expressed as an ASSOCIATION CONSTANT, $K_A = [AB]/[A][B]$ or a DISSOCIATION CONSTANT, $K_D = [A][B]/[AB]$.

equilibrium dialysis. Technique for measuring the interaction between a LIGAND (e.g., HAPTEN or substrate) and a macromolecule (e.g., antibody or enzyme). Equilibrium dialysis is used to determine the ASSOCIATION CONSTANT (or INTRINSIC ASSOCIATION CONSTANT) of such interactions. The ligand must be small enough to diffuse freely through a dialysis membrane that is not permeable to the macromolecule. In the procedure, the macromolecule is placed into one of two compartments that are separated by a dialysis membrane. The ligand is added to either (or both) compartments and allowed to diffuse until equilibrium is achieved. Equilibrium, defined as the condition in which the concentration of *free*

ligand is the same in both compartments, is usually determined by including one or more samples having no macromolecule in either compartment. A useful control, to check for 'nonspecific binding', is a set of samples containing antibody of unrelated specificity or nonspecific immunoglobulin.

After equilibrium is attained, the concentrations of free and bound ligand are determined. The concentration of free ligand is obtained by sampling the compartment that contains only ligand. The concentration of bound ligand is determined from the concentration of total ligand in the compartment containing the macromolecule by subtracting the concentration of free ligand. The concentration of total ligand is determined either by direct sampling of the 'macromolecule compartment' or by calculation from the total amount of ligand known to be added to both compartments. The SCATCHARD EQUATION (and SCATCHARD PLOT) or the SIPS DISTRIBUTION FUNCTION (and SIPS PLOT) can be used to determine the association constant.

Since the product of the association constant and the concentration of free ligand is equal to the ratio of bound to free antibody sites (*see* SCATCHARD EQUATION), determining high association constants requires measurement of small ligand concentrations. For example, to determine an association constant of $10^7 \, M^{-1}$ requires measurement of ligand concentrations in the range of $10^{-7} \, M$. Radiolabeled ligands may provide the required sensitivity. Equilibrium dialysis was used to show, for the first time, that the VALENCE of IgG antibodies is two. It remains the standard procedure for determining association constants against which other methods are calibrated.

equivalence. Proportion of antigen and antibody in PRECIPITIN REACTIONS such that neither residual antigen nor residual antibody can be detected in the supernatant. At equivalence, the amount of antibody precipitated from an antiserum is maximal or nearly maximal. *See* PRECIPITIN CURVE. *Synoymous with* optimal proportions.

erythema. Redness of the skin due to dilatation of superficial blood vessels.

erythema multiforme. Skin disease, characterized by so-called target lesions each

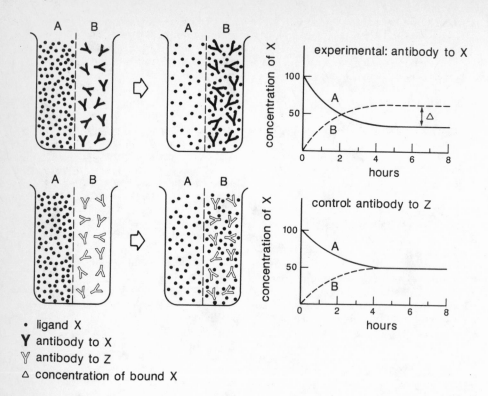

• ligand X
Y antibody to X
𝕐 antibody to Z
Δ concentration of bound X

equilibrium dialysis

with an erythematous (red) centre surrounded by a ring of pale edema and a peripheral ring of ERYTHEMA. Erythema multiforme is usually a manifestation of drug allergy or systemic infection. The lesions are infiltrated with lymphocytes and macrophages. In severe forms of erythema multiforme, there is erosion and sloughing of the mucous membranes, the so-called Stevens–Johnson syndrome.

erythema nodosum. Disease characterized by painful erythematous (red), slightly raised nodules (0.5–2 cm in diameter) usually appearing on the shins, but also occasionally on the forearms and head. Erythema nodosum may occur alone but is usually a manifestation of some underlying disease such as INFLAMMATORY BOWEL DISEASE, tuberculosis, leprosy, SARCOIDOSIS or histoplasmosis. It may occur after administration of certain drugs. The nodules of erythema nodosum have been attributed to deposition of antigen–antibody complexes in small venules. However, there is little evidence for this, and it is more likely that it

results from a .DELAYED-TYPE HYPERSENSITIVITY reaction in the venules. The nodules consist of an infiltration of the subcutaneous fat with NEUTROPHILS, LYMPHOCYTES and macrophages and exudates of blood proteins. Clots are found in small venules.

erythroblastosis fetalis. *Synonym for* HEMOLYTIC DISEASE OF THE NEWBORN.

erythrocyte. Red blood cell.

essential mixed cryoglobulinemia. Syndrome characterized by hemorrhages into the skin (purpura), joint pains, RAYNAUD'S PHENOMENON and GLOMERULONEPHRITIS, which progresses to renal failure. Granular deposits of polyclonal IgG, IgM, and COMPLEMENT are found on the basement membrane of renal glomeruli. In most cases, hepatitis B antigen is found in the serum cryoprecipitates in addition to IgG and IgM. The syndrome is usually a complication of hepatitis B. *See* CRYOGLOBULINEMIA.

euglobulin. A GLOBULIN that is not soluble in water, as distinct from a PSEUDOGLOBULIN, which is slightly soluble in water.

exchange transfusion. Procedure in which blood is removed from an individual and replaced by blood from another individual. Exchange transfusion is used in the treatment of HEMOLYTIC DISEASE OF THE NEWBORN to remove anti–Rh antibodies.

exocytosis. Process whereby the contents of intracellular vesicles are released to the external environment. In exocytosis, vesicles move to the plasma membrane, the membrane of the vesicle fuses with that of the plasma membrane, and the contents of the lumen of the vesicle are released into the external medium. Exocytosis may occur constitutively (e.g., secretion of IMMUNOGLOBULINS from PLASMA CELLS) or it may occur in response to a signal (e.g., degranulation of MAST CELLS, with release of HISTAMINE and other mediators of anaphylaxis). *See* ENDOCYTOSIS, ENDOPLASMIC RETICULUM, GOLGI COMPLEX.

exon. Segment of an interrupted gene or primary RNA transcript that is represented in mature RNA. Exons are separated by INTRONS.

exotoxin. Toxin released by living bacteria. Exotoxins are proteins and can usually be inactivated by heat, acid, or proteolytic enzymes. Chemical treatment (e.g., with formaldehyde) is used to convert exotoxins to TOXOIDS, which are used for prophylactic immunization. The genes encoding exotoxins are usually found in bacteriophages or in PLASMIDS, rather than in the bacterial chromosome. Many exotoxins are enzymes. Some (e.g., alpha-toxin of *Clostridium perfringens*) are phospholipases and damage cell membranes. Other toxins (botulinum, tetanus) block synaptic transmission in the central nervous system. Still other toxins exert their effects within the cell. For example, several toxins transfer ADP–ribose from NAD to specific host proteins, inactivating an elongation factor (EF2) involved in protein synthesis (diphtheria toxin) or activating host adenyl cyclase, causing increased fluid secretion into the intestine (cholera toxin). Toxins that act within the cell usually have two subunits,

called A and B; subunit B binds to a specific receptor on a cell membrane and subunit A carries the enzymatic activity, which is not expressed until it is released inside the cell.

experimental allergic encephalomyelitis (EAE). Autoimmune disease of the central nervous system in laboratory animals characterized by VASCULITIS and demyelination. EAE is induced by injection of brain or spinal cord tissue in complete Freund's adjuvant. Nine to fourteen days later the animal develops paralysis and infiltrates of LYMPHOCYTES and MONONUCLEAR PHAGOCYTES around blood vessels of the white matter of brain and spinal cord. Progression of EAE to a chronic phase is characterized by demyelination. EAE can be transferred to an unprimed recipient by lymphocytes but not by antibodies. EAE is mediated by the reaction of T LYMPHOCYTES with an organ-specific antigen, called myelin basic protein (M_r 18,000). Immunization with myelin basic protein or peptides derived from this protein also causes EAE. It is an experimental model for MULTIPLE SCLEROSIS and post-vaccination encephalitis.

experimental allergic neuritis. Experimental AUTOIMMUNE DISEASE induced in rats by immunization with peripheral nerve in complete FREUND'S ADJUVANT. The disease involves the sciatic nerve, which becomes infiltrated by LYMPHOCYTES and MACROPHAGES, resulting in paralysis. *See* EXPERIMENTAL ALLERGIC ENCEPHALOMYELITIS.

experimental thyroiditis. AUTOIMMUNE DISEASE of the thyroid, produced in experimental animals by immunization with thyroid extracts in complete FREUND'S ADJUVANT; a disease resembling CHRONIC LYMPHOCYTIC THYROIDITIS results. A spontaneous form of the disease occurs in the obese strain of chickens and in the Buffalo strain of rats.

expression vector. Cloning VECTOR constructed to express the protein product encoded by a particular gene in a prokaryotic or eukaryotic cell. Such vectors typically contain a strong promoter upstream from the cloning site that functions in the appropriate host. Sequences for transcription termination are typically located downstream from the cloning site. Vectors for expression in bacteria may also contain the initiation codon, AUG, and sequences that promote binding to bacterial ribosomes (SHINE–DALGARNO SEQUENCE). Eukaryotic DNA can either be inserted directly into a vector containing a Shine–Dalgarno sequence or it can be expressed as part of a fusion protein whose amino-terminal end is encoded by bacterial sequences. Since introns of foreign genes are not removed in bacteria, it is necessary to utilize cDNA copies of any genes containing such an intron. The expression of genes in eukaryotic cells permits the splicing of RNA transcripts (to remove introns), and the processing of the expressed proteins (e.g., glycosylation). The stability of expressed foreign proteins varies; they might aggregate or be degarded by proteases. Fusion proteins may be either more or less stable than the native protein. Lymphoid (e.g., myeloma) cells are efficient in expressing rearranged immunoglobulin genes because such cells recognize necessary regulatory elements (e.g., promoters and enhancers).

extended haplotype.   Group of linked alleles in the human MAJOR HISTOCOMPATIBILITY COMPLEX that are in positive LINKAGE DISEQUILIBRIUM. These genes lie between and include HLA-DR and HLA-B (i.e., HLA-DR, C2, Factor B, C4A, C4B, HLA-B). HLA-DR3, COMPLOTYPE SC01, and HLA-B8 is an extended haplotype.

F

f allotype. Allotype associated with the heavy (α) chain of a subclass of rabbit IgA. Five f allotypes, all products of allelic genes at the *f* locus, have been identified: f69, f70, f71, f72, and f73. Each allotype has several ALLOTYPIC DETERMINANTS, some of which may be shared with other f allotypes. *See* g ALLOTYPE.

F protein. Cytoplasmic protein (M_r 42,000) from the liver cells of mice. F protein exists in two allelic forms (F.1 and F.2) in different INBRED STRAINS. The F protein has been used to show that macrophages can present both self and non-self proteins to T lymphocytes.

Fab fragment. Fragment antigen binding. Fab is obtained by digestion of immunoglobulins (typically IgG) with the enzyme papain. Two Fab fragments, each containing one site for binding antigen, are obtained from one IgG molecule; the molecular weight of Fab is approximately 47,000. Since Fab is UNIVALENT it cannot cross-link and precipitate or agglutinate antigen. However, it can bind to and prevent the precipitation or agglutination of antigen by untreated BIVALENT antibody. Papain cleaves IgG in the HINGE REGION, usually on the amino-terminal side of the disulfide bridge(s) joining the two heavy chains. Each Fab fragment consists of one complete light chain and about one half of the heavy chain, held together by a single disulfide bridge and noncovalent interactions. The heavy chain piece in Fab is known as Fd and consists of the two amino-terminal domains (V_H and C_H1) and part of the hinge region. In human IgG1, the major site of papain cleavage is probably between histidine and threonine residues at positions 224 and 225. Fab-like fragments can also be obtained by treating immunoglobulins with enzymes other than papain (for example, by digesting IgM with

trypsin at 60°C). *See* Fab' FRAGMENT, F(ab')₂ FRAGMENT, Fc FRAGMENT.

Fab' fragment. Fragment obtained by reduction of the disulfide bridge(s) joining the two heavy chain pieces in the F(ab')₂ FRAGMENT. Two Fab' fragments are obtained from each F(ab')₂ fragment. Each Fab' consists of a complete light chain and the Fd' PIECE of the heavy chain. Fab' is UNIVALENT and can bind but not precipitate or agglutinate antigen. Fab' prepared from rabbit IgG or human IgG1 is slightly larger than the Fab FRAGMENT (i.e., the Fd' piece is slightly larger than the Fd PIECE). The difference is a few additional residues in the HINGE REGION of the heavy chain.

F(ab')₂ fragment. Antigen-binding fragment obtained from immunoglobulins (typically IgG) by digestion with the enzyme pepsin at pH 4.0–4.5. The F(ab')₂ fragment, which has a molecular weight of approximately 95,000, retains both of the antibody combining sites of the parent IgG molecule. Since F(ab')₂ is BIVALENT, it can cross-link and precipitate or agglutinate antigens. However, it does not retain the EFFECTOR FUNCTIONS of the intact antibody (e.g., complement fixation by the classical pathway, binding to cell membranes). Pepsin digests IgG just carboxy-terminal to the HINGE REGION. (In human IgG1 and in rabbit IgG, the site of cleavage is between two leucine residues at positions 234 and 235 of the heavy chain.) Therefore, the disulfide bridge(s) between the heavy chains is retained and each F(ab')₂ fragment consists of both light chains and a little more than half of both heavy chains, all still cross-linked by disulfide bonds. The heavy chain piece in F(ab')₂ is known as Fd'; it consists of V_H, C_H1 and the hinge region. Pepsin degrades the C_H2 domain into smaller peptides, but leaves the C_H3 domain intact.

Fragments obtained from rabbit IgG by enzymatic digestion

The two C_H3 domains remain noncovalently associated and constitute the pFc' FRAGMENT. *See* Fab FRAGMENT, Fab' FRAGMENT.

Fabc fragment. Fragment obtained after limited digestion of IgG with the enzyme papain so that only one heavy chain is cleaved (in the hinge region). It consists of one Fab FRAGMENT covalently attached to one Fc FRAGMENT (i.e., an IgG molecule from which one Fab fragment has been removed). Fabc retains only one binding site for antigen. Since it is UNIVALENT, it cannot precipitate or agglutinate antigens.

Facb fragment. Fragment antigen and complement binding. It is obtained by digestion of acid-denatured IgG with the enzyme plasmin and consists of an IgG molecule from which both C_H3 domains have been removed. The Facb fragment is BIVALENT and can therefore still precipitate and agglutinate antigens. It also retains all the complement-fixing ability of the parent IgG molecule.

Factor B. Heat-labile serum protein of the ALTERNATIVE PATHWAY OF COMPLEMENT. Factor B is a single polypeptide chain of 739 amino acid residues, which binds to C3b and is cleaved, in the presence of Mg^{2+}, by FACTOR D. Factor D cleaves an arginine–lysine bond (position 234–235) to form the amino-terminal fragment Ba, which is released, and the carboxy-terminal fragment Bb, which remains bound to the C3b. The complex, C3bBb, is the C3 CONVERTASE of the alternative pathway and the complex C3bBb3b, is the C5 CONVERTASE of the alternative pathway; the active site of the enzyme is in the Bb fragment, which is homologous with other serine proteases. Factor B contains three short homologous repeats of approximately 60 amino acid residues found in proteins that bind to C3 and/or C4. (*See* CONSENSUS SEQUENCE OF C3/C4 BINDING PROTEINS). It has four sites for attachment of N-linked oligosaccharides (two asparagines at positions 97 and 117 in the Ba fragment and two at positions 260 and 350 in the Bb fragment).

In humans, there are two common alleles: *BfS* (for *s*low electrophoretic mobility) and *BfF* (for *f*ast electrophoretic mobility). This difference is due to a glutamic acid or valine residue at position 18. The gene encoding Factor B has been mapped to the MAJOR HISTOCOMPATIBILITY COMPLEX on the short arm of chromosome 6 in humans and to chromosome 17 in mice. *Synonym for* C3 proactivator, glycine-rich beta glycoprotein (GBG).

Factor D (EC 3.4.21.46). Serine protease of the ALTERNATIVE PATHWAY OF COMPLEMENT. Factor D is a single polypeptide chain of 222 amino acid residues. It cleaves FACTOR B to form the fragments Ba and Bb. Factor D may have a zymógen form of 239 amino acid residues. *Synonym for* C3 activator convertase, GBGase.

Factor D deficiency. Very rare genetic deficiency possibly inherited as an X-linked or autosomal recessive. Affected individuals have less than 1 percent of the normal amount of FACTOR D in serum and they are susceptible to recurrent neisserial infections. Heterozygotes have half-normal amounts of Factor D in serum and are clinically normal.

Factor H. Serum protein that binds to C3b and promotes the dissociation of the ALTERN-ative PATHWAY OF COMPLEMENT C3 CONVERTASE, C3bBb, into C3b and Bb. In the presence of Factor H, FACTOR I cleaves C3b. (COMPLEMENT RECEPTOR 1 may also act as a co-factor for the cleavage of C3b by Factor I.) Human Factor H is a single-polypeptide chain of 1231 amino acid residues, consisting of 20 short homologous repeats of approximately 60 residues found in proteins that bind to C3 and/or C4. *See* CONSENSUS SEQUENCE OF C3/C4 BINDING PROTEINS. Mouse Factor H is composed of 1216 amino acid residues and has approximately 60 percent identity with human Factor H. Factor H has nine sites for attachment of N-linked oligosaccharides. In humans, the gene encoding Factor H has been mapped to chromosome 1q3.2. *Synonym for* beta-1H globulin. *See* RCA LOCUS.

Factor H deficiency. Very rare genetic deficiency inherited as an autosomal recessive. Affected individuals have less than 1 percent of the normal amounts of FACTOR H in serum and they are susceptible to recurrent PYOGENIC INFECTIONS. Heterozygotes have half-normal amounts of Factor H in serum and are clinically normal. The consequences of Factor H deficiency are very similar to those of FACTOR I DEFICIENCY.

Factor I (EC 3.4.21.45). Serine protease that cleaves the alpha chains of C3b and C4b to produce C3bi and C4bi, respectively. In the presence of FACTOR H OR COMPLEMENT RECEPTOR 1, Factor I cleaves a peptide of 17 amino acid residues, called C3f, from the alpha chain of C3b, which is thereby converted to C3bi. In the presence of complement receptor 1 (or Factor H), Factor I again cleaves the alpha chain of C3bi, which is thus converted to C3c and C3dg. In the presence of the C4 BINDING PROTEIN, Factor I cleaves the alpha chain of C4b, which is thereby converted to C4bi. A second cleavage in the alpha chain of C4bi results in the products C4c and C4d.

Factor I is a heterodimer but is synthesized as a single chain (prepro I), which is composed of a signal sequence of 18 amino acid residues, an alpha chain of 317 residues, a connecting peptide of four residues (Arg–Arg–Lys–Arg) and a beta chain (240 residues). The active site of the serine esterase is in the beta chain. There are three sites for attachment of N-linked oligosaccharides in each of the chains. After excision of the connecting peptide, the alpha and beta chains remain linked by a single disulfide bond. The heavy chain of Factor I contains one short homologous repeat of approximately 60 amino acids (position 71–136) found in proteins that bind to C3 and C4. *See* CONSENSUS SEQUENCE OF C3/C4 BINDING PROTEINS. In humans, the gene encoding Factor I is located on chromosome 4. *Synonym for* KAF, C3b/C4b inactivator.

Factor I deficiency (C3b inactivator deficiency). Rare genetic deficiency inherited as an autosomal recessive. Affected individuals have less than 1 percent of the normal amount of FACTOR I in serum and are susceptible to recurrent PYOGENIC INFECTIONS. Serum of Factor I deficient individuals is also deficient in FACTOR B and C3, because these components are rapidly cleaved *in vivo* by the ALTERNATIVE PATHWAY C3 CONVERTASE (C3bBb), which is normally inhibited by Factor I and FACTOR H. C3a, which causes release of HISTAMINE, is constantly being generated *in vivo* by the cleavage of C3 so that URTICARIA is a symptom of the deficiency. Heterozygotes have half-normal levels of Factor I in serum and are clinically normal.

Farr test. Measure of the antigen-binding capacity of an antiserum. The test can be used only to measure the binding of antigens (e.g., albumin) that are soluble in solutions of ammonium sulfate (~40 percent saturation) that precipitate antibodies. The antiserum is reacted with a radiolabeled antigen, and bound antigen is separated from free antigen by precipitating the antigen–antibody complexes with ammonium sulfate. The dilution of antiserum required to precipitate a portion (e.g. 33 per cent) of the ligand is a measure of the antigen binding capacity.

Fb fragment. Fragment obtained by digestion of IgG with the enzyme subtilisin. Fb consists of the C_L and C_H1 domains (i.e., the constant domains of the Fab FRAGMENT).

Fc fragment. Fragment crystallizable. Fc is obtained by digestion of immunoglobulin (typically IgG) with the enzyme papain. One Fc fragment is derived from each IgG molecule; its molecular weight is approximately 50,000. Fc consists of the carboxy-terminal halves of both heavy chains (the C_H2 and C_H3 domains plus part of the HINGE REGION) held together by one or more disulfide bridges and noncovalent interactions. Since Fc is derived entirely from the heavy chain constant region, all Fc fragments obtained from immunoglobulin molecules of the same isotype and allotype are identical. This accounts for the crystallizability of Fc, even when derived from pooled heterogeneous IgG. Fc-like fragments can also be obtained from IgM, usually by treating with trypsin at 60°C. The Fc fragment cannot bind antigen but it is responsible for the EFFECTOR FUNCTIONS of antibodies (e.g., COMPLEMENT FIXATION, binding to cell membranes, placental transport). *See* Fab FRAGMENT, Fc' FRAGMENT.

Fc receptor. Receptor on a variety of cell types for the Fc segment (*see* Fc FRAGMENT) of immunoglobulins. Fc receptors for IgG (FcγR) and for IgE (FcεR) have been defined. Other Fc receptors for IgM, IgD and IgA have not yet been characterized. *See* Fcγ RECEPTORS, Fcε RECEPTORS.

Fc' fragment. Minor fragment produced by digestion of IgG (or Fc or pFc') with the enzyme papain. It consists of most of the two C_H3 domains (probably extending from the 14th to about the 105th amino acid residue of both heavy chains, counting from the carboxy-terminal end), which form a noncovalently bonded dimer. Fc'-like fragments have been found in human urine.

Fcγ receptor (FcγR). Receptor for the Fc FRAGMENT of IgG. FcγRs are found on MONONUCLEAR PHAGOCYTES, POLYMORPHONUCLEAR LEUKOCYTES, PLATELETS, NATURAL KILLER CELLS, B LYMPHOCYTES and T LYMPHOCYTES. The binding of immune complexes to these receptors triggers a variety of cell responses such as PHAGOCYTOSIS, increased oxygen consumption and generation of activated oxygen metabolites (e.g., H_2O_2), synthesis and release of LEUKOTRIENES, PROSTAGLANDINS and neutral proteases, and modulation of antibody production. Three distinct human Fcγ receptors have been identified: FcγRI, FcγRII (CD32) and FcγRIII (CD16). Receptors homologous to FcγRI and FcγRII have been found in mice.

FcγRI is a high-affinity receptor on mononuclear phagocytes that binds monomeric IgG1 and IgG3 in humans and IgG2a and, to a lesser extent, IgG_1 and IgG_3 in mice. FcγRI consists of a single polypeptide chain (M_r 72,000 in humans; M_r 67,000 in mice); it is relatively trypsin-resistant. Expression of FcγRI is increased up to tenfold by interferon gamma.

FcγRII and FcγRIII are low-affinity receptors for IgG. FcγRII (M_r 40,000), is found in the membranes of NEUTROPHILS, EOSINOPHILS, MONOCYTES, B lymphocytes and platelets. In humans, it binds IgG SUBCLASSES ($IgG1 > IgG2 = IgG4 >> IgG3$). In mice, FcγRII ($M_r$ 47,000–60,000) is polymorphic and is detected by antibodies to Ly 17. It binds IgG2a, IgG2b and IgG1. In mice one form of this receptor (FcγRII.1) or mononuclear phagocytes is composed of 261 amino acid residues including a signal sequence of 30 residues, an extracellular region of 185 residues, a putative transmembrane segment of 20 residues and an intracytoplasmic domain of 26 residues. There are four sites for attachment of N-LINKED OLIGOSACCHARIDES in the extracellular region. The extracellular region is composed of two domains, which have approximately 30 percent amino acid sequence identity with constant region-like domains of members of the IMMUNOGLO-BULIN SUPERFAMILY. On mononuclear phagocytes and lymphocytes there is a second form of this receptor (FcγRII.2). The extracellular regions of the two forms are 95 percent identical in amino acid sequence; there is no identity in the signal sequences, the transmembrane segments and cytoplasmic domains.

Human FcγRIII (M_r 50,000–70,000), which is found in the membrane of neutrophils, eosinophils, natural killer cells, MACROPHAGES (but not monocytes) and some T lymphocytes, bind IgG1 and IgG3. Human neutrophils have 135,000 FcγRIII/cell (it is the most abundant FcγR in blood). When IMMUNE COMPLEXES bind to FcγRIII, the receptor is shed from neutrophils. There are two genes encoding FcγRIII, which are expressed on different cell types. FcγRIII on neutrophils is a glycosyl phosphatidyl inositol linked membrane protein (see THY-1, PAROXYSMAL NOCTURNAL HEMOGLOBINURIA) with two extracellular immunoglobulin-like domains. There are two allotypes, designated NA1 and NA2 (NA = neutrophil antigen). FcγRIII on macrophages and natural killer cells encodes a similar protein, which has transmembrane and cytoplasmic domains. FcγRIII is deficient on the membranes of neutrophils from patients with PAROXYSMAL NOCTURNAL HEMOGLOBINURIA.

Fcε receptor (FcεR). Receptor on MAST CELLS and various LEUKOCYTES for the Fc FRAGMENT of IgE. The binding of immune complexes to these receptors triggers a variety of cell responses such as release of mediators of IMMEDIATE HYPERSENSITIVITY (e.g., HISTAMINE, SEROTONIN) and modulation of antibody production. Two Fcε receptors have been identified: FcεRI and FcεRII (CD23).

FcεRI is a high-affinity receptor on mast cells and BASOPHILS that binds monomeric IgE. FcεRI has been studied most extensively in the rat. It consists of an alpha chain (M_r 35,000), a beta chain (M_r 27,000) and two gamma chains (each M_r 7,000). The alpha chain is composed of 245 amino acid residues, including a signal sequence of 23 residues, an extracellular region of 180 residues, a putative transmembrane segment of 20 residues and a cytoplasmic segment of 22 residues. There are seven sites for attachment of N-LINKED OLIGOSACCHA-RIDES in the extracellular region. The extracellular region is composed of two domains, which have approximately 30 percent amino acid sequence identity with constant region-like domains of members of the IMMU-NOGLOBULIN SUPERFAMILY. The beta chain is composed of 243 residues; it has no signal sequence. The beta chain contains four transmembrane segments; both the amino- and carboxy-termini are in the cytoplasm. The beta chain has 3 sites for attachment of N-linked oligosaccharides, but none appear to be used. The gamma chain is composed of 80 residues, including a signal sequence of 18 residues, an extracellular segment of 5 residues, a transmembrane segment of 21 residues and a cytoplasmic domain of 36 residues. The gamma chain, has no sites for attachment of N-linked oligosaccharides. The two gamma chains are linked by a disulfide bridge. The beta and gamma chains are unrelated in sequence to other known proteins.

FcεRII is a low-affinity receptor on MONO-NUCLEAR PHAGOCYTES, EOSINOPHILS, PLATE-LETS and B LYMPHOCYTES. The number of FcεRII on these cells is increased in individuals with elevated amounts of IgE in serum. FcεRII is a single polypeptide chain of 321 amino acid residues, including a 23 residue amino-terminal segment, which is in the cytoplasm, a transmembrane segment of 24 residues and an extracellular domain of the carboxy-terminal 274 residues; there is one site for attachment of an N-linked oligosaccharide. FcεRII is homologous with an asialoglycoprotein receptor, which also has an N-terminal cytoplasmic segment. Protease(s) cleave a lysine–leucine bond (position 147–148) and an arginine–methionine bond (position 149–150), releasing, respectively, the carboxy-terminal 174 or 172 amino acid residues. These segments are identical to the IgE-binding proteins previously identified in serum. When these segments are *not* combined with IgE, they are growth factors for immature B lymphocytes. This growth factor activity is abolished by the binding of IgE.

Fd piece. Heavy chain segment in the Fab FRAGMENT. Fd consists of V_H, C_H1, and part of the HINGE REGION. The exact number of amino acid residues in Fd depends on the heavy chain ISOTYPE and the V_H domain; it is approximately 225 residues. *See* Fd′ PIECE.

Fd′ piece. Heavy chain segment in the $F(ab')_2$ (or Fab′) FRAGMENT. Fd′ consists of V_H, C_H1, and the HINGE REGION of the heavy chain. The precise number of amino acid residues in Fd′ depends on the heavy chain isotype and V_H domain; it is approximately 235 residues. *See* Fd PIECE.

FDNB (1-fluoro-2,4-dinitrobenzene). *See* DNFB.

Felty's syndrome. Form of RHEUMATOID ARTHRITIS, characterized by an enlarged spleen and extreme LEUKOPENIA.

feral mouse. WILD MOUSE that was once a COMMENSAL MOUSE, but has reverted to a more wild existence.

ferritin labeling. Attachment of ferritin (an electron-dense iron-containing protein) to antibodies, allowing visualization by electron microscopy of the labeled antibodies in cells or tissues. The coupling of ferritin to antibodies may be accomplished by the addition of a cross-linking reagent, (e.g. toluene-2,4-diisocyanate). The labeled antibodies may be applied directly to the specimen or (the indirect technique) ferritin-labeled anti-immunoglobulin is prepared and reacted with the specific antibodies that are bound to the antigen. *See* IMMUNOFLUORESCENCE.

fibronectin. Glycoprotein of connective tissue, plasma and the surfaces of normal cells that promotes the adhesion of cells to surfaces. It is absent from the surfaces of tumors or transformed cells. It polymerizes into insoluble matrices and binds to fibrin, collagen, HEPARIN, C1q and cell surfaces. Fibronectin is composed of two subunits (each $M_r \sim 250,000$), linked by disulfide bridges near their carboxy-terminal ends. The number of amino acid residues in the subunits varies from 2145 to 2445, due to alternative RNA SPLICING whereby different groups of EXONS are represented in the final product. Therefore fibronectin is a group of closely related proteins. The amino acid sequence of fibronectin consists of repeated sequences of three types; usually each repeat is encoded by a single exon. A sequence (Arg–Gly–Asp–Ser) within one type of repeat mediates the binding to cell surfaces. The repeats are assembled into a series of tightly folded DOMAINS defined by the action of proteolytic enzymes, which cleave the polypeptide chains only in the extended regions between domains. Each domain is responsible for one of fibronectin's binding functions (i.e. to bind to fibrin, collagen, heparin, C1q or cell surfaces). Matrices formed by polymerized fibronectin guide the movement of cells in embryos and in wound healing. Fibronectin may also be an OPSONIN. Cold-insoluble globulin is the plasma form of fibronectin.

FIGE (field inversion gel electrophoresis). *See* PULSED FIELD GRADIENT GEL ELECTROPHORESIS.

fingerprinting. Technique in which a macromolecule (e.g., protein, RNA) is fragmented by specific enzymatic or chemical cleavage, followed by separation (e.g., by chromatography and/or ELECTROPHORESIS) of the fragments. The pattern obtained is characteristic of the macromolecule and can be used as a means of identifying it. Fingerprinting is a sensitive method for comparing two molecules and for detecting small differences in PRIMARY STRUCTURE.

flagellin. Major protein in the flagella of bacteria (e.g., Salmonella). Monomers of flagellin from various bacteria range in M_r from about 25,000 to 60,000. In the filaments of flagella, the monomers are assembled in helical chains wound around a central hollow core. Polymeric flagellin is a highly IMMUNOGENIC, THYMUS-INDEPENDENT ANTIGEN. The central portion of a flagellin monomer is variable in sequence and appears to be the site of MUTATIONS that alter ANTIGENICITY. *See* H ANTIGEN.

flocculation. Reaction between soluble antigen and antibody in which precipitation is obtained only over a narrow range of antibody–antigen ratios, evidently because soluble complexes are formed in both ANTIBODY EXCESS and ANTIGEN EXCESS. Flocculation reactions are obtained only with certain antisera (e.g. horse antisera to diphtheria toxin, sera from some patients with chronic lymphocytic thyroiditis). *See* PRECIPITIN REACTION.

fluorescein isothiocyanate. *See* IMMUNOFLUORESCENCE.

fluorescence enhancement. Enhancement of fluorescence of certain LIGANDS (e.g. derivatives of anilinonaphthalene sulfone) when they bind to an antibody. The increase in fluorescence results from the transfer of the ligand from an aqueous environment to the relatively hydrophobic environment of the ANTIBODY COMBINING SITE.

fluorescence quenching. Quenching or damping of fluorescence of an antibody molecule by its reaction with a LIGAND whose absorption spectrum overlaps the fluorescence emission spectrum of the antibody; the wavelength of maximum emission is about 345 nm. The quenching is the result of energy transfer from excited tryptophan residues to the bound ligand. Fluorescence quenching can be used to determine associa-

tion constants of antibodies for appropriate ligands. An assumption that is usually made is that the extent of quenching is directly proportional to the number of antibody combining sites interacting with ligand.

fluorescence-activated cell sorter (FACS). Apparatus for analysing and separating particles (e.g., cells) according to their fluorescence and light-scattering properties. A cell suspension containing a subpopulation of cells labeled with a fluorescent reagent (e.g., fluorescein isothiocyanate) is directed through a rapidly vibrating nozzle (~40,000 cycles per second). Tiny droplets are produced (40,000 per second), some of which contain a single cell. A laser beam is directed at the stream just before it breaks up into droplets and the fluorescence intensity of each cell is measured by a photocell. A second photocell detects scattered light, which provides a measure of cell size. If the two signals (i.e., fluorescence and light-scattering) meet certain preselected criteria, the liquid stream, just as the droplet is forming, is given a charge (either positive or negative); the droplet retains this charge and is deflected as it passes between a pair of charged metal plates. Thus, positively charged cells, negatively charged cells, and uncharged cells are all separated and each population can be collected. About 18 million cells can be sorted per hour. Data from the FACS can be displayed in two ways: (1) as a dot-plot that records the fluorescence intensity and size of each cell on two axes; (2) as a profile histogram with the fluorescence intensity or light scattering plotted on one axis against the number of cells on the second axis. Cells are not damaged by passage through the FACS.

The FACS has been used to study the functions of different lymphocyte populations in the immune response. Cells can be separated after differential labeling of surface antigens with fluorescent reagents. For example, CD4+ T lymphocytes can be reacted with a MONOCLONAL ANTIBODY to the T4 antigenic determinant, followed by reaction with fluorescein-labeled antibodies to mouse immunoglobulin. After application to the FACS, the CD4+ T lymphocytes (containing mostly HELPER T LYMPHOCYTES) are separated and can be used in subsequent experiments.

fluorescent antibody technique. *See* IMMU-
NOFLUORESCENCE.

fluorography. Technique in which fluorescent compounds are used to increase the
sensitivity of detection of radiolabeled substances that have been separated by gel
electrophoresis. The gel is impregnated with
a fluor, which is stimulated to emit photons
when it is exposed to the radioisotope. The
photons can be detected by placing the dry
gel in contact with X-ray film in the dark.

follicle. Structure in LYMPHOID tissues characterized by lymphocytes in very close prox-
imity. Follicles are situated in the superficial
cortex of LYMPH NODES and in the white pulp
of SPLEEN and contain mainly B LYM-
PHOCYTES. Resting lymph nodes contain so-
called primary follicles, which consist of
accumulations of small and medium-sized B
lymphocytes. Following antigenic stimulation, secondary follicles appear, which
contain many large dividing B lymphocytes
in the center (germinal center). Germinal
centers also contain MACROPHAGES that may
have engulfed nuclear debris (tingible body
macrophages) and FOLLICULAR DENDRITIC
CELLS. ANTIGEN–ANTIBODY COMPLEXES are
trapped and accumulate in germinal centers
where they remain for several days.

follicular dendritic cell. Cell located in the
FOLLICLES of LYMPH NODE and SPLEEN characterized by the presence of many thin
cytoplasmic extensions between closely
packed B LYMPHOCYTES. The cytoplasm contains few organelles and few endocytic vesicles. ANTIGEN–ANTIBODY COMPLEXES are
trapped and retained on the surface of the
follicular dendritic cells and do not appear to
undergo ENDOCYTOSIS. The adherence of
antigen–antibody complexes to follicular
dendritic cell correlates with the formation
of germinal centers. Follicular dendritic cells
are difficult to isolate. Limited studies indicate that these cells lack CLASS II HISTO-
COMPATIBILITY MOLECULES, but have Fc
RECEPTORS and COMPLEMENT RECEPTORS 1
and 3.

footprinting. Technique for determining
the segment(s) of DNA to which a protein
binds. Double-stranded DNA, which has
been labeled (e.g., with ^{32}P) at one of its
termini, is allowed to react with the putative

binding protein. The DNA–protein complex
is then digested with an endonuclease so that
most molecules are cut randomly and only
once. The digested test DNA and a control
sample of DNA – which has been treated the
same way except that no protein is added –
are subjected to POLYACRYLAMIDE GEL ELEC-
TROPHORESIS, under conditions that allow
separation of fragments that differ in length
by a single nucleotide. After autoradiography, a ladder of bands is seen, the rungs of
which represent the staggered DNA fragments. However, in the region of protein
binding, the DNA is 'protected' and there is
no digestion by the nuclease; the corresponding bands are missing (as compared to
the control). If a DNA sequencing gel is run
in parallel, the exact location of the protected region can be determined.

formyl–methionyl–leucyl–phenylalanine (F–
Met–Leu–Phe). Potent CHEMOTACTIC PEP-
TIDE that induces migration of LEUKOCYTES
and degranulation of NEUTROPHILS at a concentration of 10 pM. A compound similar to
F–Met–Leu–Phe is present in bacterial cultures and may be the molecule responsible
for generating an acute influx of neutrophils
in INFLAMMATION. When F–Met–Leu–Phe
binds to a receptor on neutrophils, Ca^{2+} flux
increases and activates microfilament function (*see* CYTOSKELETON) so as to facilitate
migration of leukocytes. F–Met–Leu–Phe
brings about an increase in the number of
COMPLEMENT RECEPTOR 3 molecules in the
membranes of neutrophils.

Forssman antigen. Glycolipid antigen(s)
found on the red blood cells of many species
(horse, sheep, dog, cat, mouse, chicken),
but not on the red blood cells of other
species (rat, rabbit, cow, pig). Forssman
antigen is also found in certain other tissues
(e.g., guinea-pig kidney) and in some
bacteria; thus, it is a HETEROPHILE ANTIGEN.
When injected into rabbits, Forssman antigen elicits antibodies that mediate
complement-dependent lysis of sheep red
blood cells. Although humans were originally thought to be Forssman-negative, Forssman antigen is found on the gastrointestinal
mucosa of some people, i.e., it is an ALLOAN-
TIGEN in humans. The complete antigen is a
ceramide pentasaccharide; individuals who
are Forssman-negative make a precursor
that lacks the terminal *N*-acetylgalactosa-

mine. However, tumors of the gastrointestinal tract of Forssman-negative individuals produce the complete antigen, which is therefore a TUMOR-ASSOCIATED ANTIGEN in these individuals. Forssman antigen is closely related to A blood group substance of humans (*see* ABO BLOOD GROUP).

framework region. Segment of a VARIABLE REGION that is less variable in amino acid sequence than is a HYPERVARIABLE REGION. The framework regions in an antibody DOMAIN form two opposing beta-pleated sheets, which are the basic structural elements of the domain. The strands of the beta sheet are connected by loops of polypeptide chain some of which contain the hypervariable regions. *See* IMMUNOGLOBULIN FOLD.

Freund's adjuvant. Water-in-oil emulsion used to stimulate IMMUNE RESPONSES. There are two forms of Freund's adjuvant, depending on the presence or absence of killed Mycobacteria. Complete Freund's adjuvant contains *Mycobacterium tuberculosis*, or other strains of Mycobacteria. It induces strong GRANULOMA formation at the site of injection and enhances the immune response. Weak antigens may be rendered more IMMUNOGENIC when incorporated in complete Freund's adjuvant. Antigens to which an individual is ordinarily tolerant (e.g. self-antigens) may become immunogenic when administered in complete Freund's adjuvant. For example, AUTOIMMUNE DISEASES of the central nervous system or of the thyroid can be induced by injecting the appropriate antigens in complete Freund's adjuvant. Incomplete Freund's adjuvant lacks Mycobacteria and is less stimulatory.

functional affinity. ASSOCIATION CONSTANT for the reaction between a BIVALENT (or MULTIVALENT) antibody and a bivalent (or multivalent) LIGAND. The term was introduced as a contrast to INTRINSIC ASSOCIATION CONSTANT, which describes the reaction between individual sites of the interacting species. The multivalent interaction results in enhanced AFFINITY, which may be important in many antibody–antigen interactions, such as VIRUS NEUTRALIZATION. The term AVIDITY is also frequently used to describe multivalent interactions but, in contrast to functional affinity, avidity is a descriptive term without a precise meaning.

Fv fragment. Fragment variable. It consists of one V_H and one V_L domain held together by noncovalent interactions. Therefore, Fv contains one ANTIBODY COMBINING SITE, i.e., it is UNIVALENT. Fv has been obtained from only a few immunoglobulins, by digestion with pepsin.

G

g allotype. Allotype associated with the heavy (α) chain of a subclass of rabbit IgA. Four g allotypes, all products of allelic genes at the g locus, have been identified: g74, g75, g76, and g77. Each allotype has several ALLOTYPIC DETERMINANTS, some of which may be shared with other g allotypes. *See* f ALLOTYPE.

gamma (γ)-globulin. GLOBULIN that migrates in the gamma region on electrophoresis, i.e., the most positively charged (cationic) of the serum globulins – or indeed of all the serum proteins. Most gamma-globulins are IMMUNOGLOBULINS and conversely. Therefore, the term gamma-globulin was formerly used to designate the antibody-containing fraction of the serum proteins. However, since not all antibodies are gamma-globulins, the term immunoglobulin is now preferred to designate the entire family of serum proteins that may have antibody activity.

gamma heavy chain disease. Form of MYELOMATOSIS characterized by the presence in serum and urine of abnormal MONOCLONAL IMMUNOGLOBULIN GAMMA CHAINS. The gamma chains contain extensive deletions. These deletions are variable in location but frequently start near the beginning of the variable region and extend through the C_H1 domain with resumption of the normal sequence at the beginning of the HINGE REGION. There are no associated IMMUNOGLOBULIN LIGHT CHAINS. The tumors principally involve the TONSILS. Patients have weakness, malaise, fever, enlarged LYMPH NODES and edema of the soft palate and uvula. In contrast to MULTIPLE MYELOMA, the tumors do not occur in bone. The disease is progressively fatal.

gastrointestinal lymphoid tissue. *See* GUT-ASSOCIATED LYMPHOID TISSUE (GALT).

gene bank. *Synonym for* DNA LIBRARY.

gene cloning. Replicating genes or fragments of genes by RECOMBINANT DNA TECHNOLOGY.

gene mapping. General term used to describe the localization or ordering of genes. It can refer to localization of a gene with respect to other genes or to a chromosome (or band of a chromosome). It can also mean the ordering of parts of a gene. Gene mapping in humans can be accomplished by: analysis of restriction fragments (i.e., RESTRICTION MAPPING) including determination of RESTRICTION FRAGMENT LENGTH POLYMORPHISMS; *IN SITU* HYBRIDIZATION; chromosome transfer; deletion mapping; cosegregation in somatic cell hybrids; studies of gene linkages in families; determination of LINKAGE DISEQUILIBRIUM.

generalized vaccinia. Occurrence of multiple vaccinia lesions on the skin following smallpox vaccination. This complication of smallpox vaccination occurs in children who have a primary immunodeficiency of antibody synthesis (e.g., TRANSIENT HYPOGAMMA-GLOBULINEMIA OF INFANCY). It is usually a self-limited disease. However, in children with atopic dermatitis, generalized vaccinia (*see* ECZEMA VACCINATUM) is often fatal. *See* PROGRESSIVE VACCINIA.

genetic code. Correspondence, in protein synthesis, between triplets of nucleotides (*see* CODONS) and amino acid residues (or termination signals). The linear sequence of nucleotides in mRNA is translated, according to the rules of the genetic code, into a sequence of amino acid residues.

genome. Haploid set of chromosomes.

genomic DNA. Chromosomal DNA. *See* cDNA.

genotype. Genetic constitution of an organism. *See* PHENOTYPE.

germ-free mouse. Mouse raised under sterile conditions in order to minimize exposure to environmental antigens. Germ-free mice have underdeveloped LYMPHOID organs and low (~0.1 normal) levels of SERUM IMMUNOGLOBULIN. Sometimes the diet is also restricted to reduce exposure to antigens in food. *See* AXENIC, GNOTOBIOTIC.

globulin. Member of a group of proteins that are not soluble (the EUGLOBULINS), or only sparingly soluble (the PSEUDOGLO-BULINS), in water. On the basis of solubility properties, no clear distinction can be made between pseudoglobulins and ALBUMINS. Globulins are insoluble in half-saturated ammonium sulfate. The globulins are classified according to their electrophoretic mobility into alpha-, beta-, and GAMMA-GLOBULINS, the alpha-globulins being most, and the gamma-globulins least, negatively charged. Most IMMUNOGLOBULINS are serum gamma-globulins.

glomerulonephritis. Inflammatory process in the renal glomerulus, characterized by proliferation of endothelial and epithelial cells, infiltration by NEUTROPHILS and MACRO-PHAGES, and alterations of the basement membrane. These changes affect the filtration of plasma proteins and electrolytes; they may ultimately lead to the destruction of the glomerulus and to terminal renal failure. Two immunological processes may induce glomerulonephritis: (1) the deposition of ANTIGEN–ANTIBODY COMPLEXES along the basement membrane (*see* IMMUNE COM-PLEX DISEASES); (2) the fixation of antibodies to the glomerular basement membrane (*see* MASUGI NEPHRITIS, GOODPASTURE'S SYN-DROME). The antigen–antibody complexes can be identified by IMMUNOFLUORESCENCE as irregular deposits of antigen, antibody and COMPLEMENT, whereas the antibodies to the basement membrane form linear homogeneous deposits along the capillary wall. According to the histopathology, glomerulonephritis is classified into three different types; (1) membranous glomerulonephritis, characterized by antigen–antibody complexes lodged on the epithelial side of the basement membrane with little inflammatory cell infiltration; (2) proliferative glomerulonephritis, characterized by greater deposition of antigen–antibody complexes or antibodies to basement membranes accompanied by much inflammatory cell infiltration; (3) membranoproliferative glomerulonephritis, a mixture of types (1) and (2). The severity of glomerulonephritis depends on the amount of antigen–antibody complexes in the glomeruli. There are both acute and chronic forms of glomerulonephritis. *See* ACUTE POST-STREPTOCOCCAL GLOMERU-LONEPHRITIS.

gluten-sensitive enteropathy. Form of celiac disease resulting from the ingestion of gluten, a protein found in rye and wheat flour, to which patients are hypersensitive. The disease is characterized by weight loss, diarrhea and steatorrhea (foul, bulky, malodorous stools). The villi of the small intestine are flat and atrophic, resulting in poor absorption of dietary fat, and the lamina propria is infiltrated with PLASMA CELLS and LYMPHOCYTES. Lymphocytes from intestinal biopsies synthesize antibody to gluten *in vitro*, and T LYMPHOCYTES from such biopsies are CYTOTOXIC to intestinal epithelial cells in the presence of gluten. Approximately 90 percent of Caucasian patients have the EXTENDED HAPLOTYPE HLA-B8, HLA-DR3, COMPLOTYPE SCO1 and/or HLA-B44, HLA-DR7, complotype FC31. Some patients also have DERMATITIS HER-PETIFORMIS.

Gm allotype. Human IMMUNOGLOBULIN GAMMA CHAIN (or IgG molecule) carrying one or more Gm ALLOTYPIC DETERMINANTS. The Gm allotypes are products of allelic genes encoding the constant regions of gamma1, gamma2 and gamma3 chains.

Gm allotypic determinant. ALLOTYPIC DETERMINANT of heavy chains of human IgG. Gm determinants are associated with particular IgG subclasses (e.g., G1m(1) and G1m(4) are associated with IgG1, G3m(5) is associated with IgG3). Many of the Gm determinants have been correlated with particular amino acid substitutions in the CONstant regions of the different human gamma chains. Most allotypic determinants are localized to the Fc region, but G1m(4) and G1m(17) are determined by a single amino acid substitution (arginine or lysine, respectively) at position 214 of C_H1. The presence of the light chain is necessary for the expression of this determinant.

CH₂COONa
|
AuSCHCOONa

gold sodium thiomalate

aurothioglucose

Subclass	WHO nomenclature	Original nomenclature
IgG1	G1m	
	1	a
	2	x
	3	b^w or b^2
	4	f
	7	r
	17	z
	18	Rouen 2
	20	San Francisco 2
IgG2	G2m	
	23	n
IgG3	G3m	
	5	b^1 and b
	6	c
	10	b^α
	11	b^β
	12	b^γ
	13	b^3
	14	b^4
	15	s
	16	t
	21	g

Modified from Natvig, J.B. and Kunkel, H.G., *Advances in Immunology*, 16: 1–59 (1973).

gnotobiotic. Descriptive of specially reared animals in which all the ambient microbes are known. A GERM-FREE MOUSE is gnotobiotic (i.e., no ambient microbes).

gold therapy. Injection of compounds of gold to treat RHEUMATOID ARTHRITIS. The commonly used compounds are aurothioglucose and gold sodium thiomalate. *Synonym for* chrysotherapy.

Golgi complex. Organelles of eukaryotic cells, usually located near the nucleus, and composed of stacks of flattened membranous sacs (cisternae) and associated spheri-

cal vesicles. Proteins are transported from the rough ENDOPLASMIC RETICULUM to the Golgi complex, where they are processed and then directed to different cellular locations. Proteins routed and sorted in the Golgi include: (1) membrane proteins; (2) proteins that are constitutively secreted (e.g., IMMUNOGLOBULINS); (3) proteins that are packaged into secretory granules and released in response to an external signal (e.g., COMPLEMENT RECEPTOR 3); (4) lysosomal enzymes.

A Golgi stack consists of at least three groups of morphologically and functionally different cisternae, designated *cis*, medial and *trans*; different enzymes have been localized to each of these groups. Proteins synthesized in the rough endoplasmic reticulum enter the Golgi at its *cis* face and may subsequently be modified as they pass through the cisternae, e.g., by proteolysis, glycosylation (*see* N-LINKED OLIGOSACCHARIDES and O-LINKED SACCHARIDES), fatty acid addition, phosphorylation, and sulfation. Fully processed proteins exit from the *trans* face. It is thought that proteins are transported from the endoplasmic reticulum to the different cisternae of the Golgi and then to their final destinations by successive steps of budding and fusion of membrane vesicles.

Goodpasture's syndrome. AUTOIMMUNE DISEASE in which there is severe GLOMERULONEPHRITIS and hemorrhagic pneumonia caused by AUTOANTIBODIES to the basement membranes of renal glomeruli and pulmonary alveoli. Linear, homogeneous deposits of IgG are seen in the glomeruli with fluorescein-conjugated anti-IgG. The syndrome occurs predominantly in males, is of sudden onset and results in progressive

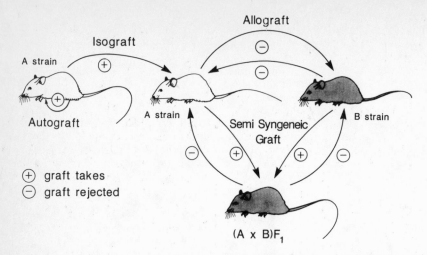

Isograft
A strain
$\oplus$
Autograft
$\oplus$

Allograft
$\ominus$
$\ominus$

A strain

B strain

Semi Syngeneic
Graft

$\ominus$ $\oplus$ $\oplus$ $\ominus$

$(A \times B)F_1$

$\oplus$ graft takes
$\ominus$ graft rejected

graft

loss of kidney function. The cause of the autoantibody formation is not known.

GPLA. MAJOR HISTOCOMPATIBILITY COMPLEX (MHC) of the guinea-pig. It consists of two loci of limited polymorphism encoding CLASS I HISTOCOMPATIBILITY MOLECULES (*GPLA-B* and *GPLA-S*); a locus encoding CLASS II HISTOCOMPATIBILITY MOLECULES (*GPLA-Ia*) and loci encoding the complement proteins FACTOR B, C2 and C4. The order of the genes is *BF* (Factor B), *C2, C4, Ia, B* and *S*.

graft. Transplantation of an organ or tissue from its usual site of residence to another.

graft rejection. Immunological reaction directed to HISTOCOMPATIBILITY MOLECULES in GRAFTS that results in the elimination or rejection of the graft. First-set rejection refers to the rejection of a graft placed in a non-immune individual; second-set rejection refers to the rejection of a graft placed in an IMMUNE individual. The rapidity of first-set rejection depends on the degree of histoincompatibility between the graft and the host. Differences in the MAJOR HISTOCOMPATIBILITY COMPLEX result in rejection within the first two weeks. Differences in one or a few MINOR HISTOCOMPATIBILITY ANTIGENS result in a slower rejection process. The first stage in graft rejection is the IMMUNIZATION of the host by cells (passenger leukocytes contain-

ing class II histocompatibility molecules) of the graft. The host subsequently produces HELPER and CYTOTOXIC T LYMPHOCYTES that recognize histocompatibility molecules of the graft, and antibodies to antigens of the graft. Thus, graft rejection is a combination of cell-mediated immunity and antibody-mediated immunity. Second-set rejection occurs within a week. Grafts can be rejected at a very accelerated rate (within hours) if implanted in an individual highly immune to the histocompatibility antigens of the graft (*see* WHITE GRAFT). Microscopically, graft rejection is characterized by damage to the endothelium of arterioles and venules and by formation of thrombi (clots) within these blood vessels. The graft is infiltrated with LYMPHOCYTES, MACROPHAGES and NEUTROPHILS and contains deposits of IgG.

graft-*versus*-host disease (GVH disease). Disease that results from the transplantation of immunocompetent, ALLOGENEIC T LYMPHOCYTES into a recipient that is unable to eliminate them. The recipient may be unable to eliminate the transplanted cells because of (1) IMMUNOSUPPRESSION by irradiation or drug therapy, (2) immunological immaturity (e.g., neonatal mice); or (3) TOLERANCE (e.g., inability of an F_1 animal to reject parental cells). GVH disease is characterized by fever, skin rash, enlargement of liver and SPLEEN, diarrhea, weight loss and aplasia of BONE MARROW CELLS. Microscopically affected organs are infiltrated by

LYMPHOCYTES and MACROPHAGES. The lymphocytes are of donor origin and are activated when they recognize allogeneic histocompatibility molecules of the recipient. These lymphocytes in turn activate host macrophages and incite INFLAMMATION. GVH disease can be acute or chronic. Chronic GVH disease in mice has been called runt disease, secondary disease or wasting disease. A GVH reaction can be studied in the developing chick by implanting allogeneic T lymphocytes on the chorioallantoic membrane. The implanted T lymphocytes induce severe inflammation in the embryo. In humans, GVH disease can be a serious complication of bone marrow transplantation.

granulocyte. *Synonym for* POLYMORPHO-NUCLEAR LEUKOCYTE.

granulocytopenia. *Synonym for* AGRA-NULOCYTOSIS.

granuloma. Accumulation of MACROPHAGES in close contact with each other, forming small microscopic masses. Foreign body granulomas surround foreign, usually poorly digestible, particles (e.g., carbon particles, surgical sutures, silica dust). Immune granulomas surround particulate antigens (e.g., fungi, parasites, intracellular bacteria). Immune granulomas are composed of activated macrophages. Granulomas are formed when T LYMPHOCYTES recognize the antigen trapped by macrophages. These T cells secrete LYMPHOKINES that attract additional macrophages to the granuloma site where they become activated. The activated macrophages in the immune granulomas restrict the growth of the invading organism. In tuberculosis, infectious granulomas are induced by HELPER T LYMPHOCYTES reactive with *Mycobacterium tuberculosis*. Immune granulomas may contain multinucleated giant cells (Langhans cells) formed by the fusion of macrophages and EPITHELIOID CELLS. T lymphocytes and a few NEUTRO-PHILS and EOSINOPHILS may be present. When the immune granuloma enlarges, the center may develop NECROSIS.

Graves' disease. AUTOIMMUNE DISEASE that results in hyperthyroidism (overactivity of the thyroid gland). Patients with Graves' disease may have an IgG AUTOANTIBODY to the thyroid-stimulating hormone (TSH) receptor. The binding of autoantibody to the receptor inhibits the binding of TSH, but mimics its action. This antibody is therefore called the long-acting thyroid stimulator (LATS). LATS may cross the placenta and cause self-limited Graves' disease in the newborn infant of an affected mother. Graves' disease is more common in females than in males.

Guillain–Barré syndrome. *See* IDIOPATHIC POLYNEURITIS.

gut-associated lymphoid tissue (GALT). Lymphoid tissue of the oropharynx (e.g., tonsils) and the gastrointestinal tract and its appendages (e.g., appendix in mammals, BURSA OF FABRICIUS in birds). In the mucosa of the gastrointestinal tract, lymphoid cells are distributed diffusely and also occur as nodules with FOLLICLES and germinal centers (Peyer's patches). Peyer's patches are rich in B LYMPHOCYTES that are precursors of IgA-synthesizing PLASMA CELLS. After antigenic stimulation, these B lymphocytes migrate, via the mesenteric LYMPH NODES and THORA-CIC DUCT, to the blood stream and eventually home to the gut or localize in other secretory tissue. Peyer's patches are more numerous in the ileum than in the jejunum or duodenum. In rabbits, the lymphoid tissue of the terminal portion of the ileum is called the SACCULUS ROTUNDUS. GALT is responsible for local immunity in the gut to bacteria, viruses and parasites.

H

H antigen. Flagellar antigen of motile Gram-negative enteric bacilli. The designation H (German '*Hauch*', breath) was used because these bacteria form a film on AGAR plates, resembling that found after breathing on a glass plate. The H antigens are used in the KAUFFMANN–WHITE SCHEME for classifying Salmonella. There are two major types of H antigen, called phase 1 and phase 2. These correspond to different FLAGELLINS, the products of non-allelic genes. An individual cell produces flagellin of only one or the other type. Phase variation is the abrupt switch from one type to the other and may occur as often as once every 1,000 bacterial divisions. This switching is controlled by the reversible inversion of a segment of DNA near the *H2* gene. Phase 1 antigens are more specific (i.e., shared by only a few Salmonella strains) than are phase 2 antigens. *See* O ANTIGEN.

H₁, H₂ blocking agents. *See* ANTIHISTAMINE.

H-2. MAJOR HISTOCOMPATIBILITY COMPLEX of mice. H-2 occupies a segment of approximately 0.5–1 centiMorgans on chromosome 17. The H-2 complex contains four regions: K, I, S and D. Genes in the K region encode CLASS I HISTOCOMPATIBILITY MOLECULES, K. Genes in the I REGION encode CLASS II HISTO-COMPATIBILITY MOLECULES, I-A AND I-E. Genes in the S REGION encode the CLASS III MOLECULES, C4, C2, Factor B and P-450 cytochrome (21-hydroxylase). Genes in the D region encode the class I histocompatibility molecules, D and L. The genes encoding class I and class II histocompatibility molecules are highly polymorphic.

Hageman factor. Plasma glycoprotein consisting of a single polypeptide chain (M_r 80,000) that initiates the cascade of the CONTACT SYSTEM and blood coagulation. Upon activation, zymogen Hageman factor is cleaved into two chains: alpha of 350 amino acid residues and beta of 243 residues which are joined by a single disulfide bond. Activated Hageman factor is a serine protease that converts prekallikrein of the con-

H-2 chart of inbred strains

H-2 haplotype	Prototype strain	H-2 haplotype	Prototype strain
a	A	m	AKR.M
an1	A.TFRI	o2	C3H.OH
ap1	B10.M(11R)	p	P/Sn
aq1	B10.M(17R)	q	DBA/1
b	C57BL/10	qp1	DA/HuSn
by1	B10.BYR	r	RIII/Wy
d	DBA/2J	s	A.SW
da	B10.D2(M504)	sq2	B10.QSR2
f	A.CA	t2	B10.S(7R)
g	HTG	t4	B10.S(9R)
h	HTH	u	PL/J
i	HTI	v	SM/J
j	JK	y1	B10.AQR
k	CBA	z	NZW

Modified from Klein, J., *Biology of the mouse histocompatibility-2 complex*, Springer-Verlag, New York, NY (1975)

tact system to KALLIKREIN. The active site of the enzyme lies in the beta chain.

hairpin loop. Region of double helix formed by base-pairing within a single-strand of DNA or RNA that has folded back on itself; the segments that form the stem of the hairpin are INVERTED REPEATS. In the original method used for cDNA cloning, a hairpin loop formed at the 3′ terminus of the first strand serves as a primer for the synthesis of the second strand. The loop of the hairpin structure can be removed with S1 NUCLEASE to allow ligation of the double-stranded cDNA into a cloning VECTOR.

Ham test. *See* PAROXYSMAL NOCTURNAL HEMOGLOBINURIA.

haploid. Descriptive of a nucleus, cell, or organism having a single set of unpaired chromosomes (i.e., one copy of each autosome and one sex chromosome). The haploid number of chromosomes in humans is 23. *See* DIPLOID.

haplotype. Specific combination of linked alleles in a gene cluster. The term is derived from 'haploid genotype' and is often used to describe a combination of alleles on one chromosome of an individual's MAJOR HISTO-COMPATIBILITY COMPLEX (e.g., H-2 or HLA). Some HLA haplotypes (e.g., HLA-A1B8) are in positive LINKAGE DISEQUILIBRIUM. *See* ALLOGROUP, COMPLOTYPE, EXTENDED HAPLO-TYPE.

hapten. Substance that can react specifically with antibodies, but that is not itself IMMUNOGENIC unless bound to a CARRIER. Usually, but not necessarily, haptens are small molecules ($M_r < 1,000$). A substance such as pneumococcal polysaccharide may be IMMUNOGENIC in some species (e.g., man, mouse) but only a hapten in other species (e.g., rabbit). A hapten coupled to a carrier may function as an ANTIGENIC DETERMINANT or as part of a determinant.

Hassall's corpuscle. Small mass or whorl of epithelial cells of unknown function in the medulla of the THYMUS.

HAT medium. Tissue culture medium containing hypoxanthine, aminopterin and thymidine, used as a selective medium to isolate HYBRID CELLS. Aminopterin is a folic acid antagonist and inhibits *de novo* synthesis of nucleic acids. However, there is a second mechanism for synthesizing nucleic acids (known as a salvage pathway) which is not blocked by antifolates. Hypoxanthine and thymidine can serve as precursors for nucleic acid synthesis in this pathway. Two enzymes required in the salvage pathway are hypoxanthine-guanine phosphoribosyl transferase (HGPRT) and thymidine kinase. Cells deficient in either of these enzymes cannot survive in HAT medium because all pathways of nucleic acid synthesis are blocked. However, hybrid cells formed from two cell lines containing different enzyme defects can grow in HAT medium, which is, therefore, used as a selective medium for such hybrid cells.

HAT medium is used in HYBRIDOMA production to select hybrids between MYELOMA cells and LYMPHOCYTES. The myeloma cell lines that are usually used lack HGPRT and cannot grow in HAT medium. Lymphocytes have the normal salvage pathway enzymes but they have only a very limited capacity to proliferate. In a hybrid formed between an HGPRT-deficient myeloma cell and a normal lymphocyte, the lymphocyte supplies the missing enzyme to the hybrid cell, which retains the proliferative capacity of the myeloma and can now grow in HAT medium.

Heaf test. Form of TUBERCULIN TEST in which a multi-pronged instrument is used to introduce TUBERCULIN into the skin. This is also called the Tine test.

heat inactivation. Destruction of biological activity by heating. In immunology, it usually refers to the destruction of COMPLEMENT activity by heating serum at 56°C for 30 minutes, conditions that inactivate C1, C2 and FACTOR B. Heating serum at 52°C for 30 minutes inactivates only Factor B, thereby destroying the ALTERNATIVE PATHWAY OF COMPLEMENT activation, but leaving the CLASSICAL PATHWAY intact. IMMUNOGLOBULINS are not inactivated by heating at 56°C for 30 minutes, except for IgE antibodies.

heavy chain. Larger polypeptide chain in a HETERODIMER. As used by immunologists, heavy chain usually refers to the heavy chain of an IMMUNOGLOBULIN molecule. *See* IMMUNOGLOBULIN HEAVY CHAIN.

helper T lymphocyte (T_H). T LYMPHOCYTE that cooperates with a B LYMPHOCYTE in antibody formation. These cells recognize protein antigens that are presented by other cells bearing CLASS II HISTOCOMPATIBILITY MOLECULES (*see* ANTIGEN PRESENTATION). Once a helper T lymphocyte has recognized antigen, it divides and differentiates. The differentiated cells secrete several LYMPHOKINES that have profound effects on the function of other cells: B lymphocytes divide and differentiate into antibody-secreting cells (PLASMA CELLS); macrophages are recruited and activated as in DELAYED-TYPE HYPERSENSITIVITY reactions; and inactive precursor cells develop into CYTOTOXIC T LYMPHOCYTES. Helper T lymphocytes have on their surface antigenic determinants recognized by monoclonal antibodies to CD4 (e.g., T4 or Leu 3 in humans, L3T4 in mice).

hemagglutination. AGGLUTINATION of red blood cells (e.g., by antibodies).

hemagglutinin. Substance (e.g., antibody to red blood cells) that agglutinates red blood cells.

hematopoietic stem cell. Undifferentiated, self-renewing cell usually found in BONE MARROW, from which cells of several lineages arise. In fetal life, hematopoietic stem cells are found in the yolk sac and subsequently in the liver.

hemolysin. Antibody to red blood cells that fixes COMPLEMENT thereby bringing about LYSIS of these cells.

hemolysis. LYSIS of red blood cells.

hemolytic anemia. Accelerated destruction of red blood cells due to: (1) an intrinsic defect in these cells (e.g., sickle cell anemia, thalassemia); or (2) infection (e.g., malaria), or (3) antibodies to membrane constituents of these cells (e.g., HEMOLYTIC DISEASE OF THE NEWBORN, AUTOIMMUNE HEMOLYTIC ANEMIA, COLD AGGLUTININ SYNDROME).

hemolytic disease of the newborn. Form of HEMOLYTIC ANEMIA in newborns caused by the transplacental passage of maternal IgG antibodies with specificity for antigens on the red blood cells of the fetus. Usually, maternal IMMUNIZATION has occurred in a previous pregnancy. Hemolytic disease of the newborn is most commonly due to fetal–maternal differences in the ABO or Rh antigens. *See* ABO BLOOD GROUP, RH BLOOD GROUP, DUFFY BLOOD GROUP, KELL–CELLANO BLOOD GROUP, LUTHERAN BLOOD.

hemolytic plaque assay. Technique for enumerating antibody-producing cells in a cell suspension. Originally this method was devised to enumerate cells synthesizing antibody to sheep red blood cells. Antibody-producing cells are mixed with a thick suspension of sheep red blood cells and the mixture is suspended uniformly in a semisolid medium (e.g., AGAR). After several hours, the agar is flooded with fresh serum as a source of COMPLEMENT. Each cell secreting IgM antibody to the sheep red blood cells is surrounded by a clear zone in the red background due to the binding of secreted antibody by the red blood cells and subsequent lysis by complement. To detect cells secreting IgG antibody to sheep red blood cells it is necessary to add anti-IgG antibodies to facilitate lysis upon subsequent addition of the complement source. The assay can be modified to enumerate cells secreting antibody to HAPTENS, polysaccharides or protein antigens by conjugating them to sheep red blood cells. The assay can also be used to determine the class of immunoglobulin secreted by an antibody-producing cell; for this purpose antibody to immunoglobulin (e.g., anti-IgG) is conjugated to the sheep red blood cells.

Henoch–Schönlein purpura. Self-limited acute bleeding disorder, occurring almost exclusively in children and adolescents. The skin, kidneys and gastrointestinal tract are the principal sites of bleeding (PURPURA). Severe abdominal pain results from gastrointestinal bleeding. The skin purpura is usually confined to the lower extremities, buttocks and lower abdomen. Joint swelling is also commonly observed. The PLATELET count is normal. Deposition of IgG in blood vessel walls and glomeruli suggests an immunological pathogenesis of the disease. The disease is seen with increased frequency in children with hereditary C2 deficiency.

heparin Complex glycosaminoglycan with anticoagulant activity, found in many tissues. It is so-named because it was originally isolated from liver. Heparin is synthesized in MAST CELLS and endothelial cells as a proteoglycan molecule consisting of at least 10 long polysaccharide chains linked via a trisaccharide galactosyl–galactosyl–xylosyl sequence to the hydroxl groups of serine residues in a polypeptide backbone containing a long sequence of alternating serine and glycine residues. Each polysaccharide chain is constructed as an oligomer of 100 to 200 disaccharide units consisting of N-acetyl-D-glucosamine and D-glucuronic acid, joined in α1-4 glycosidic linkage. This basic unit is extensively modified by deacetylation, N- and O-sulfation and epimerization, the latter reaction converting D-glucuronic to L-iduronic acid. Post-synthetic modification of the proteoglycan by an endoglucuronidase selectively cleaves the polysaccharide chains at specific sites, yielding a mixture of polysaccharides of M_r 6,000–25,000; these molecules are found in the commercially available heparin preparations. Heparin is an anticoagulant and is used clinically in the treatment of thrombosis (clots) and phlebitis (inflammation of veins). Heparin binds to the collagen-like stem of C1q and blocks the uptake of C1r and C1s. Heparin also binds to FIBRONECTIN. Its physiological role is not known.

hepatocyte stimulating factor MONOKINE that induces release of acute phase reactants (*see* ACUTE PHASE REACTION) from liver cells. It is identical to INTERLEUKIN-6.

herd immunity IMMUNITY of a sufficient number of individuals in a population, such that infection of one individual will not result in an epidemic.

hereditary angioneurotic edema (HANE or HAE). Hereditary disease, transmitted as an autosomal dominant and characterized by recurrent episodes of swelling of subcutaneous tissues, intestine and larynx. The disease is due to a genetic defect in C1 INHIBITOR so that increased cleavage of C4 and C2 occurs when C1 is activated. A KININ-like peptide generated from C2b, which enhances vascular permeability, appears to cause the symptoms. Two genetic variants of the disease are recognized: type I in which the C1 inhibitor level is low, type II in which a mutant C1 inhibitor is present in normal or elevated amounts, but is nonfunctional.

hereditary ataxia telangiectasia *See* ATAXIA TELANGIECTASIA (AT).

heteroclitic antibody. Antibody that has higher affinity for a heterologous antigen (or antigenic determinant) than for the antigen or determinant that stimulated the production of the antibody, i.e., the antibody reacts preferably with a molecule other than the IMMUNOGEN.

heterocliticity. Preferential interaction of an ANTIBODY with an ANTIGENIC DETERMINANT that is different (i.e. heterologous) from the determinant that elicited that antibody (i.e the immunogenic determinant).

heterocytotropic antibody ANTIBODY of one species that binds to MAST CELLS of another species leading to a local anaphylactic reaction (*see* ANAPHYLAXIS) when the corresponding ANTIGEN is encountered. See IgE, HOMOCYTOTROPIC ANTIBODY.

heterodimer. Protein composed of two different chains of which the larger is usually designated the alpha (or heavy) chain and the smaller the beta (or light) chain. CLASS I HISTOCOMPATIBILITY MOLECULES, CLASS II HISTOCOMPATIBILITY MOLECULES, COMPLEMENT RECEPTOR 3 and C5 are examples of heterodimers.

heteroduplex. Hybrid structure formed by annealing two DNA strands (or an RNA and a DNA strand) that have some, but not complete, complementarity in sequence. Regions of non-complementarity in a duplex (as little as one mismatched base pair) can be digested with S1 NUCLEASE. Large regions of non-complementarity can often be visualized in the electron microscope.

heterogenetic antibody. *Synonym for* HETEROPHILE ANTIBODY.

heterogenetic antigen. *Synonym for* HETEROPHILE ANTIGEN.

heterograft. *Synonym for* XENOGRAFT.

heterokaryon. Fused cell with two separate nuclei. The fusion is usually accomplished by treating a cell suspension with certain inactivated viruses (e.g., ultraviolet-treated

Sendai virus) or polyethylene glycol. *See* HYBRID CELL.

heterologous. Derived from a different source.

heterophile antibody. Antibody that reacts with a HETEROPHILE ANTIGEN. Antibodies to Forssman antigen are heterophile antibodies. Such antibodies are found in antisera to red blood cells of a variety of species (sheep, horse, mouse). Patients with INFECTIOUS MONONUCLEOSIS frequently (50–90 percent of cases) develop heterophile antibodies that agglutinate sheep red blood cells; however, these antibodies cannot be absorbed by guinea-pig kidney and therefore are not antibodies to Forssman antigen. *Synonym for* heterogenetic antibody.

heterophile antigen. Antigen (or antigenic determinant) found in a variety of tissues (e.g., red blood cells) in many species and also in bacteria. Heterophile antigens cross-react extensively with antibodies against one member of the particular heterophile group. An example of heterophile antigen is the FORSSMAN ANTIGEN. *Synonym for* heterogenetic antigen.

heterotopic. Descriptive of a tissue or organ GRAFT to a site not normally occupied by that tissue or organ.

heterozygous advantage. Condition in which the heterozygote is more fit (has selective advantage) than is either homozygote. For example, in regions of the world where malaria is endemic, there is a relatively high (up to 10 percent) incidence of a mutant gene encoding hemoglobin S (sickle cell trait). This is probably because heterozygous individuals, who have both sickle hemoglobin and normal (A) hemoglobin, have a greater chance of surviving an attack of malaria, compared to individuals who are homozygous for hemoglobin A. Homozygotes for hemoglobin S are at a disadvantage because they develop sickle cell anemia. Heterozygous advantage can lead to BALANCED POLYMORPHISM.

Heymann's nephritis. Membranous GLOMERULONEPHRITIS induced in rats by IMMUNIZATION with an AUTOLOGOUS antigen extracted from renal tubules. It is characterized by deposits of ANTIGEN–ANTIBODY COMPLEXES in glomeruli without inflammatory cells; protein is excreted in the urine. It is thought that this nephritis is an AUTOIMMUNE disease in which AUTOANTIBODIES complex with a shed antigen from the epithelial cells of the glomerulus.

high-zone tolerance. TOLERANCE induced by large amounts of protein antigens.

hinge region. Section of the IMMUNOGLOBULIN HEAVY CHAIN that lies between the C_H1 and C_H2 domains. Usually the hinge region is rich in proline and contains one or more half cystines that participate in interchain disulfide bridges. Proteolysis of IMMUNOGLOBULINS tends to occur in or near the hinge region (e.g., in production of Fab FRAGMENTS, $F(ab')_2$ FRAGMENTS, and Fc FRAGMENTS). Hinge regions are thought to impart flexibility to the immunoglobulin molecule whereby Fab domains move with respect to the Fc domain. Hinge regions are found in IMMUNOGLOBULIN GAMMA CHAINS, IMMUNOGLOBULIN ALPHA CHAINS and IMMUNOGLOBULIN DELTA CHAINS, but not in IMMUNOGLOBULINS MU CHAINS or IMMUNOGLOBULIN EPSILON CHAINS. A hinge region is usually encoded by a single short EXON. However, the hinge region of human and mouse alpha chains is encoded by the 5' portion of the C_H2 EXON, that of human gamma 3 chains by four exons, and that of human delta chains by two exons.

histaminase. Diamine oxidase, widely distributed in all tissues, that converts HISTAMINE to inactive imidazoleacetic acid.

histamine (β-aminoethylimidazole). Major mediator of IMMEDIATE HYPERSENSITIVITY and ANAPHYLAXIS in humans and guinea-pigs. Histamine is a potent dilator of small blood vessels, constrictor of smooth muscle, particularly of the bronchi and gastrointestinal tract, and inducer of secretions in the stomach. Histamine is formed by the decarboxylation of histidine by histidine decarboxylase and is mainly stored in the granules of tissue MAST CELLS and circulating BASOPHILS. Binding of histamine to H_1 receptors brings about smooth muscle contraction and increased vascular permeability; binding of histamine to H_2 receptors stimulates gastric secretion and inhibits release of mediators from basophils or mast cells and is thought to interfere with the function of SUPPRESSOR T LYMPHOCYTES. Histamine is a chemotactic attractant for EOSINO-PHILS, which release HISTAMINASE, the enzyme that degrades histamine. *See* ANTI-HISTAMINE.

$$H-C=C-CH_2-CH_2-NH_2$$
$$H-N \quad N$$
$$\backslash C /$$
$$H$$

histamine

histiocyte. Well-differentiated MACRO-PHAGE found in connective tissue, usually surrounding blood vessels.

histocompatibility Identity in CLASS I and CLASS II HISTOCOMPATIBILITY MOLECULES. There may or may not be matching at MINOR HISTOCOMPATIBILITY LOCI. The term is also used in an operational sense to mean sufficient similarity in tissue type such that GRAFTS between two individuals are accepted.

histoplasmin. Crude extract of *Histoplasma capsulatum* used to test CELL-MEDIATED IMMUNITY to the fungus.

histotope. In ANTIGEN PRESENTATION, the part of a CLASS II HISTOCOMPATIBILITY MOLECULE that interacts with the T CELLS RECEPTOR. *See* AGRETOPE, DESETOPE, RES-TITOPE.

HIV infection. Infection after exposure to HUMAN IMMUNODEFICIENCY VIRUS (HIV) as determined by the criterion of SEROCONVER-SION. Transmission of HIV occurs by three routes: sexual contact, blood (or blood product) transfusion and via the placenta. Contact with HIV does not necessarily result in infection as determined by this criterion. The infection may run the following courses: (1) approximately 15 percent of infected individuals have an acute illness, characterized by fever, rash, enlarged LYMPH NODES and meningitis within six weeks contact with HIV. Following this acute infection, these individuals become asymptomatic. (2) The remaining individuals with HIV infection are not symptomatic for years. (3) Some individuals develop persistent generalized lymphade-nopathy (PGL), characterized by swollen lymph nodes in the neck, groin and axilla. 5–10 percent of individuals with PGL revert to an asymptomatic state. (4) Any of these individuals may develop AIDS-RELATED COMPLEX (ARC); patients with ARC do not revert to an asymptomatic state. (5) Individuals with ARC, as well as those with PGL and also asymptomatic individuals eventually (months to years later) develop acquired immunodeficiency syndrome (AIDS), which inexorably leads to death.

Any time during the course of HIV infection, an individual may develop THROMBO-CYTOPENIA or neurological disease of the brain, spinal cord or peripheral nerves.

hive. *Synonym for* URTICARIA.

HLA (human leukocyte antigen). MAJOR HISTOCOMPATIBILITY COMPLEX of humans. The complex occupies a segment of 1.5–2 centi-Morgans on the short arm of chromosome 6. The HLA complex contains genes that encode CLASS I HISTOCOMPATIBILITY MOLECULES (HLA-A, HLA-B, HLA-C, and HLA-E), CLASS II HISTOCOMPATIBILITY MOLECULES, HLA-D (*see* HLA-D REGION), and CLASS III MOLECULES (C2, C4, FACTOR B and P-450 cytochrome (21–hydroxylase)). The genes encoding TUMOR NECROSIS FACTORS α and β are located between the class III genes and HLA-B. The arrangement of the genes is shown in the figure. Most of the genes in the *HLA* complex are highly poly-morphic.

HLA-D region. Segment of DNA in the MAJOR HISTOCOMPATIBILITY COMPLEX of humans (*see* HLA) that contains the genes encoding CLASS II HISTOCOMPATIBILITY MOLECULES. The HLA-D regions consists of ~ 1000 kilobases. Three clusters of genes have been identified in this region: the DP cluster includes two *DPβ* and two *DPα* genes, and a *DZα*; the DQ cluster includes *DOβ*, *DXβ*, *DXα*, *DQα* and *DQβ*; and the DR cluster includes three *DRβ*; (the middle

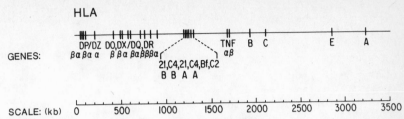

HLA

From Carroll, M., Katzman, P., Alicot, E.M., Koller, P.H., Geraghty, D.E., Orr, H.T., Strominger, G.D. and Spies, T. Proc. Nat. Acad. Sci., 84:8535, 1987. The centromere is to the left.

is a pseudogene) and a *DR*α. It is not yet known whether alpha and beta chains associate only when their respective genes are in the same cluster. Several of the genes (*DP*β, *DQ*β and *DR*β) are highly polymorphic; of the alpha genes, only the *DQ*α is highly polymorphic.

Hm-1 Major histocompatibility complex (MHC) of the Syrian hamster. The hamster MHC has very limited polymorphism, and only genes encoding class II histocompatibility molecules have been identified.

Hodgkin's disease. Malignancy of lymphoid cells of mixed cell type, involving principally lymph nodes and spleen. The Reed–Sternberg giant cell, which is diagnostic of Hodgkin's disease, is of uncertain lineage. Defects in cell-mediated immunity occur in many patients, rendering them susceptible to opportunistic infections and unreactive to skin tests for delayed-type hypersensitivity such as the tuberculin test. *See* anergy.

homing receptor. Protein on lymphocyte membranes that mediates the attachment of lymphocytes circulating in blood to high endothelial cells of post-capillary venules in lymph nodes. *See* MEL-14.

homocytotropic antibody. Antibody that binds to mast cells of the same species, leading to an anaphylactic reaction (*see* anaphylaxis) when the corresponding antigen is encountered. *See* IgE, heterocytotropic antibodies.

homodimer. Protein composed of two identical chains. The transferrin receptor is an example of a homodimer.

homograft. *Synonym for* allograft.

homology unit. immunoglobulin domain. This term is used to emphasize homology as a structural feature of the domain.

horror autotoxicus. Term introduced by Paul Ehrlich in 1901 to describe the general rule that the body does not react immunologically to its own constituents, i.e., the concept of self-tolerance.

human immunodeficiency virus (HIV). Retrovirus that causes the acquired immunodeficiency syndrome (AIDS) and related disorders. HIV is also known as HTLV-III/LAV or ARV. The virus infects mainly T lymphocytes of the CD4 subset in which the virus can be latent or lytic. HIV also infects CD4+ mononuclear phagocytes, B lymphocytes and brain cells. The virus is no more related to HTLV-I or II than it is to several other avian and mammalian retroviruses. HIV is also morphologically, genomically and taxonomically related to a group of retroviruses (lentiviruses): visna of sheep, equine infectious anemia virus and infectious arthritis virus of goats, all nononcogenic.

HIV has been isolated from blood, lymph nodes, cerebrospinal fluid and neural tissues of patients with the acquired immunodeficiency syndrome. The envelope glycoprotein (gp160) is the main antigen of HIV. It is composed of an external segment (gp120) and a transmembrane segment (gp41). gp120 interacts with the amino-terminal domain of CD4 and causes CD4+ T lymphocytes to coalesce into syncytia. Almost all antibodies to gp120 do not neutralize the virus. Attempts are being made to design a vaccine with the stable segments of gp120, which may evoke HIV neutralizing antibodies. *See* HIV infection.

humoral immunity. IMMUNITY mediated by antibodies that are in the body fluids (or 'humors') such as PLASMA or LYMPH. *See* CELL-MEDIATED IMMUNITY.

H-Y. Minor histocompatibility antigen encoded on the Y chromosome. H-Y is defined in INBRED STRAINS of mice and in HLA identical humans by various biological assays (e.g., the rejection of male skin grafts by females, or the killing of male LYMPHOID cells by female CYTOTOXIC T LYMPHOCYTES). The H-Y antigen has not yet been characterized.

hybrid antibody. Artificially constructed antibody molecule having two combining sites of different specificity. Hybrid antibodies are usually prepared by reduction and reoxidation of a mixture of $F(ab')_2$ fragments prepared from purified IgG antibodies of different specificity. A proportion of the oxidized products will be hybrid molecules and these can be purified by successive ADSORPTION and elution from immunoadsorbents containing each antigen. Hybrid antibodies are monovalent with respect to each antigen and do not precipitate with either antigen alone, although they do precipitate with a mixture of the two antigens. Hybrid antibodies have been used to visualize antigens on cell surfaces; in this application, one site is specific for a cell surface antigen and the other site for a marker that can be visualized (e.g., ferritin, an electron-dense protein that can be seen in the electron microscope).

hybrid cell. Cell produced by the fusion of two separate cells. A hybrid cell is derived from a HETEROKARYON by fusion of the two nuclei. Hybrid cells can be cloned to produce hybrid cell lines. These cell lines are often unstable and tend to lose chromosomes, a feature that makes them useful for assigning genes to chromosomes (GENE MAPPING). For example, fusions between mouse and human cells randomly lose human chromosomes, giving rise to a variety of mouse–human hybrid cell lines, each of which contains only one or a few human chromosomes. Analysis of these lines makes it possible to assign particular biochemical functions (and their associated genes) to individual human chromosomes. HAT medium is used as a selective medium to isolate hybrid cell lines.

hybridoma. Tumor derived from a HYBRID CELL. *See* B LYMPHOCYTE HYBRIDOMA, T LYMPHOCYTE HYBRIDOMA.

hydroxychloroquine (2-[[4-[(7-chloro-4-quinolyl) amino] pentyl] ethyl amino]ethanol sulfate). Drug used for the treatment and prevention of malaria. It is also used to treat SYSTEMIC LUPUS ERYTHEMATOSUS and RHEUMATOID ARTHRITIS.

hydroxychloroquine

hyper IgE syndrome. Disease characterized by extremely elevated concentrations (>0.03 mg/ml) of IgE in serum and recurrent abscesses of skin, pneumonia, sinusitis and dermatitis. The infections are mainly caused by *Staphylococcus aureus* and *Candida albicans*. The major infection caused by these microorganisms is a 'cold abscess' in the skin. These abscesses are 'cold' because IgE antibodies to the causative microorganisms do not fix COMPLEMENT and consequently little or no INFLAMMATION occurs at the site of infection.

Circulating immune complexes of IgE and IgG antibodies to IgE bind avidly to MONONUCLEAR PHAGOCYTES and release MONOKINES which cause calcium resorption from bone. Consequently, patients have frequent bone fractures as the result of osteoporosis (loss of calcium from bone).

Patients are anergic (*see* ANERGY) and their lymphocytes have markedly decreased mitogenic responses to soluble antigens. The number of CD8+ T lymphocytes in blood is decreased.

The hyper IgE syndrome occurs equally in males and females. Its onset occurs early in infancy; there is no evidence of hereditary transmission.

hyper IgM immunodeficiency. *Synonym for* IMMUNOGLOBULIN DEFICIENCY WITH INCREASED IgM.

hyperacute rejection. *See* GRAFT REJECTION.

hypergammaglobulinemia. Increased serum immunoglobulin levels. Hypergammaglobulinemia may be due to an increase in MONOCLONAL IMMUNOGLOBULIN (e.g., in MULTIPLE MYELOMA, MACROGLOBULINEMIA OF WALDENSTRÖM), or to an increase in POLYCLONAL immunoglobulin (e.g., in SYSTEMIC LUPUS ERYTHEMATOSUS, ACQUIRED IMMUNODEFICIENCY SYNDROME). Hypergammaglobulinemia also results from intensive immunization of experimental animals.

hypergammaglobulinemic purpura. *Synonym for* PURPURA HYPERGLOBULINEMIA.

hyperimmune. Having a high degree of IMMUNITY; the term usually refers to an animal that has been immunized (*see* IMMUNIZATION) repeatedly to produce large quantities of antibodies.

hyperimmunization. Repeated injection of an antigen into an animal to produce large quantities of antibodies.

hypersensitivity. State of heightened reactivity to a previously encountered ANTIGEN. Hypersensitivity is sometimes used as a synonym for ALLERGY. *See* DELAYED-TYPE HYPERSENSITIVITY, IMMEDIATE HYPERSENSITIVITY.

hypersensitivity pneumonitis. Inflammatory disease of the lung caused by antibodies to inhaled materials. Patients experience coughing, fever, chills and shortness of breath several hours after exposure to the offending inhalant. The pulmonary histopathology is characterized by alveolar and interstitial inflammation with obliterating bronchiolitis. C3 deposits are detected by IMMUNOFLUORESCENCE. The two most common forms of hypersensitivity pneumonitis are caused by antibodies to Actinomycetes spores found in hay (farmer's lung) and antibodies to IgA in pigeon droppings (pigeon fancier's lung).

hypersensitivity vasculitis. INFLAMMATION of small arterioles, capillaries and venules induced by immunological reactions to drugs, microbial antigens, or self or tumor antigens. It is a vague term.

hypervariable region. Segment of a polypeptide chain that is particularly variable in amino acid sequence when a set of equivalent sequences is compared. The term was originally used to describe segments of the VARIABLE REGIONS of IMMUNOGLOBULIN HEAVY and LIGHT CHAINS. The remaining portions of the variable regions (i.e., those that are not hypervariable) are called the FRAMEWORK REGIONS. Since most of the ANTIBODY COMBINING SITE is derived from residues in hypervariable regions, these regions are also referred to as COMPLEMENTARITY-DETERMINING REGIONS. Residues in the hypervariable regions frequently contribute to the IDIOTYPIC DETERMINANTS of immunoglobulin molecules. The degree of variability has been quantitated by an index of variability (*see* WU–KABAT PLOT).

For immunoglobulin light chains, the hypervariable regions are usually considered to be residue positions 24–34, 50–56 and 89–97. (These residue numbers conform to the immunoglobulin numbering system suggested by Kabat, E.A., Wu, T.T., Reid-Miller, M., Perry, H.M. and Gottesman, K.S.T. in *Sequences of Proteins of Immunological Interest*, U.S. Department of Health and Human Services, National Institutes of Health, 1987.) The first two and most of the third of these hypervariable regions are encoded by the V GENE SEGMENT V_κ or V_λ). Position 96 is often encoded by a codon formed from both the V and J GENE SEGMENTS and is a site for JUNCTIONAL DIVERSITY; position 97 is encoded by the J gene segment. For heavy chains, the hypervariable regions are positions 31–35, 50–65 and 95–102. The first two of these regions are encoded by the V_H gene. The third hypervariable segment is encoded by the D GENE SEGMENT and by the 5' end of the J gene segment. Utilization of a variety of D and J segments, variation at the V–D and D–J junctions, and incorporation of N REGIONS 3' and/or 5' to the D gene segment, all contribute to the diversity of the third hypervariable region of heavy chains.

The existence of hypervariable regions in the polypeptide chains of the T CELL RECEPTOR is less clear than it is in the case of immunoglobulin heavy and light chains. There does, however, appear to be some increase over the background variability at positions in the T cell receptor corresponding to the immunoglobulin third hypervariable region, possibly the result of combinatorial, junctional, and N-region diversification.

hypocomplementemia. *See* COMPLEMENT DEFICIENCY.

hypogammaglobulinemia. *See* AGAMMA-GLOBULINEMIA.

hyposensitization. *Synonym for* DESENSIT-IZATION.

I

I invariant (Ii). *See* INVARIANT CHAIN.

I region. Segment of DNA in the MAJOR
HISTOCOMPATIBILITY COMPLEX of mice that
contains the genes encoding CLASS II HISTO-
COMPATIBILITY MOLECULES. The I region consists of about 250 kilobases and is divided
into two subregions (I–A and I–E) on the
basis of frequent recombinations at the junction of the two regions. The I–A subregion
(approximately 175 kilobases) contains the
genes: pseudo $A_{\beta3}$, $A_{\beta2}$, $A_{\beta1}$ and A_{α}. The
I–E subregion (approximately 75 kilobases)
contains the genes: $E_{\beta2}$ and E_{α}. $E_{\beta1}$ straddles
the junction of the I–A and I–E subregions.
$E_{\beta3}$ is located in the S REGION. In most
INBRED STRAINS class II histocompatibility
molecules are $A_{\alpha}A_{\beta1}$ or $E_{\alpha}E_{\beta1}$. $A_{\beta2}$ and $E_{\beta2}$
are transcribed, but no protein products
have been identified. In some inbred strains
E_{β} are not expressed and only I–A molecules
are formed (e.g., C57BL/6).

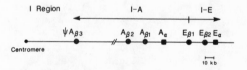

I region

Ia antigen. CLASS II HISTOCOMPATIBILITY
MOLECULE, initially defined as 'I region-
associated' antigen.

ibuprofen   ((+)-2-(p-isobutylphenyl)pro-
pionic acid).   Drug used in the treatment of
RHEUMATOID ARTHRITIS, JUVENILE RHEU-
MATOID ARTHRITIS and ANKYLOSING SPONDY-

$$(CH_3)_2CHCH_2-\!\!\!\!\bigcirc\!\!\!\!-\overset{\overset{\displaystyle CH_3}{|}}{C}HCOOH$$

ibuprofen

LITIS because of its anti-inflammatory
effects.

iC3b. *Synonym for* C3bi.

iC4b. *Synonym for* C4bi.

-id reaction. Sterile blisters of the skin
occurring during the course of fungal infections. The skin eruption is attributed to an
allergic reaction to fungal antigens.

idiopathic polyneuritis. Slowly evolving
paralytic disease that usually follows a
viral illness or vaccination, particularly
influenza vaccination. The disease resembles
EXPERIMENTAL ALLERGIC NEURITIS. Peripheral
nerves are infiltrated with LYMPHOCYTES and
MACROPHAGES, and myelin is destroyed at
these sites. The cerebrospinal fluid contains
increased amounts of protein, particularly
IgG, which is sometimes MONOCLONAL. The
number of cells in the cerebrospinal fluid is
normal or only slightly elevated. Idiopathic
polyneuritis is usually a self-limited disease,
but in some cases a chronic form of paralysis
develops. *Synonym for* Guillain–Barré syndrome.

idiopathic thrombocytopenic purpura
(ITP).   Bleeding disorder of children and
young adults caused by a loss of PLATELETS.
Patients with ITP have IgG autoantibodies
to platelets. AUTOLOGOUS or transfused
platelets are sequestered and destroyed in
the SPLEEN. ITP frequently follows the acute
viral infections of childhood (e.g., measles,
German measles).

idiotope. Epitope of an IDIOTYPE. *Synonym
for* IDIOTYPIC DETERMINANT.

idiotype. Set of IDIOTYPIC DETERMINANTS on
a particular IMMUNOGLOBULIN (or T CELL

RECEPTOR) VARIABLE REGION. Frequently, the idiotype is a unique attribute of a particular antibody in a particular animal, i.e., the product of a single CLONE (or group of closely-related clones) of B LYMPHOCYTES. Idiotypes can serve as markers for specific clones of antibody-forming cells or for gene segments encoding variable regions of IMMUNOGLOBULIN HEAVY and LIGHT CHAINS (see PUBLIC IDIOTYPIC DETERMINANTS).

idiotype network theory. See NETWORK THEORY.

idiotypic determinant. ANTIGENIC DETERMINANT characteristic of a particular VARIABLE DOMAIN of an IMMUNOGLOBULIN (or T CELL-REPTOR). Idiotypic determinants are often associated with the ANTIBODY COMBINING SITE and residues in the HYPERVARIABLE REGIONS generally form part of the determinant. However, residues in the FRAMEWORK REGIONS may also contribute to these determinants. If the idiotypic determinant is associated with the antibody combining site, a specific antigen or HAPTEN will often inhibit, at least partially, the reaction between the determinant and its corresponding antibodies. The expression of most idiotypic determinants requires the participation of residues from both the heavy and the light chains. Antibodies that recognize idiotypic determinants may be raised in another individual of the same species or in one of a different species; the antisera must be carefully absorbed to remove antibodies to ISOTYPIC or ALLOTYPIC DETERMINANTS. See IDIOTYPE.

IgA (immunoglobulin A).   Class of immunoglobulin (see IMMUNOGLOBULIN CLASS) bearing alpha chains. IgA accounts for 10–15 percent of immunoglobulins in human serum (1.5–3.5 mg/ml), where it occurs as 'monomers' of a four-chain unit or as dimers or higher multimers of such units. Each four-chain unit (M_r ~160,000), consists of two identical light chains and two identical heavy (α) chains. A form of IgA, designated secretory IgA, is the predominant immunoglobulin in the secretions of mammals (i.e., saliva, tears, colostrum, milk and fluids bathing the mucous membranes of the respiratory, gastrointestinal and genitourinary tracts); it is important in protecting

mucosal surfaces from invasion by microorganisms. Secretory IgA (M_r ~415,000) consists of two four-chain units and also contains two additional chains, J CHAIN and SECRETORY COMPONENT. J chain is probably attached to two of the alpha chains by disulfide bridges. Secretory component may or may not be joined by disulfide bridges to the alpha chains, depending on the species and subclass of IgA.

IgA is present in all mammals and has also been identified in birds. In humans, there are two subclasses of IgA: IgA1 and IgA2. IgA1 is the major subclass in serum (about 80–90 percent of the total), whereas IgA2 is somewhat more prevalent than IgA1 in secretions. There are two ALLOTYPES of IgA2: A2m(1) and A2m(2). The disulfide bridge that ordinarily connects heavy and light chains is missing in IgA2 molecules of the A2m(1) allotype. In these immunoglobulins, the two light chains may be disulfide-bonded to each other via the cysteine residue near the carboxy-terminus that ordinarily forms a bridge to the heavy chain. Secretory IgA appears to be relatively resistant to degradation by intestinal proteolytic enzymes; the presence of secretory component may contribute to this resistance, which confers protection against gut pathogens. However, IgA1 is specifically cleaved in the hinge region by enzymes secreted by certain bacteria that colonize mucosal surfaces (e.g., *Streptococcus sanguis*, *Neisseria gonorrheae* and *Neisseria meningitidis*). IgA antibodies do not fix COMPLEMENT by the CLASSICAL PATHWAY.

The alpha and light chains of IgA, as well as the J chain, are synthesized and assembled in B LYMPHOCYTES in the mucosal lamina propria of the gastrointestinal, respiratory and genitourinary tracts which are committed to IgA synthesis. In the small intestine, precursors of these IgA-specific B lymphocytes are found in Peyer's patches (see GUT-ASSOCIATED LYMPHOID TISSUE). After stimulation by antigen, these lymphocytes, which express IgA on their surfaces but do not secrete it, migrate through the mesenteric lymph nodes and the thoracic duct into the blood stream. They eventually exit from the systemic circulation by adhering to and migrating across specific endothelial cells in the walls of post-capillary venules in secretory tissue such as the lamina propria of the gastrointestinal and respiratory tracts or the interstitial tissue of exocrine glands; in these sites, the IgA-specific B lymphocytes differentiate into plasma cells that secrete IgA.

The secreted IgA, consisting of two four-chain units linked by J chain, binds to POLY-IMMUNOGLOBULIN RECEPTORS on the baso-lateral surfaces of nearby epithelial cells. The complex of IgA and receptor undergoes ENDOCYTOSIS; the receptor is then cleaved, a portion (the secretory component) remaining bound to IgA. The sIgA with attached J chain and secretory component is released at the apical portion of the cell into external secretions. This process, whereby receptors and ligands are transported across a cell, entering and exiting at opposite surfaces, is called TRANSCYTOSIS. Almost all of the IgA in secretions is derived from such local synthesis. See IMMUNOGLOBULIN ALPHA CHAIN.

IgA deficiency.   Absence of IgA1 and IgA2 (see IgA) in the blood and other body fluids. One in 700 individuals has IgA deficiency; thus, it is the most common PRIMARY IMMU-NODEFICIENCY. Most IgA-deficient individuals are clinically normal; some have increased susceptibility to PYOGENIC INFEC-TIONS, in which case there is a concomitant deficiency of IgG2 and/or IgG4 (see IgG SUBCLASS DEFICIENCY). Individuals with IgA deficiency have an increased incidence of CONNECTIVE TISSUE DISEASE compared with the normal population. IgE antibodies to IgA occur in some IgA deficients; this can result in severe, even fatal, TRANSFUSION REACTIONS when whole blood or blood plasma is given. IgA deficiency is inherited as an autosomal dominant in a few families. 70 percent of individuals with ATAXIA TEL-ANGIECTASIA have IgA deficiency. Normal numbers of B LYMPHOCYTES bearing membrane IgA (see MEMBRANE IMMUNOGLO-BULINS) are found in the blood of individuals with IgA deficiency; these mIgA-bearing B lymphocytes apparently do not terminally differentiate into IgA-secreting PLASMA CELLS.

IgA nephropathy.   IMMUNE COMPLEX DIS-EASE of the renal glomerulus, with foci of inflammatory cells and electron dense deposits containing IgA and to a lesser extent IgG, IgM and C3. IgA nephropathy usually has a benign course and is presumed to have an immunological cause.

IgD (immunoglobulin D).   Class of immunoglobulin (see IMMUNOGLOBULIN CLASS) bearing delta chains. IgD was first isolated as an unusual human MYELOMA protein; it was subsequently found to be present in normal human serum, but only at very low concentrations ($\sim$30–50 μg/ml). However, IgD is a predominant surface component of B LYMPHOCYTES.

Each IgD molecule is composed of two identical light and two identical heavy (delta) chains. The M_r of human IgD is approximately 175,000. Human IgD is highly sensitive to proteolysis, and it is difficult to isolate the intact molecule from serum. Trypsin cleaves IgD in the hinge region of the delta chain. The resulting Fab fragments are rapidly degraded, but the Fc FRAGMENTS and two peptides derived from the HINGE REGION are relatively stable to further proteolysis. Sensitivity to proteolytic digestion may be important for the biological function (as yet unknown) of IgD on the cell surface.

Immature B lymphocytes express surface IgM without IgD. As these cells differentiate, IgD is also expressed. Most mature B lymphocytes in the mouse SPLEEN have considerably more IgD than IgM on their surfaces. The IgD and IgM that are coexpressed on a particular cell share light chain type, IDIOTYPE and specificity for antigen, and presumably have the same V_L, V_H and C_L domains. After activation of B lymphocytes, surface IgD can usually no longer be detected.

No specific EFFECTOR FUNCTION is known for serum IgD. See IMMUNOGLOBULIN DELTA CHAIN.

IgE (immunoglobulin E).   Class of immunoglobulin (see IMMUNOGLOBULIN CLASS) bearing epsilon chains. IgE is a very minor component in serum ($\sim$0.1–0.3 μg/ml), but it is the major class of immunoglobulin that mediates anaphylactic reactions (see ANA-PHYLAXIS). Each IgE molecule is composed of two identical light chains and two identical heavy (epsilon) chains (M_r $\sim$190,000); it is heat-labile, being inactivated at 56°C. IgE binds tightly to Fcϵ RECEPTORS ON BASOPHILS and MAST CELLS. Cross-linking of the cell-bound IgE antibodies by antigen triggers the degranulation of these cells, releasing a variety of pharmacologically active substances. Among these are HISTAMINE and SEROTONIN, which elicit reactions of anaphylaxis, and chemicals that attract EOSINOPHILS, cells that can damage certain parasites. IgE levels in the serum may be slightly elevated in individuals with allergies such as hay fever and ASTHMA and considerably elevated in individuals with chronic parasitic infections. Before the immunoglobulin class IgE was discovered, the antibody activity associated with anaphylactic reactions was known as reagin. See IMMUNOGLOBULIN EPSILON CHAIN.

IgG (immunoglobulin G). Class of immunoglobulin bearing gamma chains. IgG is the most common IMMUNOGLOBULIN CLASS, comprising approximately three-quarters of the total immunoglobulin in mammalian serum (9–15 mg/ml). The designation IgG was chosen because these immunoglobulins migrate predominantly in the GAMMA-GLOBULIN fraction of serum (and, conversely, most of the gamma-globulin fraction is IgG). Each IgG molecule is composed of two identical light chains and two identical heavy (gamma) chains. The M_r is approximately 150,000 and the sedimentation coefficient, $s°_{20,w}$ is 7 S.

In humans, there are four subclasses of IgG (see IMMUNOGLOBULIN SUBCLASS): IgG1, IgG2, IgG3 and IgG4; they are present in serum in the following proportions: IgG1, 66 ± 8 percent; IgG$_2$, 23 ± 8 percent; IgG3, 7 ± 4 percent; IgG$_4$, 4 ± 2.5 percent. There are also four subclasses of IgG in mice (IgG1, IgG2a, IgG2b and IgG3), but there appear to be no subclasses of IgG in rabbits.

The main biological properties (i.e., EFFECTOR FUNCTIONS) of IgG antibodies are to fix COMPLEMENT, to cross the placenta, and to bind to Fcγ receptors on cell surfaces. Not all of these functions are carried out by all of the subclasses. For example, IgG4 does not activate the CLASSICAL PATHWAY OF COM-

PLEMENT. *See* IMMUNOGLOBULIN GAMMA CHAIN.

IgG subclass deficiency. Absence (or low amount) of one or more of the IMMUNOGLO-BULIN SUBCLASSES: IgG2, IgG3, IgG4 (*see* IgG). Individuals with this deficiency have a normal amount of serum IgG because IgG1 constitutes approximately 70 percent of the total IgG. Deficiency of IgG2 consistently, and deficiency of IgG3 rarely, results in susceptibility to PYOGENIC INFECTION; deficiency of IgG4 has no apparent clinical consequences. IgA DEFICIENCY, associated with susceptibility to pyogenic infections, is accompanied by deficiency of IgG2 and/or IgG4. In rare cases, IgG subclass deficiency results from deletions in C gene segments (e.g., a deletion of $C_{\alpha 1}$, pseudo C_{γ}, $C_{\gamma 2}$, $C_{\gamma 4}$ and C_{ϵ}) (*see* IMMUNOGLOBULIN GENES). It is estimated that 1–3 percent of the population is heterozygous for a deletion of some segment of the heavy chain constant gene locus.

IgM (immunoglobulin M). Class of immunoglobulin (*see* IMMUNOGLOBULIN CLASS) bearing mu chains. IgM accounts for 5–10 percent of the immunoglobulin in human serum (0.5–1.5 mg/ml). The designation IgM was chosen because this immunoglobulin has a high molecular weight and was originally called a macroglobulin. Mammalian IgM is a pentamer of four-chain units linked by disulfide bridges between heavy (mu) chains. Each of these units consists of two light chains and two heavy chains. Therefore each IgM molecule has ten heavy chains and ten light chains, and ten potential antigen-binding sites, two corresponding to each four-chain unit. All of the light chains and all of the heavy chains in each IgM pentamer are identical. In addition, each molecule of IgM contains one J CHAIN. The M_r of IgM is approximately 955,000 and the sedimentation coefficient, $s^{\circ}_{20,w}$, is 19 S. IgM can be converted by gentle reduction into the four-chain units, IgMs (sometimes called 'subunits' or 'monomers'). Because of their multivalence, the FUNCTIONAL AFFINITY of IgM antibodies for antigens is high. IgM antibodies can fix COMPLEMENT; a single molecule of pentameric IgM bound to the surface of a red blood cell can activate C1. IgM also exists as a membrane-bound molecule on the surface of B LYMPHOCYTES, where it acts as an antigen receptor. Mem-

brane IgM is a four-chain unit, and its heavy chain, μ_m, differs in its carboxy-terminus from the heavy chain, μ_s, of secreted IgM (*see* IMMUNOGLOBULIN MU CHAIN and MEMBRANE IMMUNOGLOBULIN).

IgM antibodies are typically formed early in an immune response; IgM is also the first immunoglobulin class to appear during ontogeny. IgM is found in all vertebrates and is the only immunoglobulin class in most cartilagenous and bony fish (where it is sometimes present as IgMs, the four-chain unit). In some lower vertebrates, IgM exists as a tetramer of four-chain units (bony fish) or as a hexamer of four-chain units (the South African clawed toad, *Xenopus laevis*), rather than as a pentamer of these units.

IgY (immunoglobulin Y). IMMUNOGLOB-ULIN CLASS in anuran amphibians, reptiles, and birds that is distinct from IgM. Each IgY molecule is composed of two light and two heavy chains. The evolutionary relationship of the heavy (upsilon (υ)) chains in these different classes of vertebrates to each other or to any of the immunoglobulin chains of mammals is not known. The mobility of upsilon chains in POLYACRYLAMIDE GEL ELECTROPHORESIS IN SODIUM DODECYL SULFATE is less than that of most IMMUNOGLOBULIN GAMMA CHAINS, suggesting that the upsilon chains are longer and/or richer in carbohydrate. IgY is sometimes referred to as 'low molecular weight immunoglobulin', to contrast it with IgM, the high molecular weight immunoglobulin class also present in these animals.

Ii antigens. Carbohydrate ANTIGENIC DETER-MINANTS on membranes of human red blood cells detected by IgM antibodies from individuals with the COLD AGGLUTININ SYNDROME. The i antigenic determinant is present on fetal and neonatal red blood cells and is modified during the first year of life to form the I antigenic determinant. The i antigenic determinant is composed of at least two repeats in the type 2 precursor chains of ABO BLOOD GROUPS. The I determinant is formed when galactose (β1–4) N-acetylglucosamine is attached to the galactose of the type 2 precursor chain in β1–6 linkage.

immature B cell. B LYMPHOCYTE that has IgM on its surface, but that does not secrete i: Gal $\xrightarrow{\beta1,4}$ GlcNAc $\xrightarrow{\beta1,3}$ Gal $\xrightarrow{\beta1,4}$ GlcNAc $\xrightarrow{\beta1,3}$ Gal-R

I: Gal $\xrightarrow{\beta1,4}$ GlcNAc $\xrightarrow{\beta1,3}$ Gal $\xrightarrow{\beta1,4}$ GlcNAc $\xrightarrow{\beta1,3}$ Gal-R

$\beta1,6$

GlcNAc

$\beta1,4$

Gal

R'

(Gal,D-galactose;GlcNAc,N-acetyl D-glucosamine.)

Ii antigen

immunoglobulin. This is the earliest cell of B lymphocyte lineage that can recognize antigen. The surface IgM is not polymerized into pentamers, as is secreted IgM, but is a single unit of two light and two μ_m chains. Surface IgM is an integral membrane protein; it is held in the membrane by the hydrophobic domain near the carboxy-terminus of the μ_m chain. *See* B LYMPHOCYTE, IMMUNOGLOBULIN MU CHAIN, MEMBRANE IMMUNOGLOBULIN, PRE-B CELL.

immediate hypersensitivity. Untoward immunological reactions that occur within minutes to a few hours of the introduction of antigen into an immune individual and that are mediated by antibodies. The element of time is less important than the involvement of antibodies; therefore these reactions are also called antibody-mediated hypersensitivity. In contrast, antibodies are not involved in DELAYED-TYPE HYPERSENSITIVITY. IgE antibodies (or in some species IgG1 antibodies) bound to MAST CELLS or BASOPHILS mediate ANAPHYLAXIS (e.g., penicillin reactions). Circulating IgG antibodies mediate IMMUNE COMPLEX DISEASE (e.g., ARTHUS REACTION) when they form precipitates with antigen in small blood vessels. Circulating IgG or IgM autoantibodies or alloantibodies can also mediate LYSIS of cells (e.g., HEMOLYTIC DISEASE OF THE NEWBORN).

immune. Having a high degree of natural or acquired resistance to a disease. By extension, the term indicates the altered state of an individual that results from IMMUNIZATION with any antigen. An animal or person may become immune by means of inadvertent exposure to antigen or by deliberate immunization.

immune adherence. Adherence of immune complexes or antibody-coated particles that contain bound C4b or C3b to cells bearing COMPLEMENT RECEPTOR 1 (CR1). CR1 is present on PHAGOCYTIC CELLS, B LYMPHOCYTES and some T LYMPHOCYTES of all species examined. CR1 is also present on primate red blood cells and glomerular epithelial cells. In contrast, CR1 is present on PLATELETS of other mammals, but not on their red blood cells. Immune adherence may be important for the clearance of IMMUNE COMPLEXES from the circulation but the exact mechanism by which this occurs is not known. Since red blood cells and platelets are the most abundant cells in the blood, most immune complexes adhere to them. Only a relatively small number of complexes adhere to phagocytes via CR1. It has been proposed that the bound C4b or C3b is converted to C4bi or C3bi by FACTOR I in the presence of CR1 (a cofactor for Factor I); the complexes adhering to red blood cells or platelets are then taken up by phagocytic cells via COMPLEMENT RECEPTOR 3.

immune adherence receptor. Synonym for COMPLEMENT RECEPTOR 1.

immune complex disease. Disease that results from deposition of ANTIGEN–ANTIBODY COMPLEXES in tissues. Such deposition may occur as an acute event (e.g., in ACUTE POST-STREPTOCOCCAL GLOMERULONEPHRITIS) or as a chronic phenomenon (e.g., in MEMBRANOPROLIFERATIVE GLOMERULONEPHRITIS). In immune complex disease, the antibodies are usually of the IgG class and fix COMPLEMENT, thereby inciting INFLAMMATION. In some types of immune complex disease (e.g., in SYSTEMIC LUPUS ERYTHEMATOSUS) AUTOANTIBODIES are involved. Immune complexes may form in the circulation and lodge in different vascular beds. The glomerular basement membrane is a frequent site for deposition of such complexes. Immune complexes may also form in extravascular tissues. Acute and chronic SERUM SICKNESS are experimental models for immune complex diseases.

immune deviation. The selective depression of certain IMMUNE RESPONSES with retention of others. For example, in guinea-pigs, injection of a protein antigen without ADJUVANT (or in INCOMPLETE FREUND'S ADJUVANT) results in antibody production and ARTHUS REACTIONS. When such an injection is followed by administration of the antigen in COMPLETE FREUND'S ADJUVANT, a procedure that ordinarily leads to high levels of DELAYED-TYPE HYPERSENSITIVITY and to production of IgG2, the response is blocked or 'deviated' so that there is no significant delayed-type hypersensitivity and little formation of IgG2, although total antibody remains the same.

immune elimination. Rapid removal of foreign material (antigen) from the blood as a result of its combination with antibodies. A foreign protein injected into the blood circulates with a characteristic half-life; after several days antibodies appear and the elimination of the protein is accelerated. ANTIBODY–ANTIGEN COMPLEXES bind to Fc RECEPTORS and complexes containing complement components bind to COMPLEMENT RECEPTORS of MACROPHAGES of the liver and spleen and are eliminated by PHAGOCYTOSIS.

immune hemolysis. Destruction of red blood cells by antibodies and COMPLEMENT.

immune interferon. *Synonym for* INTERFERON-GAMMA.

immune neutropenia. Immunologically mediated destruction of NEUTROPHILS by antibodies to these cells, called LEUKOAGGLUTININS. Immune neutropenia may be induced by drugs (usually penicillin derivatives) or by blood transfusions; it may also occur in AUTOIMMUNE DISEASES, such as SYSTEMIC LUPUS ERYTHEMATOSUS. Neonatal immune neutropenia results from the transplacental passage of maternal leukoagglutinins.

immune paralysis. Form of TOLERANCE in mice induced by injection of large amounts of polysaccharide, which is poorly metabolized. The immune paralysis lasts only as long as the polysaccharide persists.

immune response. Specific response of an animal to antigenic stimulation. The immune response may take the form of antibody production, CELL-MEDIATED IMMUNITY, or TOLERANCE. *See* PRIMARY RESPONSE, SECONDARY RESPONSE.

immune response (Ir) genes. Genes that control the immune response of HELPER T LYMPHOCYTES to proteins and synthetic polypeptides. Ir genes were first identified by the observation that INBRED STRAINS of mice and guinea-pigs differ in the extent of their responses to THYMUS-DEPENDENT ANTIGENS (i.e., some strains were 'responders' and others were 'non-responders'). Analysis of immune responses in CONGENIC STRAINS showed that responder status segregated with a segment of the MAJOR HISTOCOMPATIBILITY COMPLEX, called the I REGION, whose genes encode the CLASS II HISTOCOMPATIBILITY MOLECULES. Non-responder status may result from failure of processed antigen fragments (*see* ANTIGEN PRESENTATION) to bind to class II histocompatibility molecules of the non-responder strain or from failure of T CELL RECEPTORS of the non-responder strain to bind to antigen complexed to class II histocompatibility molecules (i.e., 'a hole in the T cell repertoire').

immune serum. *Synonym for* ANTISERUM.

immune serum globulin (ISG). Immunoglobulin preparation for therapeutic purposes. It is predominantly IgG and is prepared by cold ethanol fractionation of pools of human plasma derived from 500 to

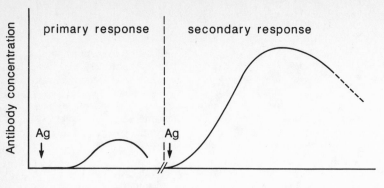

Time after immunization

immune response

1,000 donors. It is dispensed as a sterile 16.5 ± 1.5 percent solution. ISG is used as replacement therapy in IMMUNODEFICIENCY diseases and to prevent hepatitis A, measles and other viral infections. *See* IMMUNE SERUM GLOBULIN INTRAVENOUS.

immune serum globulin intravenous. IMMUNOGLOBULIN preparation for therapeutic purposes rendered suitable for intravenous administration by removal of aggregates. Sulfonation, reduction and alkylation, and acid treatment have been used to disassociate the aggregates. IMMUNE SERUM GLOBULIN (ISG) for intravenous administration is dispensed as a 5 ± 1 percent sterile solution. It is used in the treatment of IMMUNODEFICIENCY.

immune surveillance. Idea that the immune system eliminates cells that express NEOANTIGENS as a result of malignant change. According to this idea, cancer results from a failure in immune surveillance. It is currently thought that immune surveillance is carried out by NATURAL KILLER CELLS. *See* TUMOR-ASSOCIATED ANTIGEN.

immunity. State of being IMMUNE.

immunization. Administration of an ANTIGEN in order to bring about an IMMUNE RESPONSE. The term may also be used to describe the administration of antibodies to produce PASSIVE IMMUNITY.

immunoblotting. Technique in which specific antibodies are used to identify particular antigens in a mixture of proteins that

has been resolved and transferred to a membrane. The proteins are separated by an appropriate technique, usually SDS-PAGE (POLYACRYLAMIDE GEL ELECTROPHORESIS). The transfer is carried out by electroblotting to a sheet of nitrocellulose, which is then incubated with labeled antibodies specific for the antigen of interest. Either radiolabeled or enzyme-linked antibodies (*see* ELISA) can be used. Unbound antibodies are washed away, and the position of the labeled antibodies is revealed by an appropriate technique (e.g., AUTORADIOGRAPHY or addition of substrate). This technique is also known as 'Western blotting' because of similarities to SOUTHERN BLOTTING and NORTHERN BLOTTING.

immunoconglutination (IK). AGGLUTINATION of bacteria or red blood cells coated with C3bi (or C4bi) by an ANTISERUM raised against bacteria or red blood cells that have been exposed to antibody and COMPLEMENT. In effect, an antiserum to C3bi or C4bi is obtained that mimics the action of CONGLUTININ. During infection with bacteria, AUTOANTIBODIES to C3bi (or C4bi) may be made. These autoantibodies can cause immunoconglutination.

immunodeficiency (ID). Any defect of antibody function or CELL-MEDIATED IMMUNITY due to an intrinsic abnormality of B or T LYMPHOCYTES (*see* PRIMARY IMMUNODEFICIENCY) or as a consequence of loss or destruction of antibody and/or lymphocytes (*see* SECONDARY IMMUNODEFICIENCY).

immunodeficiency following hereditary defective response to Epstein–Barr virus.

Immunodeficiency that emerges during primary infection with EPSTEIN–BARR VIRUS (EBV) and usually leads to death. Before the EBV infection, patients are immunologically normal. During primary EBV infection, LYMPHOPENIA with a marked rise in NATURAL KILLER CELLS is observed. The acute stage may result in B cell LYMPHOMA, BONE MARROW failure, AGAMMAGLOBULINEMIA or death. Although originally found only in males, and therefore thought to be inherited as an X-linked recessive, a few females with this syndrome have been observed. The X-linked form of this disease has also been called Duncan's syndrome.

immunodeficiency with partial albinism. Form of COMBINED IMMUNODEFICIENCY inherited as an autosomal recessive and invariably fatal. Patients have depressed CELL-MEDIATED IMMUNITY, and NATURAL KILLER CELLS are deficient. In addition there is progressive cerebral atrophy and clumping of pigment in melanocytes.

immunodeficiency with thrombocytopenia. *Synonym for* WISKOTT–ALDRICH SYNDROME.

immunodeficiency with thymoma. Marked B LYMPHOCYTE and IMMUNOGLOBULIN deficiency in some patients with THYMOMA. In contrast to patients with X-LINKED AGAMMAGLOBULINEMIA, these patients have no PRE-B CELLS. Their CELL-MEDIATED IMMUNITY also becomes diminished as the disease progresses.

immunodiffusion. Technique for detecting antigen–antibody reactions in which antigens and antibodies are placed in a gel of AGAR (or similar material) and allowed to diffuse towards one another. A positive reaction is indicated by the presence of PRECIPITIN lines. *See* DOUBLE IMMUNODIFFUSION, IMMUNOELECTROPHORESIS, ROCKET IMMUNOELECTROPHORESIS, SINGLE RADIAL IMMUNODIFFUSION.

immunodominant site. Site on an IMMUNOGEN to which most of the IMMUNE RESPONSE is directed. A site may be immunodominant by virtue of its special location or structural properties and/or the efficient recognition and response by the host (e.g., as determined by presence of appropriate B

LYMPHOCYTES and regulatory T LYMPHOCYTES).

immunoelectrophoresis (IEP). Technique combining ELECTROPHORESIS and IMMUNODIFFUSION. It is usually carried out in a gel medium, such as AGAR. First, a mixture of antigens is placed into a well and separated by electrophoresis. Then a trough parallel to the direction of the electrophoretic separation is filled with antiserum. The separated antigens migrate radially from their positions and react with antibodies diffusing from the trough so that PRECIPITIN arcs are formed. Thus, antigens are characterized by both electrophoretic mobility and antigenic properties. The technique is very effective in identifying components in complex mixtures.

immunofixation. Technique for detecting specific antigens in a complex mixture of proteins that have been separated by ELECTROPHORESIS in an AGAROSE gel. After electrophoresis, the gel is flooded with antibodies, washed to remove soluble antigens and antibodies, and then stained to detect antigen–antibody precipitates.

immunofluorescence. Technique in which antibodies (or antigens) tagged with a fluorescent reagent are used to detect molecules of interest. Fluorescein isothiocyanate and rhodamine B isothiocyanate are the most common fluorescent reagents used for this purpose. Immunofluorescence is one of the most widely used techniques in immunology, cell biology and clinical medicine to localize antigens or antibodies on the surfaces of or inside cells and to identify pathogenic organisms in tissues or exudates. The cells or tissues to which fluorescent-tagged antibodies or antigens are bound are examined with a microscope equipped with a lamp that emits light and with a barrier filter that allows passage of the emitted fluorescent light. There are a number of variations of the technique. In the direct method, labeled antibody is reacted directly with antigen; in the indirect method, unlabeled antibody is reacted with antigen, followed by labeled antibody (second antibody) to the first antibody. The indirect method is more sensitive than the direct method. Furthermore, the indirect method is more convenient because the second antibody – e.g., fluorescein-

Direct Method — Fluorescent antibody / antigen

Indirect Method — Fluorescent (second) antibody / Unlabeled (first) antibody / antigen

immunofluorescence

Fluorescein isothiocyanate

Rhodamine B isothiocyanate

labeled anti-IgG – will react with all anti-bodies of the IgG class regardless of specificity and can, therefore, be used to detect a variety of antigens.

immunogen. Substance that is capable of inducing an IMMUNE RESPONSE (antibody response or CELL-MEDIATED IMMUNITY). Sometimes it is used as a synonym for antigen, but emphasis is on the ability to elicit a response, rather than on reactivity with antibodies. The most potent immunogens are proteins and polysaccharides, but lipids, nucleic acids, and synthetic polypeptides can also be immunogenic. See ANTIGEN, HAPTEN, IMMUNOGENIC.

immunogenic. Capable of inducing an immune response (antibody production or CELL-MEDIATED IMMUNITY). Immunogenicity is not an intrinsic property of a molecule, but is dependent both on properties of the putative IMMUNOGEN and the recipient. The necessary and sufficient conditions for a substance to be immunogenic are not known precisely. A requirement is that the immunogen be recognized as foreign (i.e., 'non-self') by the responding organism. Generally, the greater the evolutionary distance between the source of the immunogen and

the responder, the more effective the immunogen. Immunogenicity appears to be enhanced by large molecular size and molecular complexity. Factors influencing the response of an individual to immunization are the previous history (i.e., deliberate or accidental exposure to immunogens) and the repertoire of available B and T LYMPHOCYTES. See ANTIGENIC.

immunoglobulin. Protein that has antibody activity or that is antigenically related to an antibody. Most immunoglobulins are composed of heavy chains and light chains, although some may consist only of heavy chains (e.g., ALPHA HEAVY CHAIN DISEASE protein) or light chains (e.g., BENCE-JONES PROTEIN). Most immunoglobulins have antibody activity, but in some cases (e.g., MYELOMA PROTEINS), the relevant antigens are not known. See IMMUNOGLOBULIN HEAVY CHAIN, IMMUNOGLOBULIN LIGHT CHAIN.

immunoglobulin alpha (α) chain. Heavy chain of IgA (M_r ~58,000; ~470 amino acid residues). In addition to a variable region (V_H domain), alpha chains have a CONSTANT REGION composed of three domains (C_H1, C_H2 and C_H3) and a hinge region between C_H1 and C_H2. In contrast to the IMMUNOGLO-

BULIN GAMMA and IMMUNOGLOBULIN DELTA CHAINS, the HINGE REGIONS of humans and mouse alpha chains are not encoded by separate exons, but by the 5'-end of the exon that also encodes C_H2. At the carboxy-terminal end of the alpha chain, there is an 'extra' segment of 18 amino acid residues that is not part of a domain and that is unrelated in sequence to the rest of the chain (see discussion in IMMUNOGLOBULIN MU CHAIN). This segment contains, at its penultimate position, the cysteine residue that forms a disulfide bridge to J CHAIN.

In humans, there are two ISOTYPES of alpha chain (alpha1 and alpha2), corresponding to the two subclasses (see IMMUNOGLOBULIN SUBCLASS) of IgA (IgA1 and IgA2); there are two ALLOTYPES of the alpha2 chain: A2m(1) and A2m(2). The constant region of human alpha1 chains contains 353 amino acid residues; the constant regions of both alpha2 allotypes contain 340 amino acid residues. Relative to the alpha1 chain, there is a 13-residue deletion in the alpha2 hinge region. At 18 positions (in C_H1, the hinge region, and C_H2), there are subclass-specific residues where both alpha2 chains are identical but different from the alpha1 chain. At seven positions (two in C_H1 and five in C_H3), the two alpha2 chains differ from each other; at all of these positions, the A2m(1) chain is identical to the alpha1 chain. This suggests that the A2m(1) allele is a hybrid gene produced by recombination between the alpha1 and alpha2 genes.

A segment of eight amino acid residues is duplicated exactly in the alpha2 hinge region. Certain bacterial proteases (e.g., from *Streptococcus sanguis*, *Neisseria gonorrheae* and *Neisseria meningitidis*) cleave IgA1 specifically within this duplicated hinge segment. Five O-LINKED SACCHARIDES are attached to serines in the alpha1 hinge region. One of these consists only of *N*-acetylgalactosamine and the other four of galactose in β-1,3 linkage to *N*-acetylgalactosamine. The alpha2 hinge region has no carbohydrate. The number of *N*-linked oligosaccharide units is two in the alpha1 chain and four and five in the alpha2 chains of the A2m(1) and A2m(2) allotypes, respectively; all are of the complex type.

The pattern of interchain disulfide bridges is different in the two allotypes of alpha2 chains, although there is no difference in number or location of half-cystine residues.

In the A2m(1) allotype, there is no disulfide bridge between heavy and light chains, and the two light chains are often disulfide bridged to each other. In the A2m(2) allotype, a disulfide bridge connects each light chain to a heavy chain, as in other immunoglobulin molecules. This difference in disulfide bridging is probably related to two amino acid substitutions near the carboxy-terminal end of the C_H1 domain. At position 212, the replacement of proline (in A2m(1)) by serine (in A2m(2)) creates an additional carbohydrate acceptor site (i.e., the sequence asparagine–proline–serine is replaced by asparagine–serine–serine); there is indeed an N-linked oligosaccharide unit attached to asparagine 211 in A2m(2). At position 221, proline in A2m(1) is replaced by arginine in A2m(2), perhaps also contributing to a difference in conformation between the two allotypes. Two cysteine residues in C_H2 form disulfide bridges with cysteines in another heavy chain of the same subunit. All three varieties of human alpha chain have an extra intradomain disulfide bridge in C_H2. In addition, the alpha1 and alpha2 chains of the A2m(1) allotype have an extra intradomain bridge in C_H1. A cysteine residue in C_H2 may participate in disulfide bridging between IgA subunits.

The carboxy-terminal segment of the membrane form of the alpha chain is encoded by two (human) or one (mouse) exons (see IMMUNOGLOBULIN MU CHAIN, MEMBRANE IMMUNOGLOBULIN).

immunoglobulin class. Set of IMMUNOGLOBULINS that have similar or identical heavy chain CONSTANT REGIONS (i.e., that share one or more ISOTYPIC DETERMINANTS of the heavy chain constant region). Each immunoglobulin class (and the constant region of its heavy chain) is an ISOTYPE and is present in all members of a particular species. Usually, all the immunoglobulins in a species share the same set of light chains, and it is the differences in heavy chains that distinguish the different classes. In humans, the heavy chain constant regions of different immunoglobulin classes are only approximately 30 percent identical in amino acid sequence; they also vary considerably in carbohydrate content (see IMMUNOGLOBULIN ALPHA, DELTA, EPSILON, GAMMA and MU CHAINS). Immunoglobulin classes can be differentiated by antisera raised in another species. Within a species, the various immunoglobulin classes probably share the same repertoire of antigen-binding specificities, but they differ in their biological functions (e.g., complement fixation, membrane-binding) (*see* EFFECTOR FUNCTIONS). The human immunoglobulin classes are: IgG, IgM, IgA, IgD, IgE. An immunoglobulin class may consist of two or more subsets, called IMMUNOGLOBULIN SUBCLASSES.

immunoglobulin class switching. *See* CLASS SWITCHING.

immunoglobulin deficiency with increased IgM. ANTIBODY DEFICIENCY SYNDROME, characterized by increased levels of serum IgM and IgD. Serum IgG and IgA are very low or absent. It is usually, but not always, transmitted as an X-linked recessive disease. IgM AUTOANTIBODIES to PLATELETS, NEUTROPHILS, and other formed elements of the blood are frequently found. The B LYMPHOCYTES have only surface IgM and IgD and secrete only IgM and IgD, but can be forced to secrete IgG and IgA when CLASS SWITCHING is induced by co-culture with malignant T LYMPHOCYTES from a patient with LYMPHOMA. In addition, patients have clinical signs and symptoms of the antibody deficiency syndrome, i.e., increased susceptibility to pyogenic bacteria.

immunoglobulin delta (δ) chain. Heavy chain of IgD (human delta chain: M_r ~64,000; ~500 amino acid residues). In addition to a VARIABLE REGION (V_H domain), the human delta chain has a CONSTANT REGION (384 amino acid residues) consisting of three domains (C_H1, C_H2, and C_H3) and a long HINGE REGION of 58 residues. The mouse delta chain contains only two domains, C_H1 and C_H3, with an apparent deletion of C_H2; a hinge region is also present.

The hinge region of the human delta chain is encoded by two EXONS. The segment encoded by the first of these exons (34 amino acid residues) is rich in O-LINKED SACCHARIDES attached to serine and threonine residues and is resistant to proteolytic cleavage. There are four or five such groups in IgD MYELOMA protein Wah and seven in myeloma protein Nig-65. In protein Wah, about half of the groups have been shown to consist of galactose in β-1,3 linkage to *N*-acetylgalactosamine and the remainder

contain one or two residues of *N*-acetylneuraminic (sialic) acid. The hinge segment encoded by the second exon (24 amino acid residues), is highly charged, being particularly rich in glutamic acid and lysine; this segment is readily cleaved by proteolytic enzymes and is apparently responsible for the exquisite sensitivity of IgD to proteolysis. The hinge region of the mouse delta chain consists of 35 amino acid residues and is encoded by a single exon, which is homologous to the amino-terminal hinge segment of the human chain.

The carboxy-terminal segment of secreted human delta chain (8 residues), as well as that of mouse delta chain (21 residues), is encoded by a separate exon. In other secreted heavy chains, the carboxy-terminal segment is encoded by an extension of the exon encoding the last domain of the polypeptide chain. As in other heavy chains, there are two distinct exons encoding the membrane-specific segment of both the mouse and human delta chain. There are three N-LINKED OLIGOSACCHARIDES in the human delta chain, a high-mannose type in the C_H2 domain and two complex sugars in the C_H3 domain. A cysteine residue at the beginning of the C_H2 domain forms the interchain disulfide bridge with another delta chain in human IgD.

immunoglobulin domain. Fundamental structural unit of IMMUNOGLOBULIN HEAVY or LIGHT CHAIN. Immunoglobulin domains consist of about 110 amino acid residues. The domains are homologous in primary and three-dimensional structure. Many of the functional properties of immunoglobulins can be localized to individual domains. Immunoglobulin domains usually correspond to EXONS. *See* HOMOLOGY UNIT, IMMUNOGLOBULIN FOLD.

immunoglobulin epsilon (ε) chain. Heavy chain of IgE (M_r ~72,000; ~550 amino acid residues). In addition to a VARIABLE REGION (V_H domain), the epsilon chain has a CONSTANT REGION consisting of four domains (C_H1, C_H2, C_H3, and C_H4); there is no HINGE REGION. In the human epsilon chain, the constant region contains 428 amino acid residues. Two cysteine residues near the amino- and carboxy-terminal ends of C_H2 are thought to form inter-heavy chain disul-

Properties of human immunoglobulins*

Isotype	Chain structure	H chain designation	Approx M_r ($\times 10^{-3}$)	No. of domains in H chains†	Hinge Region	Approx M_r of H chain ($\times 10^{-3}$)	No. of saccharide units O-linked	No. of saccharide units N-linked	Approx serum conc. (mg/ml)	Approx half-life (days)
IgG1		γ1	148	4	+	51	0	1	9	21
IgG2		γ2	148	4	+	51	0	1	3	21
IgG3		γ3	159	4	+	56	0	1	1	7
IgG4		γ4	148	4	+	51	0	1	0.5	21
IgM		μ	955	5	−	72	0	5	1.2	5
IgA1		α1	160	4	+	57	5	2	2.0	6
IgA2 A2m(1)		α2	162	4	+	58	0	4		?
IgA2 A2m(2)		α2	166	4	+	60	0	5	0.5	6
IgD		δ	175	4	+	64	4–7	3	0.04	3
IgE		ε	190	5	−	72	0	6	0.0002	3

* modified from Nisonoff, A., Introduction to Molecular Immunology, 2nd edition, Sinauer Assoc., Sunderland, MA (1981).

† excluding hinge region.

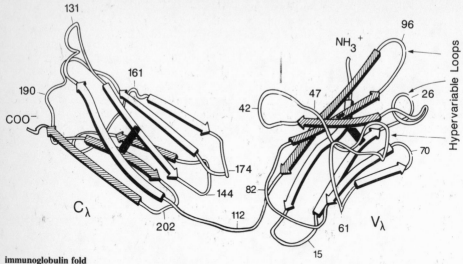

immunoglobulin fold

The white arrows form one layer of the ß-pleated sheet and the striped arrows form the second layer. The solid bars are the conserved intradomain disulfide bridges.

From Edmundson, A. B., Ely, K. R., Abola, E. E., Schiffer, M. and Panagiotopoulos, N. *Biochemistry* 14: 3953–3961 (1975)

fide bridges. An extra intrachain disulfide bridge is formed by cysteine residues near the amino-terminal ends of C_H1 and C_H2. There are six N-LINKED OLIGOSACCHARIDES: three in C_H1, one in C_H2, and two in C_H3; the one in C_H3 is high-mannose and the others are complex oligosaccharides. Human epsilon chains have no extra carboxy-terminal segment ('tail piece'); a short piece appears to be present in the mouse epsilon chain. There is less resemblance in amino acid sequence between human and mouse epsilon chain than between the IMMUNOGLOBULIN GAMMA CHAINS or the IMMUNOGLOBULIN MU CHAINS of these two species.

The carboxy-terminal segment of the membrane form of the epsilon chain is encoded by two exons (*see* IMMUNOGLOBULIN MU CHAIN and MEMBRANE IMMUNOGLOBULIN). *See* FCε RECEPTOR.

immunoglobulin fold. Basic three-dimensional structure of an IMMUNOGLOBULIN DOMAIN. The immunoglobulin fold consists of two approximately parallel BETA-PLEATED SHEETS, one containing four hydrogen-bonded, anti-parallel chain segments and the other containing three such segments. Roughly half of the amino acid residues in the domain are in the beta-

pleated sheets; the remaining residues are in the terminal segments and in loops of polypeptide chain that connect the beta-stranded segments. Invariant glycine residues occur in most of the turns. The interior of the domain, between the two sheets, is filled with hydrophobic amino acid side chains. The conserved intradomain disulfide bridge is approximately perpendicular to the sheets and connects the middle segment of the three-chain layer with one of the middle segments of the four-chain layer. Variable domains have an additional loop that has no equivalent in the constant domain. Variable and constant domains also differ in the length, shape, and chemical nature of the extended segments and bends. The FRAMEWORK REGIONS of variable domains are located in the beta-pleated sheets and the hypervariable regions are in the connecting loops.

immunoglobulin gamma (γ) chain. Heavy chain of IgG (M_r ~51,000; ~450 amino acid residues). In addition to a variable region (V_H domain) gamma chains have a CONSTANT REGION composed of three domains (C_H1, C_H2, and C_H3) and a HINGE REGION between C_H1 and C_H2. In humans, there are four isotypes of gamma chain (gamma1, gamma2, gamma3 and gamma4), corresponding to the four subclasses (*see* IMMU-NOGLOBULIN SUBCLASS), IgG1, IgG2, IgG3 and IgG4. These differ mainly in the length and sequence of the hinge region and in the number and location of interchain disulfide bridges. Excluding the hinge regions, human gamma chains are approximately 95 percent identical in amino acid sequence. The hinge region of the human gamma$_3$ chain is relatively long (62 amino acid residues) and it is encoded by four exons. The hinge regions of the other human gamma chains are 12 or 15 amino acid residues long and are encoded by a single exon. Each of the C$_H$ domains is encoded by a single exon. All of the cysteine residues that form disulfide bridges between heavy chains in human IgG are located in the hinge region; the number of such residues is two (IgG1, IgG4), four (IgG2) and 11 (IgG3). The hinge region is particularly susceptible to digestion with proteolytic enzymes (e.g. papain, pepsin) and cleavage in or near this region produces the Fab, F(ab')$_2$ and Fc FRAGMENTS. In all four isotypes, the gamma chain contains a single complex N-LINKED OLIGOSACCHARIDE in C$_H$2.

There are also four isotypes of gamma chain in mice: gamma1, gamma2a, gamma2b and gamma3. There is less resemblance in amino acid sequence among the mouse gamma chains than there is among the human gamma chains. In the rabbit, only one isotype of gamma chain has been identified. The carboxy-terminal residue in all gamma chains whose amino acid sequences have been determined is glycine; however, an additional lysine is encoded in the DNA (i.e., before the termination codon). Presumably, the terminal lysine is removed, after translation, perhaps by the activity of a carboxypeptidase.

The carboxy-terminal segment of the membrane form of each gamma chain is encoded by two exons (*see* IMMUNOGLOBULIN MU CHAIN and MEMBRANE IMMUNOGLOBULIN). *See* Fcγ RECEPTOR.

immunoglobulin gene rearrangement. Translocation of IMMUNOGLOBULIN GENES during the differentiation of B LYMPHOCYTES. There are two types of rearrangement. One type occurs in pre-B cells or unstimulated B lymphocytes and involves gene segments encoding portions of the VARIABLE REGIONS of IMMUNOGLOBULIN HEAVY and IMMUNOGLOBULIN LIGHT CHAINS; these segments, which

are separated in the germ line, become contiguous as a result of the rearrangement. After B cells are activated, a second type of rearrangement, involving only heavy chain genes, occurs.

The gene segments encoding the heavy chain variable region are the first to be rearranged. The initial event, which (in mice) usually occurs in both chromosomes, is the translocation of a *D* GENE SEGMENT to a *J* GENE SEGMENT, with deletion of intervening DNA. Next, on only one of the chromosomes, a *V* GENE SEGMENT is juxtaposed to the *D–J* segment. This step brings a PROMOTER, located 5' to the V$_H$, under the influence of a transcriptional ENHANCER, located in the INTRON between the J$_H$ and C$_\mu$ gene segments. If the rearrangement is nonproductive, a V$_H$ on the second chromosome is translocated. These events are followed by one or more rearrangements of light chain variable region gene segments, in each of which a *V* gene segment is juxtaposed to a *J* gene segment. Rearrangement of kappa gene segments occurs first. Only if V$_\kappa$ to J$_\kappa$ rearrangements on both chromosomes are not productive does a V$_\lambda$ to J$_\lambda$ rearrangement take place. In addition, it has recently been demonstrated that secondary rearrangements of V$_H$ segments can occur such that a rearranged V$_H$ segment is replaced by a germ line V$_H$ segment. It has been suggested that this replacement is mediated by a highly conserved sequence of seven nucleotides, similar to the consensus heptamer (see below), and located near the 3' end of V$_H$.

The joining or these variable gene segments (*V*, *D* and *J*) is not precise; the exact position of the crossover point between recombining segments can vary by a few base pairs, resulting in codon changes at the joints (i.e., JUNCTIONAL DIVERSITY). In addition, a few extra nucleotides may be inserted, by a non-template directed mechanism, at the V$_H$–D$_H$ or D$_H$–J$_H$ junctions (*see* N REGION). Partial rearrangements can also occur, e.g., D$_H$ to J$_H$, without a subsequent V$_H$ rearrangement; such a partially rearranged gene may give rise to a transcript and a truncated polypeptide containing the mu constant region. Rearrangements of immunoglobulin heavy chain gene segments have also been described in some T LYMPHOCYTES.

Specific sequences appear to act as joining signals for recombination of immunoglobulin gene segments. The 3' side of *V* gene

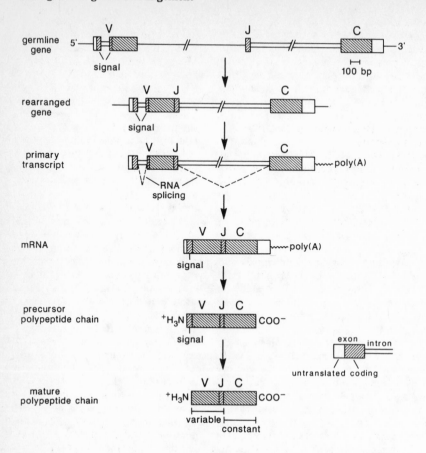

Rearrangement of Immunoglobulin λ Gene Segments

segments, 5′ side of *J* gene segments and both sides of *D* gene segments are flanked by recognition signals for DNA rearrangements. These signals consist of three components: a highly conserved palindromic heptamer (*see* PALINDROME), a somewhat less conserved A/T-rich nonamer and, between these, a non-conserved spacer sequence consisting of either 12 ± 1 base pairs (corresponding to approximately one turn of a DNA helix) or of 23 ± 1 base pairs (corresponding approximately to two turns of a DNA helix). According to the so-called 12/23-base pair spacer rule, recombination only occurs between gene segments one of which has a 12-base pair spacer and the other a 23-base pair spacer. The heptamer and nonamer sequences could form inverted stem-loop structures that juxtapose the two recombining sequences, perhaps allowing a recombin-

ase to effect the joining. Similar specific sequences, which also presumably act as joining signals, have been observed in the DNA flanking the gene segments that contribute to the variable regions of the T CELL RECEPTOR chains.

The second type of rearrangement appears to be responsible for the phenomenon of CLASS SWITCHING. A rearranged V_H–D_H–J_H gene segment, which is originally located 5′ to one C_H gene (e.g., C_μ), is translocated, as a result of one or more recombination events mediated by SWITCH REGIONS, to the region 5′ of another C_H gene (e.g., $C_{\gamma 1}$ or $C_{\alpha 1}$). This results in a change in the type of immunoglobulin produced (e.g., synthesis of IgM is replaced by synthesis of IgG1 or IgA1).

immunoglobulin genes. Genes that encode the VARIABLE REGIONS and the CONSTANT

REGIONS of IMMUNOGLOBULIN HEAVY CHAINS and IMMUNOGLOBULIN LIGHT CHAINS. The genes for heavy, kappa and lambda chains are on separate chromosomes. The chromosomal map locations of the human and mouse immunoglobulin genes are shown in the table. Immunoglobulin genes exist in two configurations, germ line and rearranged (*see* IMMUNOGLOBULIN GENE REARRANGEMENT).

In the germ line, the DNA encoding an immunoglobulin polypeptide chain is found on distinct segments of DNA that are rearranged before the gene encoding the complete polypeptide chain is expressed. Each variable region is encoded by two or three gene segments that are brought together by the rearrangement. In the case of kappa and lambda light chains, there are two segments, V and J. (1) The V GENE SEGMENT itself contains two coding regions: at the 5' end, a region (an EXON) encodes most of the SIGNAL SEQUENCE and also the 5' untranslated region of the mRNA; at the 3' end, a region (which, after rearrangement forms part of an exon) encodes the carboxy-terminal four residues of the signal sequence and the first 97 or 98 residues of the variable region. (2) The J GENE SEGMENT (also forming part of an exon after rearrangement) encodes the carboxy-terminal 12 or 13 residues of the variable region, a stretch that includes one or two residues of the third HYPERVARIABLE REGION and the fourth FRAMEWORK REGION. As a consequence of the rearrangement, the V gene segment and the J gene segment become contiguous. The resulting variable region gene contains two exons, separated by an intron usually 100–200 base pairs in length. One exon encodes most of the signal sequence and the other encodes the rest of the signal sequence and the complete variable region of the mature light chain.

The variable region of a heavy chain is encoded by three gene segments, V, D and J. (1) The V gene segment again contains two coding regions, one for most of the signal sequence and the other for the last four residues of the signal sequence and the first 98–100 residues of the variable region. (2) The D GENE SEGMENT, an additional gene segment not found in light chain genes, encodes part of the third hypervariable region. (3) The J gene segment encodes the remainder of the third hypervariable region and the fourth framework region (the J

region of a heavy chain variable region is slightly longer than the J region of a light chain variable region). Additional nucleotides may be inserted, by a non-template-directed mechanism, on either side of the D gene segment in the rearranged gene (*see* N REGION). After the rearrangement has been completed, the three gene segments are contiguous and the resulting variable region gene again contains two exons separated by an intron of about 100 base pairs. One exon encodes most of the signal sequence and the other encodes the complete heavy chain variable region.

The constant region of each immunoglobulin chain is encoded by a C GENE SEGMENT, which contains one or more exons and which is located downstream (at least 1.3 kilobases) from one or more J gene segments. The C segments retain their fixed distances from the J gene segments during the immunoglobulin gene rearrangements. The constant region of a light (kappa or lambda) chain is encoded by a single exon, C_κ or C_λ. The constant region of the heavy chain of a secreted immunoglobulin is encoded by three to seven exons. There is one exon for each domain and one to four exons for the HINGE REGION (except for the hinge region of the IMMUNOGLOBULIN ALPHA CHAIN, which is encoded at the 5' end of the C_H2 exon). The carboxy-terminal segment or 'tail-piece' of the heavy chain of a secreted immunoglobulin is encoded at the 3' end of the last C_H exon (except in the case of the IMMUNOGLOBULIN DELTA CHAIN which has a separate exon for the 'tail-piece'). Most of the constant regions of membrane immunoglobulins are encoded by the same exons as encode the secreted immunoglobulin of the same isotype except for differences at the 3' ends of the genes (carboxy-terminal regions of the chains) (*see* MEMBRANE IMMUNOGLOBULIN, IMMUNOGLOBULIN MU CHAIN). The carboxy-terminal segments (~40–70 amino acid residues) of the membrane forms are encoded by one or two additional exons, which are at least 1.4 kilobases 3' to the last exon for the secreted form of the heavy chain. In every case, the 3'-most exon also specifies a 3'-untranslated region in the mRNA.

The number and detailed organization of gene segments encoding the immunoglobulin chains differs for kappa, lambda and heavy chains. In mice, there are probably several hundred V_κ, separated by an average distance estimated to be 10–12 kilobases, and located 5' to a strip of five J_κ, four of which are functional. In humans, there appear to be fewer (probably about 80) V_κ genes and there are five J_κ; the distance from the most 3' V_κ gene segment to the J_κ is 23 kilobases. In both species, the J_κ are separated by approximately 300 base pairs and a single C_κ lies about 2.5 kilobases 3' to the last J_κ segment. It is likely that any V_κ can associate with any J_κ.

In most inbred mice, there are four J_λ and four C_λ, organized into two clusters. The gene segments in each cluster lie within about 5.5 kilobases. One of the clusters, $J_{\lambda 2}C_{\lambda 2}J_{\lambda 4}C_{\lambda 4}$, is approximately 144 kilobases 5' to the other cluster, $J_{\lambda 3}C_{\lambda 3}J_{\lambda 1}C_{\lambda 1}$. There are three V_λ gene segments: $J_{\lambda 2}$ is about 73 kilobases 5' to the '2–4' cluster and $V_{\lambda 1}$ is 19 kilobases 5' to the '3–1' cluster. A third V_λ, designated $V_{\lambda x}$, has recently been localized about 19 kilobases 3' to $V_{\lambda 2}$. Association of the V_λ with the J_λ appears to be restricted. $V_{\lambda 1}$ rearranges to $J_{\lambda 3}$ or $J_{\lambda 1}$ (resulting in a $V_{\lambda 1} J_{\lambda 3}$ $C_{\lambda 3}$ or $V_{\lambda 1} J_{\lambda 1} C_{\lambda 1}$ gene), whereas $V_{\lambda 2}$ preferentially rearranges to $J_{\lambda 2}$ (resulting in a $V_{\lambda 2}$ $J_{\lambda 2} C_{\lambda 2}$ gene). $J_{\lambda 4}$ is not used, probably because of a defect in the signal for RNA SPLICING. Occasionally, $V_{\lambda 2}$ rearranges to $J_{\lambda 3}$ (resulting in a $V_{\lambda 2} J_{\lambda 3} C_{\lambda 3}$ gene) or to $J_{\lambda 1}$ (resulting in a $V_{\lambda 2} J_{\lambda 1} C_{\lambda 1}$ gene), but a rearrangement of $V_{\lambda 1}$ to $J_{\lambda 2}$ has never been observed. To date, $V_{\lambda x}$ has been found to rearrange only to $J_{\lambda 2}$. In humans, less information is available about lambda genes, although there are also multiple (at least six) C_λ genes, each associated with its own J segment.

In the case of heavy chain genes of mice, the total number of V_H segments has variously been estimated to be 100–200 or at least one thousand. These V_H segments have been divided into a number of families on the basis of similarity in nucleic acid sequence; the members of a family are typically >80 percent identical in sequence. Nine families have been identified to date; one of these is very large (perhaps > 1000). The V_H are thought to be 5' to the D_H segments, but the distance (in mice) is not known. There are four functional J_H segments about seven kilobases 5' to the $C\mu$ gene. One D_H segment is located 696 base pairs 5' to the first J_H gene and 11 other D_H segments lie from 20 to 80 kilobases 5' to the J_H segments. In humans, the total number of V_H is thought to be 100

to 200, and there appear to be at least six families spread over 2,000–3,000 kilobases. In contrast to the V_H of mice, the V_H of different human families are highly interspersed. Six functional J_H and five D_H have been identified. Four of the D_H have been closely linked to the J_H and at least one is interspersed among the V_H. The distance from the human J_H to the nearest V_H is less than 100 kilobases.

The C gene segments encoding the different heavy chains are linked. In the mouse, the C_H are distributed over nearly 200 kilobases and are found in the following order: C_μ–C_δ–$C_{\gamma 3}$–$C_{\gamma 1}$–$C_{\gamma 2b}$–$C_{\gamma 2a}$–C_ϵ–C_α. The order of the human C_H appears to be: C_μ–C_δ–$C_{\gamma 3}$–$C_{\gamma 1}$–pseudo $C_{\epsilon 1}$–$C_{\alpha 1}$–pseudoC_γ–$C_{\gamma 2}$–$C_{\gamma 4}$–C_ϵ–$C_{\alpha 2}$. In a clone of antibody-forming cells, a particular heavy-chain variable region (encoded by a V–D–J exon) may be associated with more than one heavy-chain constant region as the result of the formation of long RNA transcripts (including more than one C_H segment) and/or translocation of the V–D–J exon from the region 5' to one C_H to the region 5' to another C_H (see CLASS SWITCHING, SWITCH REGION).

The enormous range of antibody specificities is generated by the efficient utilization of different gene segments encoding antibody variable regions. The diversification appears to result from: (1) the presence in the germ line of a variety of V, D and J gene segments; (2) combinatorial joining (i.e., the assortment of different V, D and J gene segments in variable region exons); (3) JUNCTIONAL DIVERSITY resulting from imprecision in the joining of the V, D and J segments; (4) SOMATIC MUTATION generating base substitutions in the gene segments encoding the variable region, which may lead to amino acid replacements; (5) N region diversity resulting from the insertion of N nucleotides at the junctions of V_H and D_H or D_H and J_H segments; (6) the combination of different heavy chain and light chain variable regions to form intact ANTIBODY COMBINING SITES; (7) V_H gene replacement; the substitution of a germ line V_H for an already-rearranged V_H segment. Gene conversion may also contribute to variable region diversity, as recently demonstrated for chicken light chains. See IMMUNOGLOBULIN GENE REARRANGEMENT, T CELL RECEPTOR GENES.

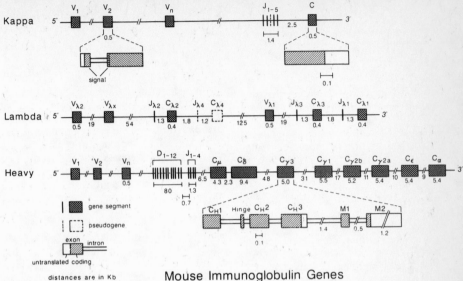

Mouse Immunoglobulin Genes

immunoglobulin genes

Chromosome map locations of immunoglobulin genes

Gene	Human	Mouse
κ	2p11	6
λ	22q11	16
H	14q32.3	12

immunoglobulin heavy chain. Larger of the two types of polypeptide chain usually found in IMMUNOGLOBULIN molecules (the smaller is the IMMUNOGLOBULIN LIGHT CHAIN). Each heavy chain (M_r ~51,000–72,000) consists of one variable domain (*see* VARIABLE REGION), usually three or four constant domains, a carboxy-terminal segment and, in some chains, a HINGE REGION (*see* CONSTANT REGION). There are several varieties of heavy chain and these define the different IMMUNOGLOBULIN CLASSES (i.e., gamma chain in IgG, mu chain in IgM, alpha chain in IgA, delta chain in IgD, epsilon chain in IgE) as well as the IMMUNOGLOBULIN SUBCLASSES (gamma1 chain in IgG1, gamma2 chain in IgG2, etc.). The constant regions of heavy chains of the different human immunoglobulin classes are about 30 percent identical in amino acid sequence. *See* IMMUNOGLOBULIN ALPHA CHAIN, IMMUNOGLOBULIN DELTA CHAIN, IMMUNOGLOBULIN EPSILON CHAIN, IMMUNOGLOBULIN GAMMA CHAIN, IMMUNOGLOBULIN MU CHAIN.

immunoglobulin heavy chain binding protein (BiP). Protein (M_r 77,000) found in the lumen of the ENDOPLASMIC RETICULUM of many cells. BiP binds transiently to some nascent secretory and membrane proteins and may be involved in their transport through the endoplasmic reticulum. BiP was discovered by virtue of its association with IMMUNOGLOBULIN HEAVY CHAINS in MYELOMAS.

immunoglobulin kappa (κ) chain. One of the two major types of IMMUNOGLOBULIN LIGHT CHAIN, the other being lambda (*see* IMMUNOGLOBULIN LAMBDA CHAIN). Each kappa chain (M_r ~23,000; ~214 amino acid residues) consists of one variable domain (*see* VARIABLE REGION) and one constant domain (*see* CONSTANT REGION). The proportion of light chains that are kappa varies among species. In humans, about two-thirds of light chains are kappa; in mice, about 95 percent are kappa. In certain other species (e.g., horse, cow, dog) almost none of the light chains are kappa. In humans and in mice there is only one kappa constant region, the product of a single *C* gene segment. In humans, there are three allotypes of kappa chain, designated Km1; Km1,2; and Km3. *See* Km ALLOTYPIC DETERMINANT.

immunoglobulin lambda (λ) chain. One of the two type of IMMUNOGLOBULIN LIGHT

Chain			*Residue at positions*		
	112	114	152	163	190
Kern⁻Oz⁺	Ala	Ser	Ser	Thr	Arg
Kern⁻Oz⁺	Ala	Ser	Ser	Thr	Lys
Kern⁺Oz⁻	Ala	Ser	Gly	Thr	Arg
Mcg	Asn	Thr	Gly	Lys	Arg

chain, the other being kappa (*see* IMMU-NOGLOBULIN KAPPA CHAIN). Each lambda chain (M_r ~23,000; ~214 amino acid residues) consists of one variable domain (*see* VARIABLE REGION) and one constant domain (*see* CONSTANT REGION). The proportion of light chains that are lambda varies among species. In humans, about one-third of light chains are lambda; in mice only about 5 percent are lambda. In certain other species (e.g., horse, cow, dog), virtually all of the light chains are lambda. In humans and in mice, there are several ISOTYPES of lambda chains, defined by their distinct constant regions. The amino acid residues that differ in four isotypes of human lambda chain are shown in the table above. Each of these constant regions is the product of a different *C* gene segment. *See* KERN ISOTYPIC DETERMINANT, Mcg ISOTYPIC DETERMINANT, Oz ISOTYPIC DETERMINANT.

immunoglobulin light chain. Smaller of the two types of polypeptide chain usually found in IMMUNOGLOBULIN molecules (the other is the IMMUNOGLOBULIN HEAVY CHAIN). Each light chain (M_r ~23,000; ~214 amino acid residues) consists of one variable domain (*see* VARIABLE REGION) and one constant domain (*see* CONSTANT REGION). There are two major types of light chain: kappa and lambda. The constant regions of kappa and lambda chains in a species (e.g., human, mouse) are about 38 percent identical in amino acid sequence. *See* IMMUNOGLOBULIN KAPPA CHAIN, IMMUNOGLOBULIN LAMBDA CHAIN.

immunoglobulin mu (μ) chain. Heavy chain of IgM (M_r ~72,000; ~570 amino acid residues). In addition to a variable region (V_H domain), mu chains have a CONSTANT REGION consisting of four domains (C_H1, C_H2, C_H and C_H4); there is no HINGE REGION. At the carboxy-terminal end of the mu chain, there is an 'extra' segment (often called 'tail piece') of 18 amino acid residues that, by homology, is not part of a domain, but that is encoded in the same exon as the C_H4 domain. This can be shown by aligning

the terminal segments of the gamma and mu chains; if one assumes that the carboxy-terminal residue of the gamma chain is lysine, there are 18 additional residues in the mu chain. (Lysine is encoded in the DNA, just before a termination codon, although it does not appear to be present in mature gamma chains (*see* IMMUNOGLOBULIN GAMMA CHAIN).) This carboxy-terminal segment of the mu chain contains, at its penultimate position, the cysteine residue that forms a disulfide bridge with J CHAIN. In those mu chains that are not directly linked to J chain, this cysteine presumably forms a disulfide bridge to another mu chain, in the same or in a different subunit (a 'subunit' of IgM is the basic four-chain unit: two mu chains and two light chains). A cysteine residue near the carboxy-terminal end of C_H2 probably forms a bridge to another heavy chain in the same subunit and a cysteine in C_H3 probably forms a bridge to another subunit. The human mu chain contains five N-LINKED OLIGOSACCHARIDES, one in C_H1, another in C_H2, two in C_H3 and one in the carboxy-terminal "tail piece". Three of these oligosaccharides are the complex type and the other two are high-mannose oligosaccharides.

The mu chain of membrane IgM (μ_m) is identical to that of secreted IgM (μ_s) except near the carboxy-terminal end of the chain. The last 20 residues of the secreted mu chain are missing and are replaced by a segment of 41 different residues, encoded by two 'membrane exons' (39 residues are encoded by one exon and the carboxy-terminal two residues by another exon). This carboxy-terminal section of μ_m includes a hydrophobic segment of 26 residues, presumably the transmembrane portion of the molecule. *See* IMMUNOGLOBULIN GENES, MEMBRANE IMMUNOGLOBULIN.

immunoglobulin subclass. Subset of IMMUNOGLOBULIN CLASS. The heavy chain CONSTANT REGIONS of immunoglobulins within a subclass are identical (except for possible differences in ALLOTYPY). Each immunoglobulin subclass (e.g., human IgG1) – and the constant region of its heavy chain – is an ISOTYPE and is present in all members of a particular species. Subclasses can differ in function (e.g., COMPLEMENT FIXATION, membrane binding). In humans, there are four subclasses of IgG; IgG1, IgG2, IgG3, IgG4, in order of decreasing concentration in serum; there are also two subclasses of IgA: IgA1 and IgA2.

The distinction between immunoglobulin classes and immunoglobulin subclasses was originally based on the degree of antigenic resemblance. A subclass of a single immunoglobulin class usually cross-reacts with antisera to another subclass that have been raised in another species and that have been rendered specific for heavy chains by absorption with light chains. However, different immunoglobulin classes are generally not cross-reactive. It is now also possible to classify immunoglobulins into classes and subclasses according to the degree of similarity in amino acid sequence of their heavy chains. The heavy chain constant regions of immunoglobulins in different subclasses within one immunoglobulin class have considerably greater similarity in sequence than those of different classes. Thus, in the four human IgG subclasses, the heavy chains are approximately 95 per cent identical in sequence (neglecting the HINGE REGION) (*see* IMMUNOGLOBULIN GAMMA CHAIN). In contrast, the constant regions of heavy chains of different immunoglobulin classes are only about 30 percent identical.

immunoglobulin superfamily. Family of proteins containing one or more DOMAINS that resemble an IMMUNOGLOBULIN DOMAIN. These domains resemble VARIABLE (V) REGIONS or domains of CONSTANT (C) REGIONS by virtue of their size, amino acid sequence, and presumably, three-dimensional structure (*see* IMMUNOGLOBULIN FOLD). A member of the superfamily may contain both V region-like and C region-like domains. Almost always the domains contain a disulfide bridge, which spans 65–75 amino acid residues in the case of variable-like domains or 55–60 amino acid residues in the case of constant-like domains.

Members of the immunoglobulin superfamily typically mediate non-enzymatic intercellular surface recognition. Molecules of immunological relevance containing only

C-related domain(s) are: CD1, CD2, CD3, CLASS I and CLASS II HISTOCOMPATIBILITY MOLECULES, BETA-2 MICROGLOBULIN, LYMPHOCYTE FUNCTION ASSOCIATED ANTIGEN-3 (LFA-3) and FcγRIII (*see* Fcγ RECEPTOR). Those containing only a V-related domain are: CD7, CD8, Thy-1 and Tp44 (CD28). The T CELL RECEPTOR has one V-related and one C-related domain in each polypeptide chain. CD4 has two V-related and one C-related domain. The POLYIMMUNOGLOBULIN RECEPTOR has four V-related and one C-related domain. In addition to these proteins, other molecules, mostly found in the nervous system, belong to the immunoglobulin superfamily: neuronal cell adhesion molecule (NCAM), myelin associated glycoprotein (MAG), P_o myelin protein, CARCINOEMBRYONIC ANTIGEN (CEA), platelet-derived growth factor receptor (PDGFR), COLONY STIMULATING FACTOR-1 receptor and link protein of basement membrane. A single serum protein (other than immunoglobulins), $\alpha_1\beta$-glycoprotein, is a member of the immunoglobulin superfamily. It is composed of five C-related domains; its function is unknown.

Most members of the immunoglobulin superfamily form HOMODIMERS or HETERODIMERS on cell membranes. There is great diversity in the transmembrane segments and cytoplasmic regions among these molecules; the cytoplasmic regions vary from 3 to 543 amino acid residues. LFA-3 and Thy-1 have phosphoglycolipid anchors in the membrane.

The genes encoding members of the immunoglobulin superfamily are scattered throughout the GENOME, excluding the sex chromosomes. However, some genes encoding molecules in the superfamily are linked. The class I and class II MHC molecules map to chromosome 6p21.3 in humans and chromosome 17 in the mouse. The genes encoding CD8 are linked to those encoding IMMUNOGLOBULIN KAPPA CHAINS in humans and mice, and map to chromosome 2p12 in humans; the genes encoding CD3 polypeptide chains are linked to the gene encoding Thy-1 and map to chromosome 11q23 in humans (NCAM also maps to 11q23). It is thought that members of the immunoglobulin superfamily evolved by gene duplication.

immunoincompetent. Incapable of mounting a normal IMMUNE RESPONSE. For example, neonatal mice or thymectomized mice are immunoincompetent; individuals with IMMUNODEFICIENCY disease are immunoincompetent. The lack of immunological competence may result from failure of B and/or T LYMPHOCYTE function.

immunologically competent cell. Cell capable of specific recognition or specific response to an antigen. The term is usually used to refer to T or B LYMPHOCYTE.

immunopotentiation. Enhancement of an IMMUNE RESPONSE by a variety of ADJUVANTS such as synthetic polynucleotides, drugs, bacterial products (e.g., LIPOPOLYSACCHARIDES, MURAMYL DIPETIDE), LYMPHOKINES and MONOKINES .

immunoprophylaxis. Prevention of disease by active or passive IMMUNIZATION.

immunosuppression. Inhibition of an IMMUNE RESPONSE by antigen, specific antibody, cytotoxic drugs, irradiation or infection of lymphoid tissue (e.g., leprosy, AIDS).

immunotherapy. *See* IMMUNOPOTENTIATION, IMMUNOSUPPRESSION.

immunotoxin. Antibody coupled to a TOXIN. Immunotoxins combine the fine specificity for antigen of the antibody molecule with the cytotoxic property of the toxin (e.g., RICIN). They can be used to target toxins to cells that bear the specific antigen. Immunotoxins are used in bone marrow transplantation to eliminate T LYMPHOCYTES from bone marrow cells to avoid GRAFT-*VERSUS*-HOST DISEASE.

in situ hybridization. Method for detecting DNA or RNA species in specific cellular locations (e.g., in cytological preparations or tissue sections), or in bacterial colonies or viral plaques. DNA segments (e.g., chromosomal DNA) must be denatured before reacting them with radiolabeled RNA or DNA probes. Cellular RNA sequences do not require denaturation. The binding sites are visualized after AUTORADIOGRAPHY. Enzyme- and fluorescent-labeled probes can also be used.

inactivated vaccine. Vaccine composed of microorganisms that have been killed by treatment with heat or chemicals (e.g., formaldehyde for influenza vaccine). *See* ATTENUATED VACCINE.

inbred strain. Population of animals that results from prolonged INBREEDING. Ideally, an inbred population is genetically identical (isogenic), but this is not possible to achieve in practice. Mice that result from 20 or more generations of brother–sister mating are considered inbred. Such mice are homozygous at most (usually at least 98 percent) of their genetic loci. Since every population harbors some deleterious genes, which are usually recessive, inbreeding allows these genes, as they become homozygous, to exert their deleterious effects. This 'inbreeding depression' may affect size, growth rate, disease susceptibility, fertility, etc. Consequently, many inbred lines do not survive beyond a certain number of generations of inbreeding. Inbred strains of mice, rats, guinea-pigs, hamsters, rabbits and chickens have been produced in the laboratory. *See* COISOGENIC STRAINS, CONGENIC STRAINS, RECOMBINANT INBRED STRAIN.

inbreeding. Mating of individuals more closely related to each other than individuals chosen at random from a population. A consequence of inbreeding is that individuals become more HOMOZYGOUS. In mice, inbreeding is usually carried out by brother–sister mating. A line that has undergone 20 or more generations of such mating is considered inbred. *See* OUTBREEDING, RANDOM BREEDING.

incomplete Freund's adjuvant. Water-in-oil emulsion used as vehicle for antigen administration. It is complete FREUND'S ADJUVANT without Mycobacteria.

index of variability. *See* WU–KABAT PLOT.

indomethacin

indomethacin (1-(4-chlorobenzylyl)-5-methoxy-2-methyl-1H-indole-3-acetic acid). Drug used for the treatment of RHEUMATOID ARTHRITIS and ANKYLOSING SPONDYLITIS. It is a potent inhibitor of PROSTAGLANDIN synthesis.

inducer T lymphocyte. T LYMPHOCYTE that recognizes conventional antigens associated with CLASS II HISTOCOMPATIBILITY MOLECULES and activates HELPER T LYMPHOCYTES, SUPPRESSOR T LYMPHOCYTES and CYTOTOXIC T LYMPHOCYTES. In contrast, helper T lymphocytes activate B LYMPHOCYTES. The mechanism of this induction of activation is not understood. In humans, inducer T lymphocytes bear a surface protein, called 2H4, a variant of the LEUKOCYTE COMMON ANTIGEN. CD4 helper T lymphocytes bear a surface molecule called 4B4. All CD4+T lymphocytes are either 4B4+ or 2H4+. The relationship between inducer and helper T lymphocytes is not known; they could be the same cell at different stages of activation. In mice, putative inducer T lymphocytes cannot be distinguished from helper T lymphocytes.

infantile agammaglobulinemia. *Synonym for* X-LINKED AGAMMAGLOBULINEMIA.

infectious mononucleosis. Acute illness of adolescents and young adults, characterized by fever, malaise, sore throat and swollen LYMPH NODES. The disease is caused by infection with the EPSTEIN–BARR VIRUS (EBV). During the acute illness, patients have NEUTROPENIA, THROMBOCYTOPENIA and LYMPHOCYTOSIS. Atypical LYMPHOCYTES, characterized by a high cytoplasm-to-nucleus ratio and cytoplasmic vacuolization, are found in the blood. These atypical cells have characteristic surface markers of T LYMPHOCYTES and are thought to be responding to EBV-infected B LYMPHOCYTES. During the recovery phase, patients develop HETEROPHILE ANTIBODIES and SUPPRESSOR T LYMPHOCYTES become transiently activated.

inflammation. Cellular and vascular changes that follow tissue injury. Inflammation is characterized by four cardinal features: calor (heat), dolor (pain), rubor (redness) and tumor (swelling). Acute inflammation takes place in minutes or hours after injury. Blood vessels become more permeable, so that blood cells and proteins leak to the extravascular space. Persistence of injury results in chronic INFLAMMATION WITH THE APPEARANCE OF LYMPHOCYTES AND MACROPHAGES FTER TISSUE INJURY THERE MAY BE REPAIR OF CONNECTIVE TISSUES WITH RESULTANT SCARRING

inflammatory bowel disease. Group of diseases of the gastrointestinal tract, of unknown cause, including ulcerative colitis and regional enteritis (Crohn's disease). These diseases are characterized by fever, abdominal pain, diarrhea and weight loss. The inflamed areas of bowel contain GRANULOMAS and are infiltrated with numerous IgA-containing LYMPHOID cells. AUTOANTIBODIES to human fetal colonic antigens can be demonstrated in serum by IMMUNOFLUORESCENCE. Normal cultured colonic epithelial cells are lysed by T LYMPHOCYTES from patients. It is not clear whether antibodies and/or T lymphocytes are involved in the pathogenesis of inflammatory bowel disease.

inflammatory macrophage. MACROPHAGE from exudates induced by non-immunological means (e.g., intraperitoneal injection of proteose–peptone broth, thioglycolate broth or mineral oil).

inoculation. Injection of an antigen to induce IMMUNITY (e.g., VACCINATION). Introduction of microorganisms into a culture medium or into the tissues of plants or animals.

instructive theory. Theory that the specificity of an antibody molecule is acquired after it encounters antigen. In one such theory, it was proposed that a non-specific progenitor antibody molecule acquires specificity by folding around an antigen, which serves as a template. This theory became untenable when it was shown that the specificity of an antibody molecule was recovered after denaturation when it was allowed to refold in the absence of the antigen. It is now known that antibody specificity is a direct consequence of the amino acid sequence of the VARIABLE REGIONS, especially of those parts of the variable region known as the COMPLEMENTARITY-DETERMINING or HYPERVARIABLE REGIONS. Additional evidence against instructive theories was the failure to find antigen in antibody-synthesizing cells (i.e., PLASMA CELLS). Instructive theories also did not explain differences between the PRIMARY

RESPONSE and SECONDARY RESPONSE to immunization. In addition, present understanding of protein synthesis and structure is not compatible with instructive theories. Instead, the CLONAL SELECTION THEORY is now believed to account for the generation of antibodies of diverse specificity.

insulin-dependent diabetes mellitus (IDDM). Heritable form of diabetes that has its onset in childhood and requires treatment with insulin. Patients with IDDM have a high incidence of HLA-DR3 (see HLA) and HLA-DR4. The EXTENDED HAPLOTYPES HLA-B8, HLA-DR3, COMPLOTYPE SCO1; HLA-B18, HLA-DR3, complotype F1C30; HLA-B26, HLA-DR4, complotype SC33; and HLA-B38, HLA-DR4, complotype SC21 have a high incidence in Caucasians with IDDM. The serum of patients may contain antibodies to cytoplasmic and membrane antigens of the islets of Langerhans of the pancreas. The islets selectively lose beta cells (insulin-producing cells) and may be infiltrated with T LYMPHOCYTES and MONOCYTES in the early phase of the disease. IDDM is also called juvenile-onset diabetes or diabetes mellitus, type 1. See B/B RAT, NOD MICE.

integrin family. Group of glycoproteins on cell membranes that act as receptors for extracellular matrix glycoproteins (e.g., FIBRONECTIN), blood proteins (e.g., C3) and other cell surface glycoproteins (e.g., LYMPHOCYTE FUNCTION ASSOCIATED ANTIGEN-3). The LIGAND for integrins is a sequence of three amino acid residues, Arg–Gly–Asp, found in proteins to which integrins bind. All integrins are HETERODIMERS.

The integrin family can be divided into three groups of proteins according to the identity of their beta chains; in each group the alpha chains are distinct. One group, LYMPHOCYTE FUNCTION ASSOCIATED ANTIGEN-1 (LFA-1), COMPLEMENT RECEPTOR 3 (CR3) and p150,95 share a common beta chain of M_r 95,000. The second group, VLA-1, VLA-2, VLA-3, VLA-4, VLA-5 (see VLA) and the chicken integrin complex share a common beta chain of M_r 130,000. The third group, the vitronectin (see S PROTEIN) receptor and glycoprotein IIb/IIIa of PLATELETS share a common beta chain of M_r 110,000.

The integrin beta chains are non-covalently linked to the alpha chains. The extracellular domains of the beta chains contain four repeats of 40 amino acid residues, which are cysteine-rich and presumably contain the binding site for the Arg–Gly–Asp sequence. The intracellular domains of the beta chains contain approximately 45 residues. The three beta chains have approximately 45 percent amino acid sequence identity. There is not sufficient amino acid sequence information to compare the structure of the alpha chains.

Integrins serve in general as transmembrane links between extracellular ligands and the CYTOSKELETON. Integrins are presumed to facilitate cell migration in embryos, wound healing, PHAGOCYTOSIS and TARGET CELL KILLING.

intercellular adhesion molecule-1 (ICAM-1). Membrane glycoprotein (M_r 90,000) of endothelial cells, dendritic cells and many other types of cells that is the ligand for LYMPHOCYTE FUNCTION ASSOCIATED ANTIGEN-1 (LFA-1). ICAM-1 is found on cells that serve as targets for CYTOTOXIC T LYMPHOCYTES, which bear LFA-1. Increased expression of ICAM-1 can be induced by TUMOR NECROSIS FACTOR, INTERLEUKIN-1, and INTERFERON-GAMMA.

interfacial test. *Synonym for* RING TEST.

interferon (IFN). Group of proteins (see INTERFERON-ALPHA, INTERFERON-BETA, INTERFERON-GAMMA) that induce resistance to viral infection in cells. Interferons do not directly kill viruses, but cause a state of resistance through the induction of host cell enzymes that affect transcription and translation of viral genes. Interferons were initially classified by their stability to heat and pH and with regard to the method of induction. Type I interferon is induced by viruses or polynucleotides and is stable both to heat (56°C) and extremes of pH (pH 2 or pH 11). Type II interferon is induced by immunological reactions or LECTINS and is heat-labile and labile to extremes of pH. Type I interferon is further subdivided into two types, depending on the cell of origin: alpha secreted by leukocytes, and beta by fibroblasts. Type II interferon is also known as interferon-gamma or immune interferon and is secreted by MITOGEN-stimulated T LYMPHOCYTES and NATURAL KILLER CELLS.

interferon-alpha   (IFN-α). INTERFERON secreted mainly by leukocytes. Secretion is induced by RNA or DNA viruses or by

single- or double-stranded polyribonucleo-
tides. Interferon-alpha inhibits virus replication. It has been used in the treatment of
tumors, notably KAPOSI'S SARCOMA in individuals with AIDS.

At least 14 genes encode interferon-alpha.
Products of these genes consist of 189 amino
acid residues including a signal sequence of
23 residues and differ from each other by as
much as 15 percent in amino acid sequences.
The genes for interferon-alpha are on
chromosome 9 in humans and chromosome 4
in mice. *See* INTERFERON-BETA, INTERFERON-
GAMMA.

interferon-beta (IFN β). INTERFERON
secreted mainly by fibroblasts. Secretion is
induced by RNA and DNA viruses or by
single- or double-stranded polyribonucleo-
tides. Interferon-beta inhibits virus replication.

Interferon-beta is encoded by a single
gene, which is linked to the genes for
INTERFERON-ALPHA on chromosome 9 in
humans and chromosome 4 in mice.
Interferon-beta consists of 187 amino acid
residues including a signal sequence of 21
residues and has approximately 30 percent
identity of amino acid sequence with the
different forms of interferon-alpha and none
with INTERFERON-GAMMA.

interferon-gamma (IFN γ). LYMPHOKINE
secreted mainly by activated T lymphocytes
and capable of inducing a wide range of
effects on many cells. Interferon-gamma is
differentiated from INTERFERON-ALPHA and
INTERFERON-BETA by its lability to extremes of
temperature and pH. The major effects of
interferon-gamma are: (1) inhibition of virus
replication in many cells; (2) induction of
expression of CLASS II HISTOCOMPATIBILITY
MOLECULES in endothelial, epithelial and connective tissue cells, allowing these cells to
become active in ANTIGEN PRESENTATION; (3)
activation of MACROPHAGES to heightened
microbicidal and tumoricidal activity and
increased expression of Fcγ RECEPTORS; (4)
inhibition of cell growth; and (5) induction of
differentiation of a number of MYELOID CELL
lines.

Interferon-gamma (M_r 40,000) is a homodimer and is encoded by a single gene that
specifies a polypeptide chain of 166 amino
acid residues, including a signal sequence of
23 residues. It contains two sites for N-
LINKED OLIGOSACCHARIDES. It is encoded by a

single gene that, in humans, is on the long
arm of chromosome 12 and in mice, on
chromosome 10.

interferon-gamma receptor. Receptor found
on all cells, except red blood cells, to which
INTERFERON-GAMMA binds. The association
constant for binding is 2×10^9 M^{-1}. The
receptor is a glycoprotein (M_r 90,000) consisting of a single polypeptide chain. In
humans, the gene encoding the interferon-
gamma receptor has been mapped to
chromosome 6q.

interleukin. CYTOKINE secreted mainly by
mononuclear cells (i.e., lymphocytes and
mononuclear phagocytes) that induces
growth and differentiation of lymphocytes
and pluripotential hematopoietic stem cells.

interleukin-1 (IL-1). MONOKINE that has
many roles in INFLAMMATION and in the
IMMUNE RESPONSE. IL-1 is secreted by MONO-
NUCLEAR PHAGOCYTES following uptake of
ANTIGEN–ANTIBODY COMPLEXES or LIPOPOLY-
SACCHARIDES, or following contact with T
LYMPHOCYTES during ANTIGEN PRESENTATION.
IL-1 may also be synthesized by epidermal
cells, NATURAL KILLER CELLS, B LYMPHOCYTES,
FIBROBLASTS and ENDOTHELIAL CELLS. Secretion of IL-1 is enhanced by INTERFERON-ALPHA
and INTERFERON-GAMMA, PHORBOL ESTERS, calcium ionophores and inhibitors of the cell
cycle that arrest cells in the G1 stage (e.g.,
hydroxyurea). IL-1 secretion can be suppressed by CORTICOSTEROIDS and PROSTAGLAN-
DINS. IL-1 induces the ACUTE PHASE REACTION,
which accompanies inflammation. IL-1
induces secretion of IL-2, which promotes
the growth of T LYMPHOCYTES after antigen
presentation. IL-1 is required for the growth
of THYMOCYTES in the presence of LECTINS.
ENDOGENOUS PYROGEN, a molecule isolated
from plasma following bacterial infection and
responsible for the production of fever, is
identical to IL-1. IL-1 also activates resorption of bone and cartilage. Another monokine, TUMOR NECROSIS FACTOR, has many
biological activities that are indistinguishable
from those of IL-1. IL-1 consists of at least
two distinct proteins, IL-1α and IL-1β. In
mice and humans, both are synthesized as
precursors of about 270 amino acid residues
(M_r 31,000). IL-1 is incorporated into the cell
membrane where it is cleaved by plasmin to
M_r 22,300 and then by elastase to the active
molecule of 159 residues (IL-1α) or 153

residues (IL-1β). There is approximately 25 percent amino acid sequence identity between IL-1α and IL-1β.

interleukin-1 receptor. Receptor for INTERLEUKIN-1 (IL-1) on T LYMPHOCYTES, fibroblasts, osteoblasts, chondrocytes and perhaps other cells. The IL-1 receptor (M_r 80,000) binds IL-1α and IL-1β equally. CD4+ T lymphocytes express more IL-1 receptors than do CD8+ T lymphocytes.

interleukin-1 receptor deficiency. Form of COMBINED IMMUNODEFICIENCY defined by the failure of T lymphocytes to absorb INTERLEUKIN-1 possibly because of the absence of an interleukin-1 receptor. Affected children have OPPORTUNISTIC INFECTIONS. The defect appears to be inherited as an autosomal recessive. After antigenic stimulation, T LYMPHOCYTES of affected children do not have a mitotic response and do not produce INTERLEUKIN-2; they have only a weak mitotic response to LECTINS.

interleukin-2 (IL-2). LYMPHOKINE (M_r 15,500) that promotes the growth of T LYMPHOCYTES (and was therefore initially called T cell growth factor). IL-2 is secreted mainly by HELPER T LYMPHOCYTES 4–12 hours following stimulation by INTERLEUKIN-1 and binding of antigen to the T CELL RECEPTOR. Binding of IL-2 to a receptor (see INTERLEUKIN-2 RECEPTOR) on T lymphocytes results in proliferation of these cells, enhanced secretion of lymphokines, heightened expression of membrane receptors for other growth factors (e.g., TRANSFERRIN RECEPTOR, insulin receptor) and CLASS II HISTOCOMPATIBILITY MOLECULES. Almost all T LYMPHOCYTE CLONES are dependent on IL-2 for growth in culture.

In humans, the gene for IL-2 has been mapped to chromosome 4. It encodes a polypeptide chain of 133 amino acid residues, plus a signal sequence of 20 residues. IL-2 contains a variable number of O-LINKED SACCHARIDES. IL-2 has been crystallized and analysed by X-ray diffraction; it contains six short helical segments (amino acid residues 11–19, 33–56, 66–78, 83–101, 107–113 and 117–133). A disulfide bridge is formed by cysteine residues at positions 58 and 105. The first, second and fifth helical segments contain the residues that contact the IL-2 receptor. Mouse IL-2 is similar to human IL-2 except for an insertion of 12 glutamine residues, starting at position 15; the functional significance of the polyglutamine stretch is not known. IL-2 synthesis and secretion are inhibited by CORTICOSTEROIDS, PROSTAGLANDINS and CYCLOSPORIN A. Although B LYMPHOCYTES may express IL-2 receptors, the effect of IL-2 on growth and differentiation of B lymphocytes is controversial. IL-2 enhances the function of NATURAL KILLER CELLS.

interleukin-2 receptor (IL-2R). Receptor for INTERLEUKIN-2 (IL-2) in the membranes mainly of T LYMPHOCYTES, B LYMPHOCYTES and NATURAL KILLER CELLS. Resting T lymphocytes have a low number of IL-2R. IL-2 secretion, which begins four hours after stimulation of T lymphocytes by interleukin-1 and the binding of antigen to the T CELL RECEPTORS, results in enhanced expression of IL-2R. Six days later, an activated T lymphocyte may express as many as 15,000 IL-2R. Five to 15 percent of IL-2R bind IL-2 with high affinity (association constant of approximately 10^{11} M^{-1}) and the remainder bind IL-2 with low affinity (association constant of approximately 10^8 M^{-1}). Binding of IL-2 to the high-affinity receptor is followed by endocytosis of the complex of IL-2 and IL-2R and activation of T lymphocytes or natural killer cells.

IL-2R is composed of two polypeptide chains (M_r 55,000 and 70,000), called p55 and p70. Together they bind IL-2 with high affinity; each chain can separately bind IL-2 with low affinity. Antigenic determinants of p55 are recognized by monoclonal antibodies (anti-Tac for humans and 7D4 for mice). Human p55 consists of 272 amino acid residues, including a signal sequence of 21 residues, a putative transmembrane segment of 19 residues and a cytoplasmic domain of 13 residues. There are two sites for attachment of N-LINKED OLIGOSACCHARIDES. The gene encoding this chain of the IL-2R has been mapped to human chromosome 10p14.

Human ADULT T CELL LEUKEMIA cells express more than 270,000 IL-2R per cell. CORTICOSTEROIDS, PROSTAGLANDINS and CYCLOSPORIN A inhibit IL-2 synthesis and secretion but do not inhibit IL-2R expression.

interleukin-3 (IL-3). See COLONY STIMULATING FACTORS.

interleukin-4 (IL-4). LYMPHOKINE (M_r 20,000) that promotes CLASS SWITCHING in mouse B LYMPHOCYTES from secretion of IgM, IgG3 and IgG2b to IgG1, IgG2a, IgA and IgE. Mouse IL-4 consists of 140 amino acid residues including a signal sequence of 20 residues and three sites for attachment of N-LINKED OLIGOSACCHARIDES. Human IL-4 consists of 153 residues and has two sites for attachment of N-linked oligosaccharides. IL-4 induces expression of CLASS II HISTO-COMPATIBILITY MOLECULES in B lymphocytes, and therefore promotes T cell–B cell interactions. In mice and humans, IL-4 is required for IgE synthesis. It also augments expression of Fcε RECEPTOR II on MONONU-CLEAR PHAGOCYTES. In addition to the requirement of IL-4 for synthesis of IgE by B lymphocytes, IL-4 promotes the growth of T lymphocytes and some T cell clones are dependent on IL-4 for growth. IL-4 promotes the growth of MAST CELLS and can act synergistically with COLONY STIMULATING FACTORS to promote the growth of hematopoietic cells. INTERFERON-GAMMA antagonizes the effects of IL-4 on B lymphocytes.

IL-4 has also been called B cell growth factor I (BCGF I) or B cell stimulating factor 1 (BSF 1).

interleukin-5 (IL-5). LYMPHOKINE (M_r 18,000) secreted by T LYMPHOCYTES that promotes the growth and differentiation of B LYMPHOCYTES into IgA secreting cells. Mouse IL-5 consists of 133 amino acid residues, including a signal sequence of 21 residues, and three sites for attachment of N-LINKED OLIGOSACCHARIDES. Human IL-5 consists of 134 amino acid residues, including a signal sequence of 22 residues and two sites for attachment of N-linked oligosaccharides.

IL-5 was first described as a factor in T CELL-CONDITIONED MEDIUM that replaces T lymphocytes in *in vitro* antibody responses to THYMUS-DEPENDENT ANTIGENS and was called thymus replacing factor (TRF). It also promotes differentiation of B LYMPHOCYTES into IgM and IgG PLAQUE-FORMING CELLS and stimulates the growth of B cell lymphomas *in vitro*; thus, it was also called B cell growth factor II (BCGF II). IL-5 augments the division of THYMOCYTES in the presence of CONCANAVALIN A; it induces differentiation of eosinophils and was called eosinophil differentiating factor (EDF).

interleukin-6 (IL-6). CYTOKINE with a wide range of biological activities secreted by MONONUCLEAR PHAGOCYTES, activated T LYM-PHOCYTES as well as some non-lymphoid cells (e.g., fibroblasts) and a variety of tumors (e.g., cardiac myxoma, bladder cell carcinoma). IL-6 was originally described as a factor that promotes the differentiation of B LYMPHOCYTES to antibody-secreting cells without inducing their proliferation. It is thought that IL-6 may be one of the factors, which, during T–B CELL COLLABORATION, promotes secretion of immunoglobulin by activated B lymphocytes. IL-6 is a growth factor for hybridomas and plasmacytomas. IL-6 also induces fever. IL-6 is a glycoprotein (M_r 21,000). The primary translation product of human IL-6 contains 212 amino acids. The mature protein contains 184 amino acid residues. It contains two sites for attachment of N-LINKED OLIGOSACCHARIDES. The gene maps to chromosome 7 in humans. IL-6 promotes release of ACUTE PHASE REAC-TANTS from liver cells, and appears to be identical to the so-called hepatocyte stimulating factor. IL-6 also promotes differentiation of HEMATOPOIETIC STEM CELLS and nerve cells.

IL-6 has been called B cell differentiation factor (BCDF) and B cell stimulating factor 2 (BSF 2).

intervening sequence. *Synonym for* INTRON.

intestinal lymphangiectasia. Dilation of the LYMPHATICS in the intestinal villi with resultant loss of protein, including IMMUNOGLOB-ULINS, and LYMPHOCYTES into the gut. This loss causes SECONDARY IMMUNODEFICIENCY. Intestinal lymphangiectasia can be primary, in which case the cause is unknown, or secondary due to obstruction of intestinal lymphatic drainage (e.g., by LYMPHOMAS of the bowel).

intrinsic affinity. *Synonym for* INTRINSIC ASSOCIATION CONSTANT.

intrinsic association constant (κ). ASSOCIATION CONSTANT that describes the equilibrium state of the reversible reaction between an individual site (S) on a macro-molecule (e.g., antibody) and a univalent LIGAND (L), i.e. $S + L \rightleftharpoons SL$. The intrinsic association constant (or microscopic association constant, the term preferred by chemists), κ, is defined by the relation:

$$\kappa = \frac{[SL]}{[S][L]}$$

where, at equilibrium, [L] is the concentration of free ligand, [SL] is the concentration of occupied sites on the macromolecule and [S] is the concentration of free sites. The intrinsic association constant is evaluated in assays (e.g., EQUILIBRIUM DIALYSIS) that establish the concentration of bound and free ligand. If all the sites are equivalent and independent, κ is defined uniquely, irrespective of the number of sites on the macromolecule or their degree of saturation with ligand. If the sites are not equivalent, an average intrinsic association constant can be defined, usually as the reciprocal of the concentration of free ligand that is required for half-saturation of the antibody sites. *See* AVERAGE ASSOCIATION CONSTANT, SCATCHARD EQUATION, SCATCHARD PLOT.

intron. Segment of a gene or primary mRNA transcript that is not represented in mature RNA. Introns (also called intervening sequences) are found in genes (and in primary transcripts) encoding proteins, ribosomal RNA and transfer RNA. Introns are located between EXONS. Introns in genes (transcripts) encoding protein generally begin with the dinucleotide GT (GU) and end with the dinucleotide AG; they also contain other unknown signals for RNA splicing.

inulin. Polymer of 20–30 fructofuranose units in α-glycosidic linkage. It is found in the rhizome of certain plants (e.g., dahlias, Jerusalem artichoke). Inulin, in solution, activates the ALTERNATIVE PATHWAY OF COMPLEMENT.

Inv allotypic determinant. *See* Km ALLOTYPIC DETERMINANT.

invariant (Ii) **chain.** Glycoprotein (M_r 31,000) associated with CLASS II HISTOCOMPATIBILITY MOLECULES. Ii is not polymorphic as are the alpha and beta chains of the class II histocompatibility molecules. In B lymphocytes and macrophages, Ii is associated with the alpha and beta chains within the cell, and is found on the plasma membrane only in small amounts. Ii molecules copre-

cipitate with class II antigens when cell lysates are incubated with antibodies to the I–A or the I–E antigens (*see* I REGION) of the mouse. The function of Ii is not known.

inverted repeat. Two segments of sequence on a single strand that are complementary, e.g., in single-stranded DNA:

5' AG GTCAA GCTAGTT TTGAC GG 3'

and in duplex DNA:

5' AG GTCAA GCTAGTT TTGAC GG 3'
3' TC CAGTT CGATCAA AACTG CC 5'

When the two halves of an inverted repeat are adjacent, the result is a PALINDROME, e.g.,

5' GTCAATTGAC 3'
3' CAGTTAACTG 5'

The two halves of an inverted repeat tend to base-pair with each other. The resulting structure formed by an inverted repeat on a single nucleic acid strand is often called a HAIRPIN LOOP, the two complementary segments forming the stem of the loop. When inverted repeats occur in duplex DNA a cruciform structure may be formed.

irradiation chimera. Animal or person who has been lethally irradiated and rescued by repopulation with cells from a donor of different genetic constitution. *See* CHIMERA.

iscom. Complex of antigen and a glycoside derived from the bark of the South American tree, *Saponaria quilaja* Moline. Iscoms (an acronym for immunostimulating complexes) are used to obtain high titers of antibodies to purified viral proteins. The glycoside forms cage-like structures, 40 nm in diameter, and binds antigen by hydrophobic interactions.

isoagglutinin. ALLOANTIBODY that AGGLUTINATES cells such as ERYTHROCYTES or LEUKOCYTES. Isoagglutinins are used to type red blood cells (e.g., type A red blood cells are agglutinated by isoagglutinin anti-A).

isoallotypic determinant. ALLOTYPIC DETERMINANT that is found as an allelic variant on one heavy-chain ISOTYPE (IMMUNOGLOBULIN CLASS or IMMUNOGLOBULIN SUBCLASS), but that is present on all molecules of another heavy-chain isotype. For example,

G1m(−1) is an allotypic determinant of the IgG1 subclass (its allele is G1m(1)), but it is present on all IgG2 and IgG3 molecules. Isoallotypic determinants are also known as 'non-markers'.

isoantibody. *Synonym for* ALLOANTIBODY.

isoantigen. *Synonym for* ALLOANTIGEN.

isoelectric focusing (IEF). Type of ELECTROPHORESIS in which molecules are separated, in a stable pH gradient, according to their ISOELECTRIC POINTS. A charged particle will migrate in the electric field until it reaches a position where it is isoelectric; at this point, its net charge is zero and it will stop moving. Usually, the pH gradient is formed by subjecting a mixture of low molecular weight amphoteric compounds ('carrier ampholytes') to electrophoresis; each component moves to its isoelectric region and remains there, stabilizing the pH gradient at that point. It is also necessary to prevent convection and the separation is usually carried out in a sucrose gradient or in a polyacrylamide gel.

isoelectric point. pH at which a protein or other amphoteric substance (i.e., a substance having both positively and negatively charged groups) has no net charge (i.e., the mean charge is zero). At pH values below the isoelectric point, a protein will be positively charged and migrate toward the cathode (negative electrode) in ELECTROPHORESIS. At pH values above the isoelectric point, the reverse is true. The value of the isoelectric point can be determined by electrophoresis or by ISOELECTRIC FOCUSING. The isoelectric point of a protein is affected by the solute (i.e. buffer) in which the measurement is carried out.

isogeneic. *Synonym for* ISOGENIC.

isogenic. Possessing identical genotypes (e.g., identical twins). *See* SYNGENEIC.

isograft. GRAFT between ISOGENIC individuals. The term isograft is also used to describe grafts between members of an inbred strain, which are not isogenic but SYNGENEIC. *See* ALLOGRAFT, XENOGRAFT.

isophile antibody. Antibody, formed in response to immunization with red blood cells, that is specific for the IMMUNOGEN and does not agglutinate red blood cells of other species. *See* HETEROPHILE ANTIBODIES.

isophile antigen. Species-specific antigen, usually of red blood cells. *See* HETEROPHILE ANTIGEN.

isoproterenol

isoproterenol (*dl*-β-(3,4-dihydroxyphenyl)-α-isopropylaminoethanol). Beta-adrenergic amine that relaxes smooth muscle, particularly of the bronchi. It is used in the treatment of ASTHMA.

isoschizomers. RESTRICTION ENDONUCLEASES that recognize the same nucleotide sequence. Some pairs of isoschizomers cut their targets at different places (e.g., *Sma* I (CCC↓GGG); *Xma* I (C↓CCGGG)). Isoschizomers may act differently according to the state of methylation of the target sequence. For example, the enzyme *Hpa* II cleaves the sequence C↓CGG, but if the second C is methylated, the site is no longer recognized. However, *Msp* I recognizes the same sequence regardless of the state of methylation and cleaves at the same position. Such enzymes are useful in studies of DNA methylation and gene expression, which may be related to the degree of methylation.

isotope. EPITOPE of an ISOTYPE. *Synonym for* ISOTYPIC DETERMINANT.

isotype. Set of ISOTYPIC DETERMINANTS generally associated with the CONSTANT REGION of an IMMUNOGLOBULIN HEAVY CHAIN (e.g., alpha1, gamma1) or IMMUNOGLOBULIN LIGHT CHAIN (kappa, lambda); alternatively, the chain (or immunoglobulin molecule) carrying these determinants. Each isotype is found in all normal members of a species. *See* ALLOTYPE, IMMUNOGLOBULIN CLASS, IMMUNOGLOBULIN SUBCLASS.

isotypic determinant. ANTIGENIC DETERMINANT of an IMMUNOGLOBULIN found in all normal members of a species. The identification of the different IMMUNOGLOBULIN CLASSES and SUBCLASSES (and their constituent heavy chains), as well as the definition of light chain types, is based on the different isotypic determinants associated with the various chains (e.g., alpha1, gamma1, kappa, lambda). Antisera that recognize isotypic determinants of an immunoglobulin from one species are raised by immunization in another species. *See* ALLOTYPIC DETERMINANT, ISOTYPE.

J

J chain. Polypeptide chain (M_r ~17,600), found in IgM and IgA, that is thought to be involved in the synthesis, polymerization and/or secretion of polymeric immunoglobulin. Since there is but a single J (joining) chain in each immunoglobulin polymer, its mass is only 2–4 percent of pentameric IgM or dimeric IgA. Human and mouse J chain are devoid of tryptophan and have a very low extinction coefficient. Despite its lower molecular weight, J chain migrates near light chains in gel filtration and in POLYACRYLAMIDE GEL ELECTROPHORESIS IN SODIUM DODECYL SULFATE (SDS-PAGE). For these reasons, the presence of J chain in polymeric immunoglobulins was overlooked for many years. Human J chain was finally identified by virtue of its rapid anionic electrophoretic migration.

Human and mouse J chains contain 137 amino acid residues and one complex N-LINKED OLIGOSACCHARIDE on asparagine 49. Three forms of this oligosaccharide, varying in sialic acid content, have been identified in human J chain and may account for the observation that this polypeptide generally migrates as a complex of three closely-spaced bands when it is analyzed in alkaline-urea polyacrylamide gels. J chain is linked by disulfide bridges to penultimate cysteine residues of IMMUNOGLOBULIN ALPHA or IMMUNOGLOBULIN MU CHAINS. The amino acid sequence of J chain does not resemble that of immunoglobulin heavy or light chains.

J chain is synthesized when a resting B LYMPHOCYTE becomes activated and differentiates into a PLASMA CELL. This stimulation of J chain expression occurs not only in plasma cells that secrete IgA and IgM, but also in cells that produce monomeric IgG and even in transformed B lymphocytes that do not produce immunoglobulin. J chain is incorporated into polymeric immunoglobulins before they are secreted from the plasma cell and appears to be necessary for the efficient TRANSCYTOSIS of such immunoglobulins across epithelial cells into external secretions (*see* IgA, POLYIMMUNOGLOBULIN RECEPTOR).

In humans and in mice, J chain is encoded by a single gene on chromosome 4q21 and chromosome 5, respectively. In the mouse, there are four EXONS; the first encodes the 5' untranslated and signal sequence, the second and third encode the amino-terminal half of the mature chain, and the fourth encodes the carboxy-terminal half of the chain as well as a large 3' untranslated sequence. Exons similar to the second, third and fourth exons of the mouse J chain have also been identified in the human gene.

J chain is not related to the *J* GENE SEGMENT.

J **gene segment.** Segment of DNA that encodes the carboxy-terminal 12–21 residues of the variable regions of immunoglobulin or T cell receptor polypeptide chains. As a consequence of IMMUNOGLOBULIN GENE REARRANGEMENT, a *J* gene segment joins (hence the symbol J) a *V* GENE SEGMENT or a *D* GENE SEGMENT to the intron 5' of the *C* GENE SEGMENT. The number and location of *J* gene segments is discussed in the definitions of IMMUNOGLOBULIN GENES and T CELL RECEPTOR GENES. See J REGION.

J region. Portion of the VARIABLE REGION of an IMMUNOGLOBULIN or T CELL RECEPTOR polypeptide chain that is encoded by a *J* GENE SEGMENT. The J region of an IMMUNOGLOBULIN LIGHT CHAIN consists of the carboxy-terminal one or two residues of the third HYPERVARIABLE REGION and the fourth FRAMEWORK REGION, i.e., the carboxy-terminal 12 or 13 residues of the variable region. The J region of an IMMUNOGLOBULIN HEAVY CHAIN is a few residues longer than that of a light chain and consists of the carboxy-terminal part of the third hypervariable region and the fourth framework region, about 15 to 20 residues in all. The J region in the T CELL RECEPTOR also comprises the carboxy-terminal section of the variable region. *See* D REGION.

Jerne plaque assay. *See* HEMOLYTIC PLAQUE ASSAY.

Jones–Mote reaction. DELAYED-TYPE HYPER-SENSITIVITY reaction in skin characterized by prominent infiltration of BASOPHILS (also named cutaneous basophil hypersensitivity). It occurs in guinea-pigs immunized with proteins in saline or in INCOMPLETE FREUND'S ADJUVANT. The reaction can be transferred by T LYMPHOCYTES.

jugular bodies. LYMPH NODE-like struc-tures, found in some higher amphibian species (e.g., ranid frogs). The jugular bodies are paired nodules, lying ventral to the external jugular veins. They are com-posed of encapsulated masses of lymphoid cells that are separated into lobules by sinu-soids lined by phagocytic cells. The jugular bodies are not part of the lymphatic system, but filter blood.

junctional diversity. Variability in amino acid sequence due to imprecise joining of gene segments that contribute to expressed variable regions. This variation in the join-ing position can change the codons at the junctions of gene segments: the $V–J$ junc-tions of immunoglobulin kappa and lambda genes and T cell receptor alpha and gamma genes; the $V–D$, $D–J$ or $D–D$ junctions of immunoglobulin heavy chain genes and/or T cell receptor beta and delta genes. Insertion of N nucleotides (*see* N REGION) also contri-butes to diversity at the junctions of these gene segments. *See* IMMUNOGLOBULIN GENES, IMMUNOGLOBULIN GENE REARRANGEMENT, T CELL RECEPTOR GENES.

juvenile onset diabetes. *Synonym for* INSULIN-DEPENDENT DIABETES MELLITUS.

juvenile rheumatoid arthritis (JRA). Per-sistent INFLAMMATION of one or more joints for at least three months in a child when there is no other known cause of arthritis. JRA is characterized by fever, rash, UVEITIS, pericarditis and RHEUMATOID NODULES. Rela-tively few of the patients (~10 percent) have RHEUMATOID FACTOR in serum. There are three main subgroups: (1) systemic Still's disease, characterized by fever, rash, enlar-gement of the liver, spleen and lymph nodes and inflammation of the pericardium; (2) pauciarticular disease (affecting one to nine joints) mainly in young females and accompanied by uveitis and antibodies to DNA; (3) polyarticular disease. Group 1 is associated with HLA-DR4 (*see* HLA) and group 2 with HLA-DR5 and DR8.

K

K562. Cell line from a patient with chronic myelogenous leukemia. K562 cells are commonly used as TARGET CELLS in assays of NATURAL KILLER CELLS.

kallikrein. Serine protease of plasma and several tissues that cleaves KININOGENS to release BRADYKININ. Plasma kallikrein is derived from a single-chain precursor molecule (M_r 88,000), prekallikrein. Activated HAGEMAN FACTOR cleaves an arginine–isoleucine (position 371–372) bond in prekallikrein to form an alpha chain of 371 amino acid residues and a beta chain of 248 residues. The enzymatic site is in the beta chain. There are two sites for N-LINKED OLIGOSACCHARIDES in the alpha chain (at asparagines 108 and 289) and three in the beta chain (at asparagines 6, 63 and 115). *See* CONTACT SYSTEM.

Kaposi's sarcoma. Malignancy of endothelial cells that appears usually as dull purple–red spots on the skin or mucous membranes. This tumor is frequently found in homosexually active males with ACQUIRED IMMUNODEFICIENCY SYNDROME.

Kaposi's varicelliform eruption. *Synonym for* ECZEMA VACCINATUM.

kappa chain deficiency. Very rare IMMUNODEFICIENCY in which kappa-containing IMMUNOGLOBULIN molecules (*see* IMMUNOGLOBULIN KAPPA CHAIN) are not detected in the serum or on the surface of B LYMPHOCYTES. This defect appears to result from point mutations in the C_κ gene at chromosome 2p11.

karyotype. Number and configuration of chromosomes in a cell. The karyotype is frequently a distinctive feature of a species. The karyotype of males and females in a species differs due to the sex chromosomes.

Kauffmann–White scheme. Systematic classification of Salmonella strains by serotyping with antibodies to O ANTIGENS and H ANTIGENS. The O antigen of each Salmonella strain has one or a few ANTIGENIC DETERMINANTS, some of which may be shared with other strains. Unabsorbed and adsorbed antisera are used to demontrate the existence of shared and specific determinants. The strains sharing a particular major determinant form a group. Additional divisions into subgroups are based on the presence of minor O determinants. The members of each O group or subgroup can be differentiated still further into SEROTYPES on the basis of their flagellar H antigens. Sixty-five O antigenic groups or subgroups and a total of about 1,500 serotypes are known.

Kawasaki's disease. Self-limited, acute, epidemic illness of infants and young children perhaps caused by a retrovirus and occurring with disproportionate frequency in Japanese. Kawasaki's disease is characterized by the occurrence of at least five days of high fever, bilateral conjunctivitis, redness of the mouth with strawberry-like swelling of the tongue, and a rash that is predominant on the extremities with pronounced redness of the palms and soles. The skin peels during the second week of the illness. Coronary artery disease, including aneurysms and thrombosis, occurs in 25 percent of cases, and may be fatal. The blood contains increased numbers of B LYMPHOCYTES, CD4+ T lymphocytes bearing CLASS II HISTOCOMPATIBILITY MOLECULES, and decreased numbers of CD8+ lymphocytes. Administration of large doses of intravenous GAMMA-GLOBULIN appears to prevent coronary artery disease.

Kell–Cellano blood group. ANTIGENIC DETERMINANTS of human red blood cells and

GRANULOCYTES detected by ALLOANTIBODIES that are the products of two alleles: *K* (Kell) and *k* (Cellano). A structure (Kx) encoded by a gene (*Xk*) on the X chromosome is modified to the Kell or Cellano antigens by the products of *K* or *k* alleles. A deletion of the *Xk* locus leads to failure of Kx expression and results in abnormal red blood cells (McLEOD PHENOTYPE) and HEMOLYTIC ANEMIA. ALLOIMMUNIZATION of mothers during pregnancy with Kell antigens can lead to HEMOLYTIC DISEASE OF THE NEWBORN.

Kern isotypic determinant. ANTIGENIC DETERMINANT of human IMMUNOGLOBULIN LAMBDA CHAINS, associated with glycine at position 152 (*see* Table in definition of immunoglobulin lambda chains). This determinant is present on some of the lambda chains of every individual. It is, therefore, not the result of genetic POLYMORPHISM.

Kidd blood group. ANTIGENIC DETERMINANTS of human red blood cells detected by ALLOANTIBODIES to the products of two alleles: *Jka* and *Jkb*. The Kidd antigens have not been biochemically characterized. ALLOIMMUNIZATION of mothers by Kidd antigens during pregnancy can lead to HEMOLYTIC DISEASE OF THE NEWBORN.

kilobase (kb). 1,000 bases or base pairs of DNA or RNA.

kinin. Peptide (e.g., BRADYKININ) derived from physiological protein precursors (KININOGENS) that dilates blood vessels, increases vascular permeability, produces edema and contracts smooth muscle.

Depending on the type of kininogen (i.e., high or low molecular weight) and the cleavage specificity of the proteases (i.e., plasma or tissue KALLIKREIN) used, four types of kinins can be generated: bradykinin, kallidin or lysyl-bradykinin, methionyl-lysyl-bradykinin and isoleucyl-seryl-bradykinin. All four kinins share a consensus sequence of nine amino acid residues, differing only in the amino-terminal residues. Kallidin, methionyl–lysyl-bradykinin and isoleucyl–seryl-bradykinin are converted to bradykinin *in vivo*. *See* CONTACT SYSTEM.

kininogen. Protein from which the potent vasoactive peptide, BRADYKININ, can be generated. In mammals, two kininogens have been identified: high molecular weight kininogen (HMK) (M_r 80,000–114,000) and low molecular weight kininogen (LMK) (M_r 50,000–68,000). In addition a third kininogen is present in rats and is called T-kininogen (M_r 68,000); it is an acute phase reactant (*see* ACUTE PHASE REACTION) in rats. HMK is a cofactor in the clotting system. LMK is an inhibitor of cysteine proteases, such as papain and cathepsins.

HMK and LMK are encoded by a single gene: the two forms result from alternative RNA SPLICING. HMK and LMK are composed of a signal sequence of 18 amino acid residues and an amino-terminal domain of 362 residues, which is followed by the nine residues of the consensus sequence (*see* KININ). LMK has a carboxy-terminal domain of 38 residues and HMK has a carboxy-terminal domain of 255 residues. After cleavage of a kinin from HMK or LMK, the amino- and carboxy-terminal domains remain linked by a single disulfide bond.

Kininogens circulate in the blood bound to prekallikrein. When the CONTACT SYSTEM is activated KALLIKREIN, which is generated from prekallikrein, cleaves bradykinin from kininogens.

Klenow fragment. Larger (M_r 68,000) of the two fragments produced by limited proteolytic cleavage of DNA POLYMERASE I (*E. coli*). The Klenow fragment retains the $5' \rightarrow 3'$ polymerase and $3' \rightarrow 5'$ exonuclease activities, but not the $5' \rightarrow 3'$ exonuclease activity of the intact polymerase. It is used in recombinant DNA procedures where only polymerization is required (e.g., to fill in cohesive ends from a recessed $3'$ terminus before addition of linkers; for second-strand synthesis in cDNA cloning; to copy single-stranded DNA in the dideoxy method of sequencing; to label $3'$-hydroxyl ends of DNA fragments).

Km allotype. Human IMMUNOGLOBULIN KAPPA CHAIN carrying one or more Km ALLOTYPIC DETERMINANTS. There are three known Km allotypes (Km1; Km1,2; and Km3), which are the products of alleles of the gene encoding the constant regions of human kappa chains; the alleles are designated *Km1*, *Km1,2* and *Km3*. The three allotypes differ at amino acid residue positions 153 and 191 (*see* Table). These two positions are near each other in the folded immunoglobulin C_κ domain. A single individual can have light chains of at most two of the three types, corresponding to an allele on each chromosome.

Chain	Residue at positions	
	153	191
Km1	Val	Leu
Km1,2	Ala	Leu
Km3	Ala	Val

Km allotypic determinant. ALLOTYPIC DETERMINANT of human IMMUNOGLOBULIN KAPPA CHAINS. Three such ANTIGENIC DETERMINANTS have been identified: (Km(1), Km(2), and Km(3)). One of the three Km ALLOTYPES carries both the Km(1) and Km(2) allotypic determinants. The Km allotypic determinants reflect variations in the PRIMARY STRUCTURE of kappa chains (at positions 153 and 191). The full expression of the Km determinants requires the presence of the IMMUNOGLOBULIN HEAVY CHAIN, presumably to maintain the proper three-dimensional configuration. Therefore, the Km alleles are examples of CONFORMATIONAL DETERMINANTS.

Küpffer cell. MACROPHAGE of the liver. Küpffer cells are derived from blood MONOCYTES that adhere to the walls of the liver sinuses and differentiate into macrophages. Küpffer cells, like all macrophages, bear Fc RECEPTORS, COMPLEMENT RECEPTORS 1 and COMPLEMENT RECEPTORS 3 and CLASS II HISTOCOMPATIBILITY MOLECULES. Küpffer cells remove particles (e.g., bacteria, ANTIGEN–ANTIBODY COMPLEXES) from the circulation by PHAGOCYTOSIS.

Kveim reaction. SKIN TEST used to diagnose SARCOIDOSIS. A saline suspension of a LYMPH NODE from a patient known to have sarcoidosis is injected intracutaneously into a person suspected of having sarcoidosis. Four to six weeks later the injection site is biopsied. A nodule at the biopsy site resembling EPITHELIOID CELL GRANULOMA is diagnostic of sarcoidosis.

L

lambda bacteriophage. Double-stranded DNA virus that infects *E. coli*. This phage has been studied in great detail and has been developed as a VECTOR for molecular cloning. Lambda DNA consists of 48,502 base pairs and codes for about 60 proteins. In the viral particle, the DNA is a linear duplex with single-stranded complementary ends of 12 nucleotides (COHESIVE ENDS). After entering the bacterial host, the DNA circularizes through pairing of the cohesive ends. Lambda can replicate lytically or as part of the *E. coli* chromosome (*see* LYSOGEN). In the lytic cycle, the circular DNA is replicated many times and a large number of bacteriophage gene products are synthesized. The DNA is packaged into mature phage particles, which are released upon lysis of the cell; the released phage can then infect other cells. In the lysogenic state, the lytic functions are repressed and the phage genome is integrated into the bacterial chromosome (it is then called a prophage) and is replicated and transmitted to progeny like any other gene on the chromosome. The host cells are not lysed. However, with a low frequency, lysogenic cells (i.e., those carrying a prophage) can spontaneously enter the lytic life cycle. Certain agents (e.g., ultraviolet light) can induce this event in virtually all of the lysogenic cells. Most laboratory stains of lambda contain a mutant repressor, which is thermolabile, so that the prophage can be induced by heat.

Lambda bacteriophage has served as the basis for the construction of a large number of cloning vectors that can accept foreign DNA inserted into a variety of restriction sites. These vectors are of two types: (1) those with a single target site into which foreign DNA is inserted (insertion vectors); (2) those with a pair of sites spanning a non-essential segment of vector DNA that can be removed and replaced with foreign DNA (replacement vectors). Since there is an upper limit on the total amount of DNA that can be packaged, insertion vectors can accommodate less foreign DNA and are used for cloning cDNA or small restriction fragments; replacement vectors are used for cloning larger pieces of DNA.

Langerhans cell (LC). Cell of the skin and lymphoid organs (where it is called a dendritic cell) characterized by multiple thin cytoplasmic processes that extend between neighboring cells. LC have a high density of CLASS I and CLASS II HISTOCOMPATIBILITY MOLECULES and are active in ANTIGEN PRESENTATION. LCs in the skin have variable amounts of CD1, Fcγ RECEPTORS and COMPLEMENT RECEPTORS 1 AND 3. Many LCs have a characteristic cytoplasmic structure, the BIRBECK GRANULE, which is a small round or rectangular vacuole of 10 nm, containing a central, irregular electron-dense mass. LCs are derived from bone marrow STEM CELLS, migrate to the epidermis and then, by way of the lymphatic circulation, into LYMPH NODES where they localize in the deep cortex or via the blood to the SPLEEN. Dendritic cells do not express CD1 and most have no Fcγ receptors. LCs appear to be highly active in DELAYED-TYPE HYPERSENSITIVITY reactions of the skin where they take up antigen and carry it to the lymph nodes. LCs appear to be identical to veiled cells isolated from lymph. *See* DENDRITIC EPIDERMAL CELL.

latent allotype. ALLOTYPE that is not expected based on the genetic constitution of the animal, i.e. an allotype different from the expected or 'NOMINAL' ALLOTYPE. This phenomenon has been described for the a (heavy chain variable region), b (kappa light chain), and d and e (gamma heavy chain constant region) allotypes of rabbit IMMUNOGLOBULINS. For example, an F_1 rabbit produced by mating a homozygous a1 rabbit with a homozygous a2 rabbit would be

Table of lectins

Lectin	Carbohydrate specificity	Mitogenic activity
Conconavalin A (jack bean)	α-D-mannosyl α-D-glucose	+
ricin	β-D-galactose N-acetyl-D-galactosamine	−
soy bean	N-acetyl-D-galactosamine D-galactose	−
wheat germ	N-acetyl-D-glucosamine	−
pokeweed	β-N-acetyl-D-glucosamine	+
phytohemagglutinin (red kidney bean)	N-acetyl-D-galactosamine	+
lima bean	α-N-acetyl-D-galactosamine	−
peanut	D-galactosyl-(β1–3)-N-acetyl-D-galactosamine	−

expected to produce heavy chains of allotypes a1 or a2. Occasionally, especially after suitable stimulation, such rabbits also produce heavy chains expressing the a3 ALLOTYPIC DETERMINANTS. Such an unexpected allotype is designated a 'latent allotype'. Latent allotypes are usually expressed at very low levels, although high levels have also been reported.

lattice theory.   Idea that antigen–antibody precipitation results from the formation of large complexes (i.e. lattices) of antigens and antibodies. To form lattices, both the antigen and the antibody must have two or more binding sites (i.e., be BIVALENT or MULTIVALENT). Complex formation is particularly efficient if a variety of antibodies recognizing different determinants of the antigen are present.

L-cell conditioned medium.   Medium from cultures of L cells (a long-term fibroblast line) that contains a potent growth factor for MACROPHAGES (M-CSF). *See* COLONY STIMULATING FACTORS.

LE cell (lupus erythematosus cell).   Neutrophil that has ingested insoluble complexes of nucleoproteins and antibodies. The complexes appear as large homogeneously-staining cytoplasmic masses. The presence of these cells, after incubation of blood for one hour at 37°C, was used as a diagnostic test for SYSTEMIC LUPUS ERYTHEMATOSUS.

leader peptide.   *See* SIGNAL SEQUENCE.

leader sequence.   *See* SIGNAL SEQUENCE.

lectin.   Protein that recognizes specific carbohydrate residues and binds to cell surface glycoproteins or glycolipids. Lectins were originally isolated from plants (especially seeds), but have subsequently been found in a variety of other organisms. Lectins can be soluble or membrane-bound; they are BIVALENT or POLYVALENT and often agglutinate cells (e.g., erythrocytes). Lectins interact with specific regions of relatively complex oligosaccharides; in some cases, their reactivity is directed to a particular monosaccharide constituent, and such lectins can be inhibited by low concentrations of the appropriate free sugar; other lectins can be inhibited only by oligosaccharides. Certain lectins (e.g. pokeweed and CONCANAVALIN A) are MITOGENS and stimulate the transformation of small, resting lymphocytes into large blast cells that may undergo mitotic division.

lepromin. Crude extract of *Mycobacterium leprae* derived from autoclaved infected human tissue. Two to four weeks after intradermal injection of lepromin into a patient with leprosy, a nodular GRANULOMA develops, indicating the presence of CELL-MEDIATED IMMUNITY to *Mycobacterium leprae*.

Leu 7. Surface antigenic determinant of human NATURAL KILLER CELLS, detected with a mouse MONOCLONAL ANTIBODY.

Leu 11. Surface antigenic determinant of Fcγ receptor III on human NATURAL KILLER CELLS, detected with a mouse MONOCLONAL ANTIBODY.

leukoagglutinin. Substance (e.g., specific antibody) that agglutinates white blood cells.

leukocyte. White blood cell. The major classes of leukocytes are: GRANULOCYTES, LYMPHOCYTES, MONOCYTES.

leukocyte adhesion deficiency (LAD). Defect in adhesion and mobility of phagocytes and lymphocytes, resulting from a deficiency of the membrane proteins p150,95, LFA-1 and COMPLEMENT RECEPTOR 3 (CR3) and leading to recurrent PYOGENIC INFECTIONS. These three proteins are not expressed on the cell surface due to defective biosynthesis of the beta chain (M_r 95,000), a subunit shared by all three proteins. Phagocytes are defective in random migration, chemotaxis and spreading on charged surfaces. C3-coated particles do not induce a respiratory burst or degranulation of phagocytes and are not ingested. These defects of phagocytes have been ascribed to the deficiency of CR3 and p150,95. T LYMPHOCYTES of patients do not proliferate normally in response to stimulation by MITOGENS, ANTIGENS or ALLO-ANTIGENS. They also do not provide adequate help for immunoglobulin production

by B LYMPHOCYTES, do not secrete INTERFERON-GAMMA and are defective in killing TARGET CELLS. These defects of lymphocytes have been ascribed to the deficiency of LFA-1. NATURAL KILLER CELLS are also defective in killing target cells, and this has also been ascribed to the deficiency of LFA-1. Patients with LAD deficiency have symptoms resulting from defects in phagocyte function (e.g., abscesses and periodontitis), but they have no clinical problems associated with the T lymphocyte deficiency. The defect is inherited as an autosomal recessive. Heterozygotes can be easily detected by their half-normal amounts of CR3 on phagocyte membranes but are clinically normal.

leukocyte common antigen (L-CA or T200). Family of major cell surface glycoproteins (M_r 180,000–220,000) found on most LEUKOCYTES, but not on other cell types. These antigens are rich in carbohydrate and comprise up to 10 percent of the total membrane proteins. Rat thymocyte L-CA (M_r 180,000) contains 1118 amino acid residues. The amino-terminal 391 residues are extracellular. There is a transmembrane segment of 22 amino acid residues and a cytoplasmic portion of 705 residues. The cytoplasmic domain includes possible phosphorylation sites and two regions of internal homology. The function of this protein is unknown, but the large intracellular segment suggests a role in interaction with the CYTOSKELETON. In mice, L-CA is identified by antibodies to the Ly5 ALLOANTIGEN. L-CA molecules show heterogeneity in size and antigenicity and different forms are specific to different lymphocyte types. Antigenic determinants include: (1) those common to all L-CA molecules; (2) those specific to B LYMPHOCYTE L-CA; and (3) those found on L-CA of B lymphocytes, CD8+ T LYMPHOCYTES and 70 percent of CD4+ T lymphocytes.

The gene encoding members of the L-CA family consists of approximately 30 exons. The heterogeneity of L-CA molecules results from variable splicing between exons 3 and 7. Removing exons 4, 5 and 6 results in the lowest molecular weight form, found on thymocytes, whereas transcription of all the exons results in the highest molecular weight form, consisting of 1281 amino acid residues, found on B lymphocytes. Of eight possible

leukotrienes

forms of L-CA, which could result from variable splicing of exons 4, 5 and/or 6, six have been identified.

leukocyte inhibitory factor (LIF). LYMPHO-KINE found in cultures of activated T LYM-PHOCYTES that inhibits the migration of blood leukocytes, mainly NEUTROPHILS, from a capillary tube. LIF differs from MIGRATION INHIBITING FACTOR (MIF) in that LIF can be inhibited by serine esterase inhibitors, whereas MIF cannot be so inhibited.

leukotriene (LT). Molecule derived from arachidonic acid by the action of enzymes called lipooxygenases. LTs are released from MAST CELLS following IgE-mediated reactions. Other cells (e.g., neutrophils) can also release LT. SLOW REACTING SUBSTANCE OF ANAPHYLAXIS has been shown to be a mixture of LTC$_4$, LTD$_4$ and LTE$_4$. These three molecules are potent constrictors of smooth muscle, particularly of the small bronchi and bronchioles (about one hundred times more potent than HISTAMINE) and may be responsible for the bronchoconstriction in ANA-PHYLAXIS of guinea-pigs and in ASTHMA. LTC$_4$ and LTD$_4$ also increase vascular permeability. Another leukotriene, LTB$_4$, is a potent CHEMOTACTIC FACTOR for NEUTROPHILS; LTB$_4$ also causes aggregation and degranulation of neutrophils.

Arachidonic acid is converted to LTA$_4$ by a 5-lipooxygenase and a dehydrase; LTA$_4$ has no biological activity. It can be hydrolyzed to LTB$_4$ or converted to LTC$_4$ by addition of glutathione. Removal of glutamic acid by a transpeptidase reaction generates LTD$_4$. Further removal of a glycine by a dipeptidase results in the formation of LTE$_4$. Leukotrienes were so named because they were first isolated from leukocytes and contained a structure with three unsaturated carbon bonds (triene).

ligand. Chemical group or molecule bound (tied) to another chemical group or molecule.

light chain. Smaller polypeptide chain in a HETERODIMER. As used by immunologists, the term light chain usually refers to the light chain of an IMMUNOGLOBULIN molecule. *See* IMMUNOGLOBULIN LIGHT CHAIN.

limiting dilution analysis. Method for estimating the frequency in a population, of responding cells of defined specificity and function, by application of the Poisson distribution. For example, to determine the frequency of a specific type of B LYMPHOCYTE in a suspension of spleen cells, aliquots containing graded numbers of the spleen

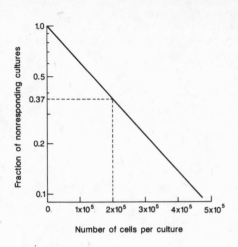

limiting dilution analysis

cells are cultured, in multiple replicas, under conditions designed to optimize the specific response. The B cells must be present in limited number (i.e., so that some cultures contain no B cells) and the cultures must be supplemented with an optimal number of any other type of cell (e.g., HELPER T LYMPHOCYTES) needed for the response. (In practice, T lymphocytes would be removed from the cell suspension that serves as the source of B cells so that the total number of T lymphocytes is limited to those that are added.) At each cell dose, the fraction of nonresponding cultures (i.e., those containing no B cells) is determined and is plotted, on a logarithmic scale, against the number of cells. A linear relation should be obtained if the responsive B lymphocyte is limiting in number and if a single such cell is sufficient for the response. From the Poisson distribution, it follows that the cell dose (i.e., 2×10^5 cells in the example shown) that yields a fraction of nonresponding cultures of e^{-1} (i.e., 0.37) probably contains one specific B lymphocyte, a frequency of one per 2×10^5 total cells. Such a frequency might be found in a primary response; the frequency of specific B lymphocytes in a secondary response is usually considerably higher. This type of analysis is also used to determine the frequency of HELPER T LYMPHOCYTES, CYTOTOXIC T LYMPHOCYTE PRECURSORS, etc.

linkage disequilibrium. Occurrence on the same chromosome of alleles of two or more genes with greater or lesser frequency than would be expected from the frequencies of these alleles in the population. Genes may display linkage disequilibrium for two main reasons: (1) there has not been sufficient time to reach equilibrium; (2) a particular combination of alleles has a selective advantage. An example of linkage disequilibrium in human populations is the frequent occurrence on the same chromosome of HLA-A1 and HLA-B8 in populations of Northern European origin. *See* COMPLOTYPE, EXTENDED HAPLOTYPE.

linked recognition. *See* MHC RESTRICTION.

lipopolysaccharide (LPS). Major constituent of the outer membrane of Gram-negative bacteria (e.g., Escherichia, Salmonella, Bacteroides, Pseudomonas). LPS is a complex molecule composed of lipid A, a core polysaccharide, and a variable polysaccharide known as O ANTIGEN. Lipid A, which is buried in the membrane, consists of two phosphorylated glucosamine residues to which are linked six long-chain fatty acids. The structure of lipid A is practically the same in all enterobacteria. Salmonella have a common core polysaccharide that contains the unusual sugars 2-keto-3-deoxyoctonic acid (KDO) and heptose; other genera (e.g. *E. coli*) have different cores. Variation in the O antigens among strains forms the main basis for the classification of the Salmonella in the KAUFFMANN–WHITE SCHEME.

The introduction of Gram-negative bacteria or of LPS lowers blood pressure, and can cause fever, NEUTROPENIA, blood clotting and shock, resulting in death. The lipid A moiety is responsible for the toxic activities of LPS. Many of these effects are indirect, i.e., LPS induces secretion of active agents by other cells, e.g., the production of INTERLEUKIN-1 and TUMOR NECROSIS FACTOR by macrophages. LPS can also activate the ALTERNATIVE PATHWAY OF COMPLEMENT; it can induce B LYMPHOCYTES of many species (but not of humans) to proliferate and differentiate into PLASMA CELLS. *See* ENDOTOXIN, SHWARTZMAN REACTION.

liposome. Synthetic lipid vesicle consisting of phospholipid bilayers (~5 nm thick) surrounding one or more aqueous compartments. Liposomes can be formed by: (1) suspending phospholipids (e.g., phosphatidylcholine (lecithin)) in an aqueous medium (with or without sonication) or (2) dispersing phospholipids in aqueous medium with detergent, followed by dialysis to remove the detergent. Liposomes are spherical or slightly elongated in shape and may be up to 1–2 mm in diameter. Small (~25 nm) liposomes are formed by sonication of larger ones and can be graded according to size by gel filtration. Liposomes may be simple unilamellar vesicles (single central aqueous compartment surrounded by a single bilayer) or they may be multilamellar (onion skin) with several shells of aqueous medium in addition to the central compartment, all separated by a series of concentric lipid bilayers. To mimic natural membranes, cholesterol and other membrane components (e.g., ionic channels) can be incorporated into the phospholipid bilayer. Solutes present in the aqueous phase when the liposome is formed become trapped inside the aqueous compartment(s).

Liposomes have been used as models for biological membranes (e.g., studies of membrane permeability or complement-mediated lysis). Antigens can be embedded in liposome membranes for induction of immune responses. Liposomes can serve as vehicles for drug delivery. The latter application depends on the ability of liposomes to adsorb to virtually any type of cell and then to release their contents. Fusion of the liposome and cell membrane may or may not occur. Liposomes may be taken up by phagocytic cells. The efficacy of liposomes as therapeutic agents is, however, limited by their inability to leave the circulatory system and by their clearance by cells of the reticuloendothelial system.

local immunity. Immunological reactions that take place mainly in the gastrointestinal or respiratory tract due to antibodies that are present locally. For example, the GUT-ASSOCIATED LYMPHOID TISSUE can mount a predominant IgA response to ingested antigens.

long-acting thyroid stimulator (LATS). *See* GRAVES' DISEASE.

long homologous repeat. *See* CONSENSUS SEQUENCE OF C3/C4 BINDING PROTEINS.

low-zone tolerance. TOLERANCE induced by very small amounts of protein antigens administered repeatedly.

Lutheran blood group. ANTIGENIC DETERMINANTS of human red blood cells detected by ALLOANTIBODIES to the products of two alleles: Lu^a and Lu^b. The Lutheran antigens have not been biochemically characterized. ALLOIMMUNIZATION of mothers by Lutheran antigens during pregnancy can lead to HEMOLYTIC DISEASE OF THE NEWBORN.

Ly antigen. ALLOANTIGEN found on the surface of mouse lymphocytes. Ly antigens are expressed to variable degrees on T and B LYMPHOCYTES and thymocytes.

Ly1 B cell. Mouse B lymphocyte containing the Ly1 (CD5) antigen on its surface. Ly1 B cells comprise no more than 5–10 percent of all B lymphocytes in the SPLEEN and LYMPH NODES. They are markedly increased in inbred strains of mice with AUTOIMMUNE DISEASES (e.g., NEW ZEALAND MICE). The relationship between Ly1 B cells and the majority of B lymphocytes is not known. *See* CD5.

Lyb. ALLOANTIGEN on the surface of mouse B lymphocytes. The structure and function of these alloantigens is not known. *See* Ly1 B CELL, CBA/N MOUSE.

lymph. Fluid of the lymphatic circulation which contains a variety of leukocytes. Most (80 percent) of the cells in lymph are small LYMPHOCYTES. There is less protein in lymph than in plasma.

lymph node. Small (normally less than 0.5 cm) encapsulated, bean-shaped secondary LYMPHOID organ, containing a mixture of LYMPHOCYTES and ACCESSORY CELLS held together in a loose reticulum, that filters the LYMPH. Lymph nodes are distributed widely throughout the body, often in groups draining a particular anatomical location (e.g. axilla, neck, groin). Lymph enters the node via afferent lymphatics and exits at the hilus via efferent lymphatics to more central lymph nodes and eventually to the THORACIC DUCT. Lymph nodes have an outer domain (cortex) and an inner domain (medulla). The cortex is subdivided into a superficial cortex composed of accumulations of B LYM-

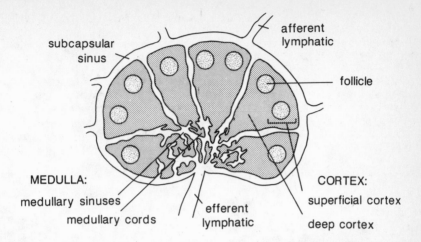

subcapsular sinus

afferent lymphatic

follicle

MEDULLA:
medullary sinuses
medullary cords

efferent
lymphatic

CORTEX:
superficial cortex
deep cortex

lymph node
Modified from Unanue, E.R. and Benacerraf, B. *Textbook of Immunology*, 2nd edition, 1984. Williams and Wilkins, Baltimore, MD.

PHOCYTES called FOLLICLES, and a deep cortex composed of T LYMPHOCYTES in no particular organized pattern of distribution. Antigen comes into the node through the afferent lymphatics and is trapped by phagocytic cells (e.g., MACROPHAGES and FOLLICULAR DENDRITIC CELLS) in the stroma. The stroma of the node is composed of reticulum cells that, in the central portions, form medullary cords and sinuses. T lymphocytes continuously circulate through the nodes; they emerge from the blood at the post-capillary venules in the deep cortex, drain into the medullary sinuses and exit in the efferent lymphatics. PLASMA CELLS are also found abundantly in the medulla. However, if T lymphocytes encounter antigen they are arrested in the lymph node. Immune responses can be initiated in lymph nodes.

True lymph nodes do not occur below the phylogenetic level of mammals. However, clusters of lymphoid cells (e.g., JUGULAR BODIES) that perform a similar function are found in some higher amphibians and birds.

lymphadenitis. Inflammation of LYMPH NODES, usually resulting from bacterial or viral infection.

lymphadenopathy. Abnormality of lymph nodes. The term frequently refers to enlargement of the lymph nodes.

lymphatic. Vessel that carries LYMPH into or out of LYMPH NODES. The lymphatics that

enter the node at its periphery are termed afferent, and those that exit at the hilus of the node are termed efferent. *See* LYMPH NODE.

lymphoblast. Large cell of LYMPHOCYTE lineage that contains a nucleolus and synthesizes DNA. *See* BLAST CELL, LYMPHOCYTE TRANSFORMATION.

lymphocyte. Cell that mediates the specificity of immune responses. Lymphocytes are spherical or ovoid cells, 8–12 µm in diameter. The nucleus is ovoid or indented into a kidney-shape; its chromatin is densely packed and stains intensely blue with most routinely used stains (e.g., Giemsa or Wright). The cytoplasm forms a thin rim around the nucleus and stains light blue; it contains few organelles. By scanning electron microscopy, lymphocytes are seen to have many surface villi covering 70–90 percent of the cell surface. Lymphocytes are divided into two major groups: B and T LYMPHOCYTES. These two groups of cells cannot be distinguished by routine staining or by morphological characteristics; the distinction between them is based on the presence of different surface molecules and on their different roles in immunological reactions. In addition to B and T lymphocytes, there is a small population of large lymphocytes (~15 µm in diameter) that have prominent granules in the cytoplasm – so called large granular lymphocytes – or

NATURAL KILLER CELLS. Lymphocytes of the thymus are called thymocytes. Lymphocytes are the most numerous cell in the body.

lymphocyte function associated antigen-1 (LFA-1, CD11a,18). Membrane glycoprotein of LYMPHOCYTES and PHAGOCYTES. LFA-1 participates in the adherence of CYTOTOXIC T LYMPHOCYTES and NATURAL KILLER CELLS to TARGET CELLS and in other cell–cell interactions. The ligand for LFA-1 on target cells is called INTERCELLULAR ADHESION MOLECULE-1 (ICAM-1). LFA-1 is composed of an alpha chain (M_r 180,000) and a beta chain (M_r 95,000), which is identical to the beta chain of p150,95 and COMPLEMENT RECEPTOR 3. The beta chain is composed of 769 amino acid residues including a signal sequence. There are six sites for N-linked oligosaccharides. The gene for the alpha chain is on chromosome 16 and the gene for the beta chain is on chromosome 21. See LEUKOCYTE ADHESION DEFICIENCY.

lymphocyte function associated antigen-2 (LFA-2). *Synonym for* CD2.

lymphocyte function associated antigen-3 (LFA-3). Cell surface ANTIGEN on all B and T LYMPHOCYTES as well as on MONOCYTES, GRANULOCYTES, PLATELETS, vascular endothelium and fibroblasts. LFA-3 is a single polypeptide chain (M_r 60,000). Mouse monoclonal antibodies to LFA-3, when bound to TARGET CELLS, inhibit cytolysis by CYTOTOXIC T LYMPHOCYTES. LFA-3 has been mapped to human chromosome 1. LFA-3 has recently been shown to be the ligand for CD2.

lymphocyte recirculation. Continuous passage of LYMPHOCYTES from blood to LYMPH NODES and SPLEEN and back to the blood via the LYMPHATICS. Lymphocytes enter the nodes and spleen from the blood; they bind to and traverse the high endothelial cells of the post-capillary venules of lymph nodes or the marginal sinuses of the spleen, and after a day or two exit into the efferent LYMPH. From the lymph, they reenter the blood stream via the THORACIC DUCT. This continuous process allows lymphocytes to sample the lymphoid tissues for antigen. The encounter of T lymphocytes with antigen interrupts the re-circulation; the T lymphocytes remain in the node, proliferate and later re-enter the circulating pool. See MEL-14.

lymphocyte transformation. Change from a small, resting lymphocyte into a large lymphocyte. This change may follow (1) stimulation by antigens or LECTINS or (2) viral infection (e.g. with Epstein–Barr virus, human T cell leukemia virus I). See TRANSFORMATION.

lymphocytic choriomeningitis (LCM). Infection caused by an arenavirus that is endemic in mice and occurs sporadically in humans and household pets. Infection of an immunocompetent host by LCM leads either to immunity or to death from the acute infection. The acute infection is characterized by enlargement of the spleen and lymph nodes and perivascular infiltration by T lymphocytes of all viscera, particularly the brain. Infection of a neonatal or immunosuppressed mouse results in a chronic carrier state. The carriers produce large amounts of anti-viral antibodies that do not eliminate the infection. These mice may develop IMMUNE COMPLEX DISEASE of the renal glomeruli, arterial walls, lungs, liver and heart. Transfer of lymphocytes from an immune donor into a carrier causes death of the carrier. The transferred CYTOTOXIC T LYMPHOCYTES recognize LCM viral antigens on the membranes of cells in the brain and meninges; this leads to severe inflammation and death. The phenomenon of MHC RESTRICTION of cytotoxic T lymphocyte cells was discovered in the LCM system.

lymphocytosis. Increased number of lymphocytes in the blood. See LYMPHOPENIA.

lymphocytotropic. Having an affinity for LYMPHOCYTES. For example, HUMAN IMMUNODEFICIENCY VIRUS and human T CELL LEUKEMIA virus are lymphocytotropic for CD4+ lymphocytes and EPSTEIN–BARR VIRUS is lymphocytotropic for B LYMPHOCYTES.

lymphoid. Referring to LYMPHOCYTES or to tissues that contain large accumulations of lymphocytes (e.g., SPLEEN, LYMPH NODES, THYMUS).

lymphokine. Polypeptide (but not an immunoglobulin) secreted by LYMPHOCYTES that affects the functions of other cells. There are many lymphokines and they have a wide range of biological activity. The first lymphokine to be studied was the MIGRATION INHIBITORY FACTOR (MIF). Well-characterized lymphokines include INTERLEUKIN-2, INTERLEUKIN-3, INTERFERON-GAMMA, INTERLEUKIN-4 and INTERLEUKIN-5. *See* MONOKINE, CYTOKINE.

lymphoma. Malignant tumor of LYMPHOCYTES (e.g., BURKITT'S LYMPHOMA, HODGKIN'S DISEASE).

lymphomatoid granulomatosis. Distinctive, usually fatal, VASCULITIS of the lung of unknown cause. All types of pulmonary blood vessels are infiltrated by atypical LYMPHOCYTES and PLASMA CELLS, which exhibit frequent mitoses. Cavities form in the lung. Nodular vasculitis occurs less frequently in the skin, kidneys and nervous system.

lymphomatosis. Multiple LYMPHOMAS in various parts of the body. Lymphomatosis occurs in HODGKIN'S DISEASE, avian leukosis, etc.

lymphopenia. Decreased number of LYMPHOCYTES in the blood. *See* LYMPHOCYTOSIS.

lymphotoxin (LT). Protein secreted by activated T LYMPHOCYTES or lymphoid cell lines that have CYTOLYTIC and/or cytostatic properties for susceptible tumor cells or tissue culture cell lines, particularly the mouse fibroblast line L-929. LT is secreted following stimulation of T lymphocytes by antigen or MITOGEN. It kills TARGET CELLS more slowly than do intact CYTOTOXIC T LYMPHOCYTES. Human LT is a protein of 205 amino acid residues, including a signal sequence of 34 residues; it has one site for an N-LINKED OLIGOSACCHARIDE (asparagine at position 62). Mouse LT is composed of 202 amino acid residues, including a signal sequence of 33 residues; it has one site for an N-linked oligosaccharide (asparagine at position 60). Human and mouse LT have 74 percent amino acid sequence identity.

It has been proposed that lymphotoxin has a role in target cell damage by cytotoxic T lymphocytes, but this has not been clearly established. Target cells, which are killed by

LT, do not have pores in their membranes, such as those induced by PERFORIN or COMPLEMENT. Susceptible target cells bind LT with high affinity ($K_d \sim 1.5 \times 10^{-10}$ M) and internalize it. Even though receptor binding of LT occurs at 4°C, LT kills target cells at 37°C by disrupting unknown metabolic processes.

LT is approximately 30 percent identical in amino acid sequence to TUMOR NECROSIS FACTOR (TNF). The gene for LT has been mapped to the MAJOR HISTOCOMPATIBILITY COMPLEX of mouse chromosome 17 and human chromosome 6. The gene encoding LT is closely linked to the gene encoding TNF; they are separated by approximately 1,100 nucleotides. LT has also been called TNFβ while tumor necrosis factor has been called TNFα.

Lyon effect. Random inactivation, early in development, of most of the gene loci on one of the two X chromosomes in each somatic cell of female mammals. This inactivated state persists stably in all the cell's descendants and can lead to mosaicism of traits encoded by genes on the X chromosome; the inactive chromosome appears as heterochromatin (condensed chromatin) and this heterochromatin is known as a Barr body. The effect was discovered by and named after Mary Lyon, a British cytogeneticist.

lysin. Substance (e.g. bacterial toxins, antibodies plus COMPLEMENT) that brings about cell LYSIS. At one time, it was thought that only a particular type of antibody had the capability of sensitizing cells for complement-dependent lysis, but it is now known that many antibodies have this capability, providing that they can fix complement.

lysis. Dissolution of cells. In immunology, lysis usually refers to destruction of cells by ANTIBODIES and COMPLEMENT or by CYTOTOXIC T LYMPHOCYTES. *See* MEMBRANE ATTACK COMPLEX.

lysogen. Bacterium carrying, in stable form, a complete set of bacteriophage genes. The phage DNA in the bacterium is called a prophage. Usually, as in the case of LAMBDA BACTERIOPHAGE, the prophage is integrated into the bacterial chromosome. Sometimes, however, as in *E. coli* phage P1, the phage genes are carried as a plasmid. In a lysogen, expression of most of the phage genes is prevented by a phage-specific repressor protein. When a lysogen carrying an integrated prophage is induced by various environmental changes, the repressor is inactivated and a lytic cycle is initiated. The prophage is excised as a single segment of DNA, which replicates and produces active phage particles.

lysozyme (muramidase; peptidoglycan *N*-acetylmuramoylhydrolase; EC 3.2.1.17). Enzyme that hydrolyses the β-1,4 glycosidic bond between *N*-acetylmuramic acid and *N*-acetylglucosamine in the peptidoglycan (mucopeptide) of bacterial cell walls, leading to the osmotic lysis of bacteria. The usual turbidometric assay for lysozyme measures the decrease in absorbance of a suspension of *Micrococcus luteus*. With Gram-negative bacteria, the outer membrane must be disrupted (e.g., by treatment with EDTA) to allow access of lysozyme to the underlying peptidoglycan layer. Lysozyme can potentiate the action of antibodies and COMPLEMENT on Gram-negative bacteria. It also enhances the phagocytic activity of MONONUCLEAR PHAGOCYTES and POLYMORPHONUCLEAR LEUKOCYTES.

Lysozyme is widely distributed, being found in bacteriophage, bacteria, fungi, plants, invertebrates and vertebrates. Four distinct classes of lysozyme have been described: (1) chicken-type lysozyme, typified by the enzyme from hen eggs (129 amino acid residues; M_r 14,000); (2) goose-type lysozyme, found in nine different orders of birds (185 amino acid residues; M_r 21,000); (3) phage-type lysozyme, described in T4, T2, and P22 bacteriophage (164 amino acid residues; M_r 18,700); (4) a bacterial lysozyme produced by *Streptomyces erythraeus*. The amino acid sequences of lysozymes within one of these families are clearly related, but there is no significant overall homology among members of different families. However, similarities in the three-dimensional structure of the first three classes of lysozyme are consistent with the hypothesis that these enzymes have evolved from a common ancestor.

In vertebrates, lysozyme is found particularly in egg white, tears, saliva and mucus; it is also secreted by mononuclear phagocytes and is found in plasma. The mammalian lysozymes that have been characterized belong to the chicken-type lysozyme family. Lysozyme was the first protein to have both its amino acid sequence and three-dimensional structure determined. It has been used as a model antigen in many immunological studies.

Lyt. ALLOANTIGEN on the surface of mouse T LYMPHOCYTES. Since many Lyt antigens are found also on the surface of B LYMPHOCYTES, the term Ly is preferred for those also found on B lymphocytes. Lyt 2 and Lyt 3 are two polypeptide chains of mouse CD8.

M

M cell. Epithelial cell of the gastrointestinal tract that transports macromolecules and microorganisms (e.g., viruses) from the lumen to the underlying Peyer's patches (*see* GUT-ASSOCIATED LYMPHOID TISSUE). M cells have broad apical surfaces with short microvilli. Macromolecules and microorganisms bind to the microvilli, are taken up into COATED PITS and are transported to the basolateral surface (*see* ENDOCYTOSIS). The basolateral surfaces are deeply invaginated and the invaginations are filled with LYMPHOCYTES and MONONUCLEAR PHAGOCYTES. Substances, transported through M cells, are exposed on the basolateral surfaces, where they can be sampled by lymphoid cells, and presumably, initiate an IMMUNE RESPONSE.

M13 bacteriophage. Filamentous bacteriophage of *E. coli* containing a single-stranded circular DNA molecule 6,407 nucleotides in length. M13 is a male-specific phage; only strains of bacteria harboring F pili are infected. When viral DNA enters the bacterial host cell, it is converted to a double-stranded replicative form (RF). The RF multiplies rapidly until there are about 100 RF molecules per cell. Replication of the RF then becomes asymmetric; only one of the two DNA strands is produced in large amount and this becomes complexed to a single-strand-specific DNA binding protein. As the DNA single strands are released from the cell, the DNA binding protein is replaced by a capsid protein. Phage particles – as many as 1,000 per cell per generation – are extruded from infected cells into the medium. Replication of phage DNA does not result in lysis of the host cell. Instead, infected cells continue to grow and divide, although more slowly than uninfected cells. The inhibition in growth of infected cells leads to the appearance of turbid plaques on a bacterial lawn.

M13 bacteriophage have been widely used as cloning VECTORS. A major advantage is that the DNA can be obtained easily either in the single-stranded or double-stranded form. The double-stranded replicative form (isolated from the bacterial cell) can be used just like plasmid DNA to make recombinants *in vitro*; the single-stranded DNA (from phage particles) can be used directly as template for DNA sequencing by the dideoxy-chain termination method. Another advantage of filamentous phages like M13 is that they are not fixed in length and can accommodate variable amounts of DNA; this flexibility is very useful in a cloning vector. A large number of vectors based on M13 have been developed.

macroglobulin. High molecular weight (M_r >400,000) GLOBULIN (e.g., IgM, alpha-2 macroglobulin).

macroglobulinemia of Waldenström. Form of MYELOMATOSIS occurring mainly in elderly males and characterized by MONOCLONAL IgM in the serum. In contrast to MULTIPLE MYELOMA, skeletal lesions do not occur. The bone marrow contains increased numbers of lymphoid cells and plasmacytoid lymphocytes, which contain cytoplasmic IgM. The elevated levels of IgM in blood increase its relative viscosity; symptoms of circulatory failure appear when the relative viscosity increases more than approximately fourfold. Anemia, cutaneous hemorrhages and diverse neurological symptoms are the most common manifestations of macroglobulinemia. Macroglobulinemia of Waldenström is a more benign disease than multiple myeloma.

macrophage. Highly differentiated MONONUCLEAR PHAGOCYTE found in various tissues.

Macrophages are more mature than MONO-CYTES.

macrophage-activating factor (MAF). LYMPHOKINE that activates MACROPHAGES. The major MAF is INTERFERON-GAMMA.

major histocompatibility complex (MHC). Chromosomal region containing genes that encode cell surface glycoproteins that regulate interactions among cells of the immune system. These genes were discovered because of their role in immunologic rejection of grafts. The MHC typically contains genes encoding CLASS I HISTOCOMPATIBILITY MOLECULES and CLASS II HISTOCOMPATIBILITY MOLECULES, which are important for the growth and differentiation of B and T LYMPHOCYTES, ANTIGEN PRESENTATION, CYTOTOXICITY, GRAFT REJECTION and MIXED LYMPHOCYTE REACTIONS. The genes encoding these molecules are the most highly polymorphic (*see* POLYMORPHISM) genes known. The MHC also contains genes encoding proteins that are not cell surface glycoproteins; CLASS III MOLECULES (components of the COMPLEMENT system (C2, C4 and FACTOR B) and P-450 cytochrome 21-hydroxylase), TUMOR NECROSIS FACTOR and LYMPHOTOXIN. An MHC has been identified in anuran amphibians, birds and mammals. The best studied MHCs are those of mice and humans. In mice the MHC consists of the H-2 complex and occupies 0.5-1 centiMorgan of chromosome 17. In humans the MHC consists of the HLA complex and occupies about 1.5–2.0 centiMorgans of the short arm of chromosome 6.

Mantoux test. Test for CELL-MEDIATED IMMUNITY to tuberculosis in which TUBERCULIN is injected intradermally.

marginal sinus. *See* SPLEEN.

mast cell. Cell found in connective tissues, especially around blood vessels and under mucosal surfaces, characterized by the presence of numerous basophilic granules. Mast cells are important in mediating IMMEDIATE HYPERSENSITIVITY reactions. Mast cells have Fc receptors for IgE (*see* Fcε RECEPTORS). Cross-linking by antigen of IgE bound to Fc receptors triggers the release of granules

from mast cells. Other methods of cross-linking the Fcε receptors (e.g., by anti-IgE, anti-idiotype or antibody to the receptor) also trigger granule release. The granules contain preformed mediators of immediate hypersensitivity: HISTAMINE and/or SEROTONIN (depending on the species), several enzymes (e.g., hexosaminidase, aryl sulphatase, glucuronidase, chymotrypsin, trypsin-like protease) and chemotactic factors for EOSINOPHILS and NEUTROPHILS. Cross-linking of Fcε receptors also induces the synthesis and release of LEUKOTRIENES, PROSTAGLANDINS and PLATELET-ACTIVATING FACTOR. The release of granules is an energy-dependent reaction that requires Ca^{2+}. Biochemical events that accompany mediator release include activation of adenylate cyclase, resulting in a rapid burst of cyclic AMP synthesis, activation of a protein kinase, methylation of phospholipids and activation of a serine esterase.

In addition, mast cells of the gastrointestinal and respiratory mucosa contain chondroitin sulfate; they synthesize and release mainly leukotriene C_4. Mast cells in connective tissue contain heparin; they synthesize and release mainly prostaglandin D_2.

mast cell growth factor-1. *Synonym for* INTERLEUKIN-3.

mast cell growth factor-2. *Synonym for* INTERLEUKIN-4.

Masugi nephritis. GLOMERULONEPHRITIS induced in experimental animals by injection of antibodies to the glomerular basement membrane. Antibodies are produced in one species by immunization with basement membranes from kidneys of the species of the prospective recipient (e.g., rats develop glomerulonephritis when injected with rabbit antibodies to rat glomerular basement membrane). The antibodies circulate briefly, bind to the glomeruli and produce injury, with an increase in glomerular permeability and infiltration of NEUTROPHILS and MONOCYTES. Masugi nephritis has been used extensively to study the mechanism of tissue injury induced by antibodies. GOODPASTURE'S SYNDROME, an autoimmune disease of humans, resembles Masugi nephritis.

maternal immunity. IMMUNITY acquired passively by a newborn from its mother (e.g., by ingestion of COLOSTRUM or transplacental passage of ANTIBODIES). Maternal immunity, is, in fact, PASSIVE IMMUNITY of the neonate and not immunity in mothers.

maturation of affinity. Progressive increase in the AFFINITY of antibodies that often occurs after IMMUNIZATION.

Mcg isotypic determinant. ANTIGENIC DETERMINANT of human IMMUNOGLOBULIN LAMBDA CHAINS, associated with asparagine at position 112, threonine at position 114, and lysine at position 163 (see Table in definition of immunoglobulin lambda chains). This determinant is present on some of the lambda chains of every individual. It is, therefore, not the result of genetic POLYMORPHISM.

McLeod phenotype. Absence of Kell or Cellano ANTIGENS (see KELL–CELLANO BLOOD GROUP) on red blood cells. The red blood cells appear under the microscope to have spikes or burrs (acanthocytes). The *Xk* gene, which encodes a precursor of the Kell or Cellano antigens, is closely linked to the gene for CHRONIC GRANULOMATOUS DISEASE on the short arm of the X chromosome. Hence, deletion in this chromosomal region (Xp21) may result in the McLeod phenotype and chronic granulomatous disease.

M-component. *See* MONOCLONAL GAMMOPATHY.

megakaryocyte. Very large cells (35–160 μm in diameter) of the BONE MARROW, from which PLATELETS are derived. The cytoplasm of megakaryocytes forms filamentous arms that break up into platelets.

MEL-14. Rat monoclonal antibody that recognizes an ANTIGENIC DETERMINANT, gp90MEL-14, of a surface glycoprotein of LYMPH NODE lymphocytes in mice. MEL-14 blocks the binding of these lymphocytes to post-capillary venules. gp90MEL-14 appears to be the homing receptor of lymphocytes that migrate preferentially to the lymph nodes rather than to the GUT-ASSOCIATED LYMPHOID TISSUE.

melphalan. (l-phenylalanine mustard). Nitrogen mustard used for the treatment of MULTIPLE MYELOMA.

melphalan

membrane attack complex (MAC). Amphiphilic macromolecular complex composed of one molecule each of C5b, C6, C7 and C8 and 12 or more molecules of C9. MAC formation is the end result of activation by the CLASSICAL PATHWAY or the ALTERNATIVE PATHWAY of COMPLEMENT. The MAC inserts into the membrane of TARGET CELLS and kills them.

When C5 is cleaved by C5 CONVERTASES, the C5b, which is formed, has a metastable binding site for C6 and C7. Complexes of C5b, C6 and C7 appear, under the electron microscope, like a leaf on a stalk, the leaf being composed of C5b and the stalk of C6 and C7. These complexes are embedded in the target cell membrane without inflicting any damage. C8 then binds to the C5b67 complex; a transmembrane channel (pore) is formed, 3 nm in diameter. The C5b678 complex can cause LYSIS of target cells, albeit very slowly. The process of lysis is rapidly accelerated, in the presence of Ca^{2+}, Mg^{2+} or Zn^{2+}, by the polymerization of C9 on C5b678 complexes. Polymerized C9 forms a cylindrical structure, 16 nm in height, with an internal diameter of 10 nm; the wall of the cylinder is 2 nm thick. The top of the cylinder is hydrophilic and is capped by a ring or an annulus, which remains outside the target cells; the other end of the cylinder is lipophilic, becomes embedded in the target cell and forms transmembrane channels. This causes a micellar rearrangement of the lipid bilayer; the pores coalesce into so-called 'leaky patches'. The target cell loses potassium, imbibes sodium and water, swells and bursts (lyses). The entire series of events leading to lysis is non-enzymatic. S PROTEIN inhibits MAC formation.

membrane immunoglobulin. Immunoglobulin that is inserted into a cell membrane and that may function as a receptor for antigen. Membrane IgM and membrane IgD are expressed on unstimulated B LYMPHOCYTES. After the B cell interacts with antigen, the cell differentiates into a PLASMA CELL, which actively secretes IgM. The switch from membrane to secreted IgM is accompanied by an

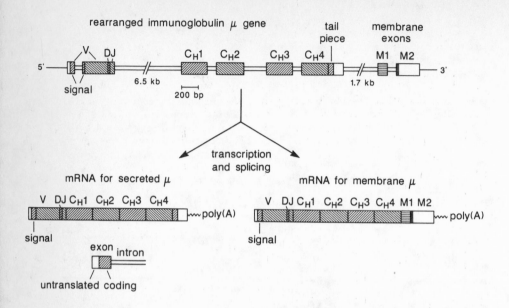

increase in the synthesis of J CHAIN. Secreted IgM is a pentamer (five four-chain units), whereas membrane-bound IgM is a monomer (a single four-chain unit). Presumably, all immunoglobulins exist in a membrane form (mIg) as well as a secreted form (sIg). Membrane immunoglobulins of the IgG and IgA classes are thought to function as antigen receptors on memory B lymphocytes. The portion of the immunoglobulin that is inserted into the membrane is a hydrophobic segment of the heavy chain near its carboxy-terminus; there is no known difference in the light chains of membrane and secreted immunoglobulins.

Information about the heavy chains of membrane immunoglobulins has been derived mainly by analysis of the genes encoding these chains. For a given ISOTYPE, the membrane form of the heavy chain is longer than the secreted form, the two differing at their carboxy-terminal ends. The two forms of heavy chain are encoded by different mRNA species that are derived from a single gene. It is thought that competition between splicing of the CH4-M1 intron and polyadenylation at a site within this intron determines which of the two mRNAs is produced. The transcript for the membrane-bound chain is longer than that for the secreted chains and includes sequences from one or two EXONS that encode the carboxy-terminal portion that is specific for

the membrane form. (Usually there are two such exons but, in the case of the mouse alpha chain, there is only one.) This longer transcript is processed so that the termination site of the mRNA for the secreted form is removed and the terminal C_H exon is spliced to the first membrane exon.

Analysis of a number of genes encoding membrane-associated heavy chains has revealed that the carboxy-terminal segments, which are unique to the membrane forms of the heavy chains range in length from 41 amino acid residues (mouse and human membrane mu chain (*see* IMMUNOGLOBULIN MU CHAIN)) to 72 residues (mouse membrane epsilon chain). These segments can be divided into three regions: (1) an acidic spacer (12–26 amino acid residues) at the amino-terminal end, which connects the terminal C_H domain to the transmembrane segment; this spacer is thought to be external to the membrane; (2) a hydrophobic transmembrane segment consisting of 26 amino acid residues, which presumably spans the lipid bilayer; this segment is highly conserved in mouse and human membrane heavy chains; (3) a hydrophilic carboxy-terminal segment (3–28 residues), which is thought to lie in the cytoplasm and which may communicate external signals to intracellular structures.

membranoproliferative glomerulonephritis (MPGN). Form of IMMUNE COMPLEX DIS-EASE of the renal glomerulus that usually progresses to renal failure. Glomeruli have enlarged lobules due to an increase in the number of cells. Subendothelial deposits contain C3, IgG and to a lesser extent IgM and IgA as detected by IMMUNOFLUORESCENCE. In a variant of MPGN, electron-dense deposits are found in the basement membrane of the glomerulus, so-called dense deposit disease. MPGN is presumed to have an immunological cause. See GLOMERULONEPHRITIS.

6-mercaptopurine (6-MP). Analogue of hypoxanthine in which the 6-hydroxyl group is replaced by 6-thiol. 6-MP is a substrate for the enzyme hypoxanthine–guanine phosphoribosyl-transferase (HGPRT); it converts 6-MP to 6-thioinosine-5'-phosphate, which inhibits several vital metabolic reactions of purines. In addition 6-MP is incorporated into DNA in the form of thioguanine. 6-MP is used in cancer chemotherapy and for IMMUNOSUP-PRESSION.

6-mercaptopurine

metaproterenol (*dl*-β-[3,5-dihydroxyphenyl]-α-isopropylaminoethanol). Beta-adrenergic amine that relaxes smooth muscle, particularly of the bronchi. It is used in the treatment of ASTHMA.

metaproterenol

methotrexate (*N*-[*p*-[[(2,4-diamino-6-pteridinyl) methyl]methylamino]benzoyl] glutamic acid). Folic acid analogue that binds to folate reductase and competitively inhibits conversion of dihydrofolate to tetra-hydrofolate, thereby inhibiting thymidine synthesis. It is used in cancer chemotherapy and for IMMUNOSUPPRESSION, particularly for the suppression of GRAFT-*VERSUS*-HOST DISEASE following BONE MARROW transplantation.

methotrexate

MHC class I deficiency. Form of SEVERE COMBINED IMMUNODEFICIENCY associated with absence of CLASS I HISTOCOMPATIBILITY MOLECULES on membranes of LYMPHOCYTES. The deficiency is inherited as an autosomal recessive trait. B LYMPHOCYTES from patients do express class I molecules when they are transformed.

MHC class II deficiency. Form of COMBINED IMMUNODEFICIENCY associated with absence of CLASS II HISTOCOMPATIBILITY MOLECULES on membranes of LYMPHOCYTES and MONOCYTES. The deficiency has been observed mainly in children from North Africa. It is inherited as an autosomal recessive trait. Transformed B LYMPHOCYTES from patients do not contain mRNA transcripts of any alpha or beta genes of the HLA-D REGION. Synthesis of BETA-2 MICROGLOBULIN and the I INVARIANT chain is normal. The amount of class I expression on lymphocytes and monocytes is also decreased. Patients have AGAMMAGLO-BULINEMIA, normal numbers of B and T lymphocytes in the circulation and a decrease in CELL-MEDIATED IMMUNITY. Diarrhea with intestinal malabsorption is the most prominent symptom observed in these patients.

The genetic defect does not map to the major histocompatibility locus. It may result from the failure of binding of a protein to the upstream promoter region of the class II histocompatibility genes.

MHC restriction. Phenomenon in which the interaction of T LYMPHOCYTES with antigen presenting cells (see ANTIGEN PRESENTATION) or with TARGET CELLS is restricted by histocompatibility molecules. CD4+ T lymphocytes proliferate when they recognize antigen presented by self CLASS II HISTOCOMPATIBILITY MOLECULES; CD8+ T lymphocytes kill target cells when they recognize antigen in association with self CLASS I HISTOCOMPATIBILITY MOLECULES. In an F_1 of two INBRED STRAINS, two distinct sets of T lymphocytes are found, each restricted by the histocompatibility molecules of one or the other parent. MHC restriction develops during maturation of lymphocytes in THYMUS where thymocytes first encounter histocompatibility molecules on the thymic stromal cells. *Synonym for* linked recognition.

mid-piece. Obsolete term for the COMPLEMENT components found in the EUGLOBULIN fraction of SERUM. It is now known that this fraction contains all of the C1, no C2, and some of the remaining complement components. *See* END-PIECE.

migration inhibitory factor (MIF). LYMPHOKINE that inhibits the movement of MONOCYTES and MACROPHAGES. A test for MIF is carried out by placing a capillary tube containing macrophages, usually from peritoneal exudates, in a culture dish. During incubation, the macrophages move out of the tube, and the extent of migration can be estimated by measuring the area occupied by the cells. Addition of a culture supernatant from activated T LYMPHOCYTES, containing MIF, reduces the area of migration usually by 25–75 percent. INTERFERON-GAMMA has MIF activity, but it is not clear whether there are additional proteins with this property. The MIF test became popular as a test to measure CELL-MEDIATED IMMUNITY, but it has largely been superseded by more direct and quantitative assays. The biological significance of MIF is not known; perhaps it serves to minimize the migration of cells out of areas of immune reactivity.

minor histocompatibility antigen. Transplantation antigen that is not encoded in the major histocompatibility locus (*see* MINOR HISTOCOMPATIBILITY LOCUS). Each minor histocompatibility antigen plays a weak role in GRAFT REJECTION, but since there are many such antigens (~50), their aggregate effect may be considerable. *See* H-Y, SKIN SPECIFIC HISTOCOMPATIBILITY ANTIGEN.

minor histocompatibility locus. Genetic locus encoding an antigen that provokes a relatively weak immunological response to grafts. The response is weak compared to the response to antigens encoded by the MAJOR HISTOCOMPATIBILITY COMPLEX because there are fewer CYTOTOXIC T LYMPHOCYTE precursors specific for the minor antigens. Typically, grafts transplanted across a single minor histocompatibility difference are rejected slowly, i.e., in more than three weeks, rather than one to two weeks for grafts transplanted across a single difference in the major histocompatibility complex.

However, the effects of differences in minor antigens can be cumulative, so that many differences may result in rapid graft rejection. In contrast to products of the major histocompatibility complex, which can be recognized by T LYMPHOCYTES and serve as restricting elements in recognition of foreign antigens, minor histocompatibility antigens are recognized by T lymphocytes only in the context of major histocompatibility complex molecules. The molecular nature and function of the minor histocompatibility antigens are not known; they are probably membrane-bound and are usually present in a number of tissues. It is difficult to produce antibodies to minor histocompatibility antigens and they cannot usually be detected by serological assays. In contrast to the major histocompatibility complex-associated antigens, the minor antigens are not highly polymorphic (*see* POLYMORPHISM). *See* H-Y.

mitogen. Substance that induces mitosis of cells. As used by immunologists, the term refers to substances that induce TRANSFORMATION of diverse (polyclonal) lymphocytes. Some LECTINS (e.g., phytohemagglutinin) transform T LYMPHOCYTES; other lectins (e.g., pokeweed) transform both T and B LYMPHOCYTES. LIPOPOLYSACCHARIDES transform mouse, but not human, B lymphocytes.

mixed connective tissue disease. Disease in which patients have clinical features of SYSTEMIC LUPUS ERYTHEMATOSUS, SYSTEMIC SCLEROSIS and POLYMYOSITIS. Patients have high serum titers of ANTINUCLEAR ANTIBODY, with specificity for nuclear ribonucleoproteins.

mixed lymphocyte culture (MLC). *See* MIXED LYMPHOCYTE REACTION.

mixed lymphocyte reaction (MLR). Reaction that takes place upon culture of two sets of ALLOGENEIC leukocytes. The HELPER T LYMPHOCYTES (mouse or human CD4-bearing T cells) in either set recognize allogeneic CLASS II HISTOCOMPATIBILITY MOLECULES of the other set and undergo proliferation and differentiation, releasing a variety of LYMPHOKINES. In the 'one-way MLR', one set of cells is irradiated or treated with inhibitors of DNA synthesis and the cells therefore serve only as stimulators to the helper T lymphocytes in the other set. The mixed lymphocyte reaction is important in transplantation biology to study differences in histocompatibility antigens between donor and recipient. The degree of T cell proliferation, measured by the incorporation of [³H]-thymidine into DNA gives an estimate of the degree of HISTOINCOMPATIBILITY.

MNSs blood group. ANTIGENIC DETERMINANTS of the glycophorins of human red blood cell membranes detected by ALLOANTIBODIES. Red blood cell membranes have two types of glycophorins: glycophorin A (M_r 31,000) and glycophorin B (M_r 11,000). Glycophorin A bears the M (serine at position 1 and glycine at position 5) or the N (leucine at position 1 and glutamic acid at position 5) ALLOANTIGENS. Glycophorin B bears the S (methionine at position 29) or the s (threonine at position 29) alloantigens. The *MN* alleles and *Ss* alleles are on chromosome 4 and are linked. ALLOIMMUNIZATION by MNSs alloantigens can cause HEMOLYTIC DISEASE OF THE NEWBORN.

molecular hybridization probe. Nucleic acid molecule that is made detectable by a labeling procedure (e.g., radiolabeling, fluorescent labeling) and that is used to detect nucleic acid molecules of complementary sequence by molecular hybridization.

molecular mimicry. Sharing of an ANTIGENIC DETERMINANT by mammalian cells and microorganisms. For example, the M protein of streptococci shares antigenic determinants with membranes of human heart cells.

monoclonal. Related to or derived from a single CLONE.

monoclonal antibody. Antibody derived from a CLONE of B LYMPHOCYTES. Usually a monoclonal antibody is obtained from a B LYMPHOCYTE HYBRIDOMA, which is a clone from a single B lymphocyte that was fused with a myeloma cell. Monoclonal antibodies are therefore homogeneous in structure. These antibodies are useful in structural studies and immunoassays (e.g., amino acid sequence analysis of antibodies, identification of single antigens in complex mixtures, identification of cell surface molecules, and measurement of drugs and hormones). *See* MONOCLONAL IMMUNOGLOBULIN, POLYCLONAL ANTIBODIES.

monoclonal gammopathy. Presence in serum of a MONOCLONAL IMMUNOGLOBULIN (sometimes called 'M-component'), as in MULTIPLE MYELOMA, MACROGLOBULINEMIA OF WALDENSTRÖM, BENIGN MONOCLONAL GAMMOPATHY and certain other diseases.

monoclonal immunoglobulin. IMMUNOGLOBULIN that is the product of a CLONE of B LYMPHOCYTES or plasma cells (e.g., MYELOMA PROTEIN, MONOCLONAL ANTIBODY).

monocyte. Circulating immature cell of the MONONUCLEAR PHAGOCYTE lineage. Monocytes are considered to be more immature than MACROPHAGES because their cytoplasm contains fewer organelles and enzymes, their membranes have fewer receptors, and they are less active in pinocytosis.

monogamous bivalency. ANTIGEN–ANTIBODY COMPLEXES in which each BIVALENT antibody molecule combines with two determinant groups on a single antigen molecule or particle, rather than cross-linking two different antigen molecules or particles. Such monogamous binding requires that the antigens have repeating determinants that are suitably spaced to accommodate both Fab arms (*see* Fab FRAGMENT) of a single antibody molecule. If this requirement is met, binding of the first Fab arm places the second Fab arm in a favorable position for forming the second bond. The FUNCTIONAL AFFINITY of such interactions is very high; therefore, these binary complexes are extremely stable. A similar situation may occur if a single IgM antibody binds to several determinants on a multivalent antigen particle; this would be 'monogamous multivalency'.

monokine. Polypeptide, secreted by monocytes and macrophages, that affects the functions of other cells (e.g., INTERLEUKIN-1, TUMOR NECROSIS FACTOR). *See* LYMPHOKINE, CYTOKINE.

mononuclear phagocyte. Widely distributed cell characterized by its high rate of uptake of soluble and particulate materials (*see* PHAGOCYTOSIS). Mononuclear phagocytes derive from stem cells found in large numbers in the bone marrow and in other tissues. The young differentiated cells in this lineage are monocytes, which circulate in blood for 24–48 hours. The fully differentiated cells are macrophages, which are found in different tissues usually in a perivascular distribution. Monocytes and macrophages do not proliferate. Macrophages of liver are known as Küppfer cells, those in the central nervous system as microglia, those in the lung alveoli as alveolar macrophages and those in the connective tissue as histiocytes. Macrophages derive from stem cells found in the tissues and from the migration of blood monocytes. The contribution of one or the other source appears to vary among different tissues. The localization of macrophages to sites of inflammation results mostly from the emigration of blood monocytes. The multiplication of the stem cells is regulated by COLONY STIMULATING FACTOR-1 (CSF-1) a specific mitogen that is abundantly secreted in cultures of fibroblasts.

Mononuclear phagocytes have receptors for carbohydrate (mannose and fucose), for the heavy chains of IgG and IgE (Fcγ and Fcε RECEPTORS), for C3 (COMPLEMENT RECEPTOR 1 and COMPLEMENT RECEPTOR 3) and for denatured proteins. Through these receptors they are able to bind proteins, cells and microorganisms. Monocytes and macrophages express CLASS II HISTOCOMPATIBILITY MOLECULES and can serve as antigen-presenting cells. Expression of these molecules is in part stimulated by INTERFERON-GAMMA, a LYMPHOKINE produced by activated T LYMPHOCYTES. Mononuclear phagocytes secrete a wide range of molecules such as eicosanoids (e.g., PROSTAGLANDINS, thromboxane and LEUKOTRIENES), complement proteins (C2, C3, C4 and FACTOR B), enzymes (e.g., LYSOZYME, collagenase, elastase) and CYTOKINES (e.g., INTERLEUKIN-1, TUMOR NECROSIS FACTOR, INTERLEUKIN-6). Many of these molecules are only released following stimulation by microbial products (e.g., lipopolysaccharide) or lymphokines.

Monocytes and macrophages participate in immunity by presenting antigen (*see* ANTIGEN PRESENTATION) to T lymphocytes and in host defense after activation by lymphokines (*see* ACTIVATED MACROPHAGES).

monospecific antiserum. ANTISERUM containing antibodies against only one antigen or antigenic determinant.

monovalent. *Synonym for* UNIVALENT.

monovalent antiserum. *Synonym for* MONOSPECIFIC ANTISERUM.

moth-eaten mouse. Mouse of a mutant strain (me/me) derived from the INBRED STRAIN, C57BL/6J, characterized by patchy loss of hair, susceptibility to infection and AUTOIMMUNE DISEASE. Moth-eaten mice develop POLYCLONAL HYPERGAMMAGLOBULINEMIA, impaired CELL-MEDIATED IMMUNITY and an autoimmune disease, characterized by deposition of immune complexes in the kidney.

MRL/1pr mouse. Mouse of a mutant strain, characterized by profound changes in LYMPHOID tissues. MRL/1pr mice have marked hyperplasia (excess tissue formation) of all lymphoid organs, produce multiple AUTOANTIBODIES and deposit immune complexes in the kidney. The lymphoid hyperplasia is due to a proliferating cell derived from the thymus that bears little Thy-1 and no L3T4 (*see* CD4) or Lyt2,3 (*see* CD8).

mu heavy chain disease. Form of MYELOMATOSIS, characterized by the presence in serum of abnormal MONOCLONAL IMMUNOGLOBULIN MU CHAINS and in urine of BENCE-JONES PROTEIN. Mu chain disease is a rare complication of CHRONIC LYMPHOCYTIC LEUKEMIA or of reticulum cell sarcoma. PLASMA CELLS, found in the bone marrow, produce immunoglobulin mu chains with extensive deletions and IMMUNOGLOBULIN LIGHT CHAINS. The deletions in the mu chains are variable in location but usually start near the beginning of the variable region and extend through the C_H1 domain with resumption of the normal sequence in the C_H2 domain.

mucocutaneous lymph node syndrome. *Synonym for* KAWASAKI'S DISEASE.

multiple myeloma. Malignant disease of PLASMA CELLS occurring most frequently in elderly men. Widespread tumors of plasma cells usually develop in bone marrow and cause destruction of bone. Myeloma cells usually secrete MONOCLONAL IMMUNOGLOBULIN (myeloma protein) of the IgG, IgA, IgE or IgD class and/or BENCE-JONES PROTEIN. The frequency distribution of immunoglobulin classes found in multiple myeloma is the same as the relative concentration of the immunoglobulin classes in normal serum. In very rare cases, a patient may have two myeloma proteins, derived from a single clone, and differing only in their heavy chain CONSTANT REGIONS. Presumably this occurs because the cell that became transformed was in the process of switching from the production of one immunoglobulin class to production of another class (*see* CLASS SWITCHING). More frequently, two or more unrelated myeloma proteins are produced as a result of TRANSFORMATION of two or more distinct plasma cells. Patients with multiple myeloma frequently have impaired B LYMPHOCYTE function and susceptibility to infection with pyogenic organisms (*see* PYOGENIC INFECTIONS).

multivalent. Having more than two binding sites. *See* UNIVALENT, BIVALENT.

multivalent antiserum. ANTISERUM containing antibodies against more than two antigens.

muramyl dipeptide (MDP, *N*-acetylmuramyl-L-alanyl-D-isoglutamine). Synthetic peptide that can replace killed mycobacteria in COMPLETE FREUND'S ADJUVANT in the induction of antibodies and cell-mediated immunity. A number of derivatives of MDP have also been shown to have adjuvant activity. Some of these derivatives may be suitable for use in human vaccination.

mutant. Descriptive of a MUTATION (adjective). Gene, protein, cell or individual bearing a mutation (noun).

mutation. Heritable change in the genome of an organism. Mutations are alterations in the sequence of DNA; they may occur either in germ cells or somatic cells. A mutation occurring in a germ cell can be inherited by subsequent generations; a mutation in a somatic cell is inherited in the descendents produced by mitotic division of that cell. Mutations range from changes in a single base pair (point mutation) to gross changes in a chromosome (e.g., duplication, translocation, inversion, deletion). Point mutations in the DNA encoding a protein may not be expressed (because of ambiguity in the genetic code) or they may result in an amino acid substitution (missense mutation) or in chain termination (nonsense mutation). The insertion or deletion of one or a few base pairs (not multiples of three) leads to a frameshift. Mutations occur spontaneously at a low level; the mutation rate can be increased by mutagens (e.g., X-irradiation; chemicals

such as nitrous acid, alkylating agents, acridines). Most mutations are deleterious or neutral, although some mutations may be advantageous and be selected during evolution.

myasthenia gravis. AUTOIMMUNE DISEASE of young adults characterized by fluctuating muscle weakness due to faulty neuromuscular transmission. Patients with myasthenia gravis have IgG AUTOANTIBODIES to acetylcholine receptors at the neuromuscular junction, resulting in a decrease in the number of functional receptors. The disease is often ameliorated by THYMECTOMY. Infants of mothers with myasthenia gravis may also develop the disease due to passive transfer of maternal IgG antibodies to acetylcholine receptors.

***myc* oncogene.** v-*myc* is a retroviral ONCOGENE (from avian myelocytomatosis virus) that encodes a protein found in the nucleus of infected cells. c-*myc* is the related proto-oncogene found in normal eukaryotic cells; c-*myc* has been mapped to chromosome 8q24 in humans and to chromosome 15 in mice. In human BURKITT'S LYMPHOMA and in mouse MYELOMAS, there are reciprocal rearrangements between one copy of the chromosome bearing c-*myc* and the chromosomes bearing IMMUNOGLOBULIN GENES; these translocations deprive the *myc* gene of its normal transcriptional regulatory sequences (e.g., promoter, enhancer) and replace these with sequences from the immunoglobulin gene. This translocation deregulates the gene, its expression is enhanced and contributes to the neoplastic transformation of the cell. The c-*myc* gene may also become deregulated by the nearby integration of a retrovirus.

myelocyte. Immature cell of bone marrow that is the precursor of POLYMORPHONUCLEAR LEUKOCYTES. The most immature cells of this lineage are called myeloblasts. Myeloblasts are approximately 18 μm in diameter; the nucleus is large and has finely dispersed chromatin and two prominent nucleoli. The cytoplasm is sparse and stains intensely with basophilic dyes. As myeloblasts mature, large azurophilic (blue staining) PRIMARY GRANULES appear in the cytoplasm (promyelocyte stage) and, subsequently, specific or SECONDARY GRANULES appear (myelocyte stage), the nuclear chromatin begins to form dense clumps and the nucleoli disappear. As this process of nuclear condensation continues, the cells lose their capacity to divide (metamyelocyte stage); the nucleus elongates into a sausage shape (band stage) before turning into the characteristic trilobed structure of polymorphonuclear leukocytes.

myeloid cell. Undifferentiated cell of the BONE MARROW from which are derived PLATELETS, MONOCYTES, NEUTROPHILS, EOSINOPHILS, BASOPHILS and red blood cells.

myeloma. Neoplastic proliferation of a CLONE of PLASMA CELLS, particularly in bone marrow. Myelomas are found in the human disease MULTIPLE MYELOMA and can be induced experimentally in certain susceptible INBRED STRAINS of mice (e.g., BALB/c) by the injection of mineral oil into the peritoneal cavity. Myelomas can occur spontaneously in mice, rats, cats, dogs and other species.

myeloma protein. MONOCLONAL IMMUNOGLOBULIN produced by a CLONE of neoplas

tic PLASMA CELLS (e.g., in MULTIPLE MYELOMA or in the experimentally induced disease MYELOMATOSIS in mice). Before HYBRIDOMAS became available, myeloma proteins were the chief source of homogeneous immunoglobulins and were widely used in structural studies. *See* MYELOMA.

myelomatosis. Disease characterized by PLASMA CELL proliferation (e.g., MULTIPLE MYELOMA, MACROGLOBULINEMIA OF WALDENSTRÖM, ALPHA, GAMMA and MU HEAVY CHAIN DISEASE).

myeloperoxidase (MPO) **deficiency.** Absence of myeloperoxidase from NEUTROPHILS and MONOCYTES. MPO (M_r 116,000) constitutes 7 percent of the weight of neutrophils and is found in PRIMARY GRANULES. It is a deep green color due to a heme ring, which accounts for the color of pus. The deficiency is inherited as an autosomal recessive and causes a mild form of CHRONIC GRANULOMATOUS DISEASE. Infections with *Candida albicans* are particularly common in MPO deficiency.

N

N nucleotide. *See* N REGION.

N region. Short portion of a VARIABLE REGION of an IMMUNOGLOBULIN or T CELL RECEPTOR polypeptide chain that is not encoded by the germ line gene segments, but rather by short nucleotide (N) insertions at the recombinational junctions. Such 'N nucleotides' have been found both 3′ and 5′ to the *D* GENE SEGMENT of rearranged immunoglobulin heavy chain genes and also at the *V–J*, *V–D–J* and *D–D* junctions of T cell receptor variable region genes. Before the insertion of N nucleotides, a few bases at these junctions may be removed by an exonuclease. It is thought that the N nucleotides are inserted at random by a non-template directed mechanism, perhaps catalysed by the enzyme DNA NUCLEOTIDYLEXOTRANSFERASE (terminal transferase).

naproxen (2-naphthaleneacetic acid, 6 methoxy-α-methyl). Drug used in the treatment of RHEUMATOID ARTHRITIS, JUVENILE RHEUMATOID ARTHRITIS and ANKYLOSING SPONDYLITIS because of its anti-inflammatory effects.

naproxen

natural antibodies. Antibodies that are not the result of known IMMUNIZATION. These antibodies may be the result of cryptic immunization (e.g., antibodies to the A and B blood group in humans).

natural killer (NK) **cell.** LYMPHOID cell capable of killing a variety of nucleated cells in the absence of antigenic stimulation. NK cells have been identified as distinct cells capable of expressing 'natural cytotoxicity'. NK cells are found in the blood (approximately 10 percent of the total lymphocytes) and in lymphoid tissues, including those of athymic individuals (e.g., NUDE MICE, neonatally thymectomized mice, SCID MICE and in infants with SEVERE COMBINED IMMUNODEFICIENCY). They are about 15 μm in diameter, bear a kidney-shaped nucleus, and two or three large granules in the cytoplasm (hence, the term large granular lymphocytes). NK cells can kill some, but not all tumor cells, some virus-infected cells and most nucleated cells coated with antibody. In the latter group, the killing takes place because of the adherence of the NK cells, which have an Fcγ RECEPTOR, to the opsonized target (a phenomenon termed antibody-dependent cell-mediated cytotoxicity (ADCC)). Cells that mediate ADCC have been called killer (or K) cells but are thought to be the same as NK cells. NK cells may represent a first line of defense against spontaneously arising tumor cells and against viral infections. In experimental animals, there is a correlation between the number of NK cells and the degree of natural resistance to tumors. NK cells are distinct from monocytes, B lymphocytes and T lymphocytes and, hence, may represent a distinct lineage. It is noteworthy that some strongly activated CYTOTOXIC T LYMPHOCYTES can show natural cytotoxicity (i.e., kill some tumor cells unrelated to the cellular antigens that induced them).

necrosis. Death of tissue.

neoantigen. Newly expressed ANTIGENIC DETERMINANT. For example, a neoantigen may emerge: (1) upon conformational change in a protein; (2) as a newly expressed determinant on the surface of a transformed cell; (3) as the result of complex formation of two or more molecules or, (4) as a result of cleavage of a molecule with resulting expression of new determinants. TUMOR-ASSOCIATED ANTIGENS are examples of neo-antigens.

network theory. Theory that views the immune system as a network of lymphocytes bearing IDIOTYPES to which are directed corresponding lymphocytes bearing anti-idiotypes. Antigen disrupts the balance of this network resulting in the increased production of certain idiotypes and the consequent increased production of the corresponding anti-idiotypes, which may then modulate the response. Anti-idiotypes have been found in the course of immunization with some antigens. When isolated and injected into experimental animals, such anti-idiotypes may inhibit the response to that antigen. The binding site of some anti-idiotypes resembles the immunizing ANTI-GENIC DETERMINANT and is therefore called the internal image of the antigenic determinant. Not all anti-idiotypes are internal images. Immunization with anti-idiotypes bearing an internal image may result in the production of antibodies that bind the original antigen. Thus, anti-idiotypes have been used to protect mice against certain viruses. Anti-idiotypes may also bind to cellular receptors for the original antigen and have been used to isolate such receptors.

neutralization test. Test of capacity of an antibody to neutralize the biological activity of an antigen or of an organism (e.g., a virus) bearing an antigen.

neutropenia. Decrease in the number of NEUTROPHILS in the blood.

neutrophil. Type of POLYMORPHONUCLEAR LEUKOCYTE, characterized by SECONDARY GRANULES that stain pink with Wright or Giemsa stains. Neutrophils constitute approximately 60 percent of the white cells of blood; they are the most numerous phagocytes of blood.

New Zealand mice. TWO INBRED STRAINS – the New Zealand black (NZB) and the New Zealand white (NZW) – used in the study of AUTOIMMUNE DISEASE. NZB develop AUTOIM-MUNE HEMOLYTIC ANEMIA and low titers of ANTI-NUCLEAR ANTIBODIES. NZB mice have spontaneously activated B LYMPHOCYTES and abnormalities of T LYMPHOCYTES, the nature of which is not clear. It is not known which abnormality is the primary defect. Several genes appear to be responsible for the manifestations of AUTOIMMUNITY. NZW mice are asymptomatic, but the offspring of NZW × NZB matings develop a severe immune complex disease, which resembles SYSTEMIC LUPUS ERYTHEMATOSUS, characterized by high titers of anti-nuclear antibodies and GLOMERULONEPHRITIS.

nick translation. Term referring to the movement ('translation') of a nick along a duplex DNA molecule. A nick is a discontinuity in one strand of the duplex; at the nicked site there is a free 3'-hydroxyl and a free 5'-phosphoryl group, but no loss of nucleotides. Nicks are introduced at widely separated random sites in DNA by very limited treatment with DEOXYRIBONUCLEASE I. In the presence of DNA-DIRECTED DNA POLYMERASE I (*E. coli*), nucleotides are progressively removed from the 5'-terminus of the nick (by virtue of the $5' \rightarrow 3'$ exonuclease activity of this enzyme), and other nucleotides are added to the 3'-hydroxyl terminus; i.e., the nick translates along the duplex in the $5' \rightarrow 3'$ direction. If the reaction is carried out in the presence of one or more radio-labeled nucleoside triphosphates (e.g., $[\alpha\text{-}^{32}P]\text{-dNTP}$), preexisting nucleotides in the DNA strand are replaced by labeled ones. It is possible to prepare ^{32}P-labeled DNA with a specific activity greater than 10^8 counts per minute per microgram.

nitroblue tetrazolium (NBT) **dye test.** Quantitative blood test for the diagnosis of CHRONIC GRANULOMATOUS DISEASE (CGD). NBT is a clear yellow dye that is taken up by neutrophils and monocytes during PHAGOCY-TOSIS. NBT is reduced within the phagocytes to an insoluble deep purple dye. A negative test, the failure of NBT reduction, is diagnostic of CGD.

NK 1.1. ALLOANTIGEN found on NATURAL KILLER CELLS (NK) of some INBRED STRAINS of mice (e.g., C57BL/6).

N-linked oligosaccharide. Oligosaccharide attached covalently to asparagine residues of many proteins. All N-linked oligosaccharides have a branched core structure consisting of two residues of *N*-acetylglucosamine and three residues of mannose. Three main types, differing in their outer branches, are distinguished: (1) high-mannose oligosaccharides, which typically have two to six additional mannose residues linked to the pentasaccharide core; (2) complex oligosaccharides, which contain two to five terminal branches composed of *N*-acetylglucosamine, galactose, usually *N*-acetylneuraminic acid (sialic acid), and sometimes other sugars such as fucose; (3) hybrid molecules, having features of both high-mannose and complex oligosaccharides.

The pentasaccharide core is derived from a branched precursor containing two residues of *N*-acetylglucosamine, nine of mannose, and three of glucose, linked by a pyrophosphoryl group to dolichol, a long-chain unsaturated lipid. This structure is transferred, by the enzyme oligosaccharide transferase on the luminal side of the rough ENDOPLASMIC RETICULUM, to a nascent polypeptide chain at a tripeptide acceptor sequence, asparagine–X–serine or asparagine–X–threonine (X is any amino acid residue except possibly proline or aspartic acid). Soon after transfer, while the polypeptide is still in the rough endoplasmic reticulum, the three glucose residues and at least one of the mannose residues are removed. The polypeptide is usually now transported to the GOLGI COMPLEX. Here, the high-mannose oligosaccharides may be trimmed further by removal of mannose. Extensive modification to form the complex and hybrid oligosaccharides takes place in the Golgi complex; additional mannose residues are removed and the branched arms are constructed by stepwise transfer from nucleotide sugar precursors, catalysed by individual glycosyl transferases. Fucose and *N*-acetylglucosamine may be added to the core.

IMMUNOGLOBULINS of all classes contain N-linked oligosaccharides. These are usually attached to the constant region of the heavy chain, although some variable regions having a tripeptide acceptor sequence may also contain such oligosaccharides. Most of the oligosaccharides are of the complex type, but the mu, delta and epsilon constant regions also contain high-mannose oligosaccharides. The number of N-linked oligosaccharides varies from one in the constant region of human gamma chains to six in the constant region of human epsilon chains. Sialic acid is the only sugar residue of immunoglobulins that bears a charge (negative), and variations in content of sialic acid can lead to charge heterogeneity even of homogeneous immunoglobulins such as MYELOMA PROTEINS and MONOCLONAL ANTIBODIES.

The function of N-linked oligosaccharides differs for different glycoproteins. They may play a role in maintaining protein stability, and they may be important for movement within cells, for secretion, or for mediating clearance of glycoproteins from the blood. In some, but not all classes of immunoglobulins, glycosylation seems to be important in maintaining the conformation necessary for assembly and secretion. The presence of carbohydrate may protect immunoglobulins from proteolytic degradation. Removal of carbohydrate has variable impact on the effector functions of antibodies (e.g., COMPLEMENT activation, binding to Fc RECEPTORS). *See* O-LINKED SACCHARIDES.

NOD mouse. Mouse of a mutant strain, characterized by the early onset of autoimmune INSULIN-DEPENDENT DIABETES MELLITUS. The NOD mutation is inherited as an autosomal recessive. Pancreatic islets of Langerhans in NOD mice are infiltrated with LYMPHOCYTES and β cells of the islets are destroyed. NOD is an abbreviation for *non-obese diabetic*.

nominal allotype. ALLOTYPE that is expected according to the genetic constitution of the animal. The term nominal allotype is used in contrast to LATENT ALLOTYPE.

non-adherent cell. Cell that does not adhere to surfaces *in vitro* (e.g., LYMPHOCYTE). *See* ADHERENT CELL.

non-precipitating antibody. Antibody that does not precipitate with antigen. However, such antibodies may coprecipitate with insoluble complexes formed by antigen and other (precipitating) antibodies. Antibodies may be non-precipitating because of low AFFINITY for antigen, or because they do not cross-link different molecules or particles of antigen. *See* MONOGAMOUS BIVALENCY.

non-secretor. Person whose secretions (e.g., gastric juice, saliva, tears, ovarian cyst mucin) do not contain the ABO BLOOD GROUP substances. Non-secretors are homozygous for the gene *se*; they constitute approximately 20 percent of the population. *See* SECRETOR.

non-specific. Not involving specific immune recognition.

Northern blotting. Technique for detecting specific RNA sequences within a population of RNA molecules that have been separated by gel electrophoresis. Either the RNA is denatured with glyoxal or dimethylsulfoxide before electrophoretic separation, or methylmercuric hydroxide or formaldehyde is added to the gel to achieve denaturation of the RNA. Following electrophoresis, the RNA is transferred, by 'blotting' (or electrophoresis), to diazobenzyloxymethyl (DBM) paper (no longer much used) or to nitrocellulose or nylon membranes, and is hybridized with a probe (eg. radiolabeled DNA or RNA). The term Northern blotting or transfer was coined because the method is similar to the technique for transferring and detecting DNA fragments which had been described by and named after E.M. Southern. *See* IMMUNOBLOTTING, SOUTHERN BLOTTING.

nude mouse. Mutant mouse, characterized by the complete absence of hair and THYMUS. These mice are homozygous for an autosomal recessive mutation (v) which maps to chromosome 11. The relationship between the absence of thymus and hair is not clear. Nude mice are used extensively to study the immunological effects of thymus deprivation. Nude mice cannot reject homografts (*see* ALLOGRAFT), do not express CELL-MEDIATED IMMUNITY, and do not make antibodies to most antigens. They lack T LYMPHOCYTES but have normal NATURAL KILLER CELLS and B LYMPHOCYTES.

null cell. LYMPHOCYTE that cannot be identified as a T or B LYMPHOCYTE or a NATURAL KILLER CELL.

O

O antigen. Oligosaccharide antigen of the cell envelope of Gram-negative bacteria. The designation O (German, '*ohne Hauch*', 'without breath') was used because the non-motile bacteria, which contain O but not H antigens, do not form a film on agar plates (*see* H ANTIGEN). The O antigen is the highly variable portion of the LIPOPOLYSACCHARIDE (LPS) molecule, the major surface constituent of the cell envelope of these bacteria. It is composed of up to 40 repetitions of a unit consisting of a linear trisaccharide or a branched tetra- or pentasaccharide, often including unusual 3,6-dideoxyhexoses (abequose, tyvelose, paratose, colitose); the resulting chain is attached to a core polysaccharide which, in turn, is linked to lipid A. In each strain, the repeating oligosaccharide units are the same, although the length of the chains varies. The O antigens form the main basis for classification of strains of Salmonella in the KAUFFMANN-WHITE SCHEME. The antigenic determinants consist of groups of sugar residues; dideoxyhexoses have an immunodominant role in many of these determinants. The O antigen is also known as the somatic (or cell-bound) antigen of these bacteria, in contradistinction to the H or flagellar antigen.

old tuberculin (OT). Heat-concentrated filtrate from broth cultures in which *Mycobacterium tuberculosis* was grown. It was formerly used in TUBERCULIN skin tests.

oligoclonal. Related to or derived from a few CLONES.

O-linked saccharide. Sugar residues attached to the hydroxyl groups of serine, threonine or, sometimes, hydroxylysine residues of certain proteins. In most plasma proteins and in glycoproteins of mucinous secretions, the linking sugar residue is N-acetylgalactosamine and it is attached to serine or threonine. O-linked saccharides of plasma proteins usually consist of one to four residues. In addition to N-acetylgalactosamine, they frequently contain galactose and N-acetylneuraminic acid (sialic acid). The O-linked oligosaccharides in blood group substances are considerably larger and may contain more than a dozen saccharides. The sugar residues are added one at a time by different glycosyl transferases in the GOLGI COMPLEX. There is no known acceptor sequence for O-linked saccharides, but proline is often found adjacent to glycosylated serine or threonine residues and may promote beta turns in the polypeptide chain. In collagen and C1q, galactose (the linking residue) and glucose are attached to hydroxylysine residues.

Only two constant regions of human immunoglobulin chains contain O-linked saccharides. The hinge region of the alpha1 chain contains four disaccharides consisting of N-acetylgalactosamine and galactose and one monosaccharide, N-acetylgalactosamine, all linked to serine. The hinge region of the delta chain contains four to seven saccharides linked either to serine or threonine; these consist of N-acetylgalactosamine and galactose and, sometimes, one or two sialic acid residues. *See* N-LINKED OLIGOSACCHARIDE.

oncofetal antigens. Antigens normally expressed in fetal life that reappear in tumors. *See* ALPHA-FETOPROTEIN, CARCINOEMBRYONIC ANTIGEN.

oncogene. Gene that brings about or contributes to the neoplastic TRANSFORMATION of cells. The term may refer to: (1) genes, originally of cellular origin, that have been incorporated into retroviral genomes and, in the process, have acquired the ability to

161

transform cells (e.g., v-*src* in Rous sarcoma virus, v-*abl* in ABELSON MURINE LEUKEMIA VIRUS, v-*myc* in avian myelocytomatosis virus); (2) genes from tumors that have arisen spontaneously or from cells that have been transformed by chemical carcinogens and that are responsible for maintenance of the neoplastic state; (3) genes from DNA viruses (e.g., polyoma, adenovirus) that can induce cellular transformation.

Retroviral and cellular oncogenes arise from cellular genes called proto-oncogenes (e.g., c-*src*, c-*abl*, c-*myc*), which play a role in normal growth and differentiation. An alteration in a growth regulatory signal (e.g., due to an increase in the amount of gene product or in its structure) may induce neoplastic transformation. This may occur by several different mechanisms: (1) as already noted, acquisition by a retrovirus, which places the cellular gene under the control of viral transcriptional promoters and enhancers; (2) nearby integration of a retrovirus; (3) gene amplification; (4) chromosomal translocation with resulting loss of normal regulation (e.g. translocation of the c-*myc* proto-oncogene from chromosome 8 to one of the chromosomes containing IMMUNOGLOBULIN GENES); (5) mutation of protein-encoding sequences, which may occur as the only change responsible for mutagenesis or which may accompany the other mechanisms, contributing to the oncogenic transformation.

More than 20 cellular proto-oncogenes are known. Their products have been classified according to cellular location: secreted, cell surface, cytoplasmic, and nuclear. Some (e.g., c-*src* and c-*abl*) encode protein kinases that phosphorylate tyrosine residues of specific cellular proteins; c-*ras* genes encode proteins that bind tightly to guanine nucleotides and possess GTPase activity. Some oncogenes have been identified as growth factors or growth factor receptors; c-*sis* encodes one chain of the platelet-derived growth factor; c-*erb*B encodes part of the epidermal growth factor receptor; c-*fms* encodes the receptor for the macrophage COLONY STIMULATING FACTOR, CSF-1.

open reading frame (ORF). Stretch of DNA or RNA that may encode a protein or part of a protein. Open reading frames must not contain termination CODONS. A complete open reading frame would begin with the initiation codon ATG (AUG) and end at a termination codon (TAA (UAA), TAG (UAG), or TGA (UGA)). The identification of an open reading frame may be the first indication for the existence of a previously unknown protein. *See* UNIDENTIFIED READING FRAME (URF).

opportunistic infections. Infections that occur mainly in patients with defects in CELL-MEDIATED IMMUNITY (e.g., ACQUIRED IMMUNODEFICIENCY SYNDROME and SEVERE COMBINED IMMUNODEFICIENCY). Microorganisms causing opportunistic infections include *Pneumocystis carinii*, *Candida albicans*, *Mycobacterium avium intracellulare*, Toxoplasma, Cryptosporidia and herpes virus.

opsonin. Substance in serum that binds to particles (e.g. red blood cells or bacteria) and increases their susceptibility to PHAGOCYTOSIS. The term has been used to describe the following: (1) antibodies specific for ANTIGENIC DETERMINANTS of the particles. The Fc FRAGMENT of the bound antibody attaches to Fc RECEPTORS of phagocytic cells, thereby facilitating phagocytosis of the particle. Antibodies are known as heat-stable opsonins. (2) Products of complement activation. C3b or C3bi, bound to particles by transacylation with the thiolester of C3, attach to COMPLEMENT RECEPTOR 1 or COMPLEMENT RECEPTOR 3, respectively, on phagocytic cells. C3b and C3bi are known as heat-labile opsonins. (3) Certain other substances that bind to particles (e.g., FIBRONECTIN).

opsonization. Deposition of OPSONINS onto particles, such as red blood cells or bacteria, thereby facilitating their PHAGOCYTOSIS.

optimal proportions. *Synonym for* EQUIVALENCE.

original antigenic sin. Tendency to react to IMMUNIZATION by producing antibodies to a determinant on the stimulating antigen that resembles a determinant on an antigen encountered previously. Antibodies that cross-react with the original antigen are produced preferentially. The term was first used to describe the response to reinfection with influenza when the host makes a SECONDARY IMMUNE RESPONSE to the strain of influenza of a previous infection. In the interval between infections, the influenza virus has undergone antigenic change. *See* ANTIGENIC DRIFT, ANTIGENIC SHIFT.

orthotopic.   Descriptive of a tissue or organ GRAFT to a site normally occupied by that tissue or organ.

osteoclast-activating   factor   (OAF). Activity found in the cultures of antigen-stimulated lymphocytes that induces resorption of bone *in vitro*. Several molecules have been identified as having OAF activity including LYMPHOTOXIN elaborated by T LYMPHOCYTES and TUMOR NECROSIS FACTOR, INTERLEUKIN-1 and PROSTAGLANDINS all elaborated by MACROPHAGES. OAF activity may be responsible for bone resorption found in patients with lymphoid cell malignancies

such as MULTIPLE MYELOMA or T cell LYMPHOMAS.

outbreeding.   Mating of individuals less closely related than individuals chosen at random from a population. Outbreeding tends to promote genetic diversity in a population. *See* INBREEDING, RANDOM BREEDING.

overlap syndrome.   *Synonym for* MIXED CONNECTIVE TISSUE DISEASE.

Oz isotypic determinant.   ANTIGENIC DETERMINANT of human IMMUNOGLOBULIN LAMBDA CHAINS associated with lysine at position 190 (*see* Table in definition of immunoglobulin lambda chain). This determinant is present on some of the lambda chains of every individual. It is, therefore, not the result of genetic POLYMORPHISM.

P

p150,95 (CD11c,18). One form of COMPLE-MENT RECEPTOR 4 composed of an alpha chain (M_r 150,000) (CD11c) and a beta chain (M_r 95,000) (CD18). The beta chain is identical to the beta chain of LYMPHOCYTE FUNCTION ASSOCIATED ANTIGEN-1 (LFA–1) and of COMPLEMENT RECEPTOR 3 (CR3).

palindrome. Group of letters (word or sentence) that read the same forward or backward, (e.g., 'able was I ere I saw Elba'). In duplex DNA a palindrome is a sequence that is the same when each strand is read in the 5′→3′ direction, e.g.,

5′ CATATG 3′
3′ GTATAC 5′

See INVERTED REPEAT.

parabiotic intoxication. Disease that occurs when two outbred animals are surgically anastomosed or joined (parabiosis). The interchange of blood can result in GRAFT-VERSUS-HOST DISEASE in one or both animals.

paraprotein. Homogeneous immunoglobulin (*see* MONOCLONAL IMMUNOGLOBULIN) derived from an expanded CLONE of PLASMA CELLS and unrelated to known antigenic stimulation e.g., MYELOMA PROTEIN.

paratope. *Synonym for* ANTIBODY COMBINING SITE.

paroxysmal cold hemoglobinuria. Form of HEMOLYTIC ANEMIA in which patients have hemoglobin in their urine (hemoglobinuria) after they have been exposed to cold temperatures. A HEMOLYSIN, called the Donath–Landsteiner antibody, binds to red blood cells only in the cold, and the red cells subsequently lyse in the presence of COMPLEMENT when rewarmed to 37°C. Although classically associated with syphilis, Donath–Landsteiner antibodies can also appear following acute viral illnesses. Patients with these antibodies experience severe hemoly-

tic episodes with fever and chills, in addition to hemoglobinuria.

paroxysmal nocturnal hemoglobinuria (PNH). Form of HEMOLYTIC ANEMIA that results from a clonal defect expressed in some ERYTHROCYTES, PLATELETS and NEUTROPHILS. The affected cells are abnormally sensitive to lysis by COMPLEMENT. PNH cell membranes lack the DECAY ACCELERATING FACTOR, which downregulates the formation of the classical pathway C5 CONVERTASE on the cell membrane and the formation of the membrane attack complex. The membranes of PNH erythrocytes are deficient in all glycophospholipid anchored proteins (e.g., decay accelerating factor, LFA-3 and FcγRIII). Increased lysis of PNH red blood cells in acidified serum (Ham test) is used to diagnose the disease. For unknown reasons the hemolysis occurs predominantly at night.

partial lipodystrophy. Loss of subcutaneous fat from the upper half of the body with concomitant obesity of the lower half of the body. C3 NEPHRITIC FACTOR, an AUTOANTIBODY to the ALTERNATIVE PATHWAY C3 CONVERTASE (C3bBb), is present in the serum of patients with this syndrome. Most of the patients develop MEMBRANOPROLIFERATIVE GLOMERULONEPHRITIS. Partial lipodystrophy is presumed to be an IMMUNE COMPLEX DISEASE, but its cause is unknown.

passenger leukocyte. LEUKOCYTE present within an ALLOGRAFT and contributing to the IMMUNIZATION of the host because it has CLASS II HISTOCOMPATIBILITY MOLECULES. Passenger leukocytes include MONOCYTES, MACROPHAGES, B LYMPHOCYTES, LANGERHANS CELLS.

passive agglutination. AGGLUTINATION, by antibodies to a soluble antigen, of particles bearing the same antigen bound to their surfaces. Attachment of the antigen may be covalent or noncovalent (i.e., by adsorption). It is a very sensitive test for antibodies. *See* PASSIVE HEMAGGLUTINATION.

passive cutaneous anaphylaxis (PCA). Type of ANAPHYLAXIS induced in the skin after intradermal injection of antibodies (e.g., IgE) that bind to MAST CELLS (*see* Fcε RECEPTOR). The test animal is injected intravenously with antigen and a dye, such as Evans blue, hours or days after the intradermal injection of antibodies. A positive reaction is indicated by the leakage of the dye at the site of the antigen–antibody interaction, resulting in a circumscribed area of blue skin.

passive hemagglutination. AGGLUTINATION, by antibodies to a soluble antigen, of red blood cells bearing the same antigen bound to their membranes. *See* PASSIVE AGGLUTINATION.

passive hemolysis. Lysis of derivatized red blood cells by COMPLEMENT that has been activated by the combination of antibodies with antigens bound to the red blood cell membrane.

passive immunity. IMMUNITY acquired by the administration of antibodies from immune individuals (e.g., the immunity of newborns that results from the transfer of antibodies across the placenta or the ingestion of COLOSTRUM, the immunity that results from administration of ANTITOXINS or ANTIVENOMS). *See* ACTIVE IMMUNITY, ADOPTIVE TRANSFER.

passive transfer. Transfer of an IMMUNE RESPONSE, or some component of it, from one individual to another by means of cells or serum. The transfer by means of cells is called ADOPTIVE TRANSFER. LYMPHOCYTES from an immunized mouse are transferred to a recipient mouse which, upon challenge with an appropriate antigen develops a secondary antibody response or DELAYED-TYPE HYPERSENSITIVITY. For successful passive transfer of cells, inbred animals should be used. Irradiation of the recipients may also be important perhaps because it reduces LYMPHOID mass that could interfere with the homing of lymphocytes. Antibodies are given to recipients for the passive transfer of HUMORAL IMMUNITY. Passive transfer has

been invaluable in identifying the functions of lymphocytes and of antibodies.

patch test. Method for establishing the cause of ALLERGIC CONTACT DERMATITIS. The suspected provoking substance is applied to a small piece of linen, cotton, filter paper or aluminum foil, and placed on the skin for 24 to 48 hours. After removal of the patch, the skin is examined for ERYTHEMA, vesiculation and edema, which indicate a positive result.

patching. LIGAND-induced redistribution of membrane proteins into clusters as a result of cross-linking by BIVALENT or MULTIVALENT antibodies or LECTINS. Such redistribution can occur because the lipid bilayer is fluid and proteins can diffuse freely within the plane of the membrane. Redistribution into patches is a passive process and does not require energy, but it can be prevented by chemically 'fixing' the cell membrane so that its proteins are immobilized. The distribution of membrane proteins can be visualized by reacting them with fluorescent-labeled or ferritin-labeled ligands followed by light or electron microscopy, respectively. Since a bivalent or multivalent ligand can itself induce redistribution, the organization of membrane proteins in the native state should be examined by attaching the label to a monovalent ligand (e.g., the Fab FRAGMENT of an antibody).

Paul–Bunnell test. Test for HETEROPHILE ANTIBODIES in individuals suspected of having INFECTIOUS MONONUCLEOSIS. Test serum is absorbed with guinea-pig kidney to remove antibodies to FORSSMAN ANTIGEN. The titer of heterophile antibodies in test serum is then determined by the degree of AGGLUTINATION of sheep red blood cells.

pBR322. *E. coli* PLASMID under relaxed control (can exist in high copy-number) that contains both ampicillin- and tetracycline-resistant genes and a number of convenient restriction sites and that is widely used as a cloning VECTOR. pBR322 consists of 4,363 base pairs. It was derived by methods of genetic engineering from naturally-occurring *E. coli* plasmids.

pediatric AIDS. Form of ACQUIRED IMMUNODEFICIENCY SYNDROME (AIDS) in infants due to intrauterine or intrapartum infection with HUMAN IMMUNODEFICIENCY VIRUS (HIV). Infected infants usually develop symptoms between three weeks and 24 months of age. Like adults with AIDS, affected infants have enlarged lymph nodes, fever, THROMBOCYTOPENIA and elevated numbers of circulating B LYMPHOCYTES and a marked increase in the serum concentration of IgG, IgM and IgD. Unlike adults with AIDS, they are prone to infections with EPSTEIN–BARR VIRUS resulting in interstitial pneumonia and inflammation of the salivary glands, have normal numbers of T LYMPHOCYTES in the blood, and frequent blood stream infections with pyogenic bacteria (e.g., pneumococci or *Hemophilus influenzae* b). Affected infants only rarely have KAPOSI'S SARCOMA and OPPORTUNISTIC INFECTIONS that are typical of adult AIDS. Growth and development of these infants are retarded. Pediatric AIDS is almost always fatal.

pemphigoid. Blistering disease of the skin, differentiated from PEMPHIGUS by the absence of acantholysis (intraepidermal bullae). The bullous formation in pemphigoid is subepidermal, and linear deposition of IgG can be detected by IMMUNOFLUORESCENCE in the basement membrane zone. IgG antibodies to basement membrane of skin are present in the serum. Pemphigoid is seen most frequently in the elderly.

pemphigus. Blistering AUTOIMMUNE DISEASE of the skin, characterized by intraepidermal bullae, so-called acantholysis. Deposition of IgG, C1q, C4 and C3 is detected by IMMUNOFLUORESCENCE in the skin lesions. The disease is caused by AUTOANTIBODIES to antigens in the intercellular spaces of the skin. The cause of autoantibody formation is not known. Pemphigus is improved by treatment with CORTICOSTEROIDS. Pemiphigus occurs at all ages.

penicillin allergy. Allergy (HYPERSENSITIVITY) to penicillin or to its breakdown products or to contaminants in penicillin preparations. Some derivatives (e.g., penicilenic acid) become conjugated to proteins, forming penicilloyl derivatives, and act as HAPTENS in inducing an allergic response, which may be antibody-mediated (*see* IMMEDIATE HYPERSENSITIVITY) or cell-mediated (*see* DELAYED-TYPE HYPERSENSITI-

VITY). Antibody-mediated reactions include ANAPHYLAXIS (due to IgE antibodies), SERUM SICKNESS (rash, fever, joint pains) and HEMOLYTIC ANEMIA. Cell-mediated reactions may be manifest as ALLERGIC CONTACT DERMATITIS; this is quite common in individuals (e.g., nurses, pharmacists) who handle penicillin. PATCH TESTS with penicillin are used to detect cell-mediated reactions to the drug. Penicilloyl–polylysine may induce a wheal and flare response (URTICARIA) when injected into the skin of individuals who have IgE antibodies to penicilloyl–protein conjugates; this reagent, which does not appear to be IMMUNOGENIC, has been used to test for immediate hypersensitivity to penicillin derivatives.

perforin. Protein (M_r 75,000) isolated from the cytoplasmic granules of NATURAL KILLER CELLS (NK) and CYTOTOXIC T LYMPHOCYTES that is thought to mediate the lysis of TARGET CELLS. Following intimate contact of the NK cells or cytolytic T lymphocytes with target cells, intracellular granules are released with subsequent polymerization of perforin in the presence of Ca^{2+}. Polymerized perforin inserts into the membranes of target cells causing depolarization, abnormal ion flux and cell LYSIS. The membranes of target cells have characteristic round lesions, resembling those seen in COMPLEMENT-dependent lysis (*see* MEMBRANE ATTACK COMPLEX). Antibodies to complement component C9 cross-react with perforin.

periarteritis nodosa. *Synonym for* POLYARTERITIS NODOSA.

peripolesis. Clustering of cells around a different type of cell (e.g., LYMPHOCYTES around a MACROPHAGE).

pernicious anemia (PA). AUTOIMMUNE DISEASE characterized by AUTOANTIBODIES to intrinsic factor and to gastric parietal cells. Parietal cells normally secrete a heat-labile substance, called intrinsic factor (M_r 60,000), which binds dietary vitamin B12 and facilitates its absorption in the distal small intestine. Pernicious anemia results from a deficiency of vitamin B12. For unknown reasons pernicious anemia is a frequent complication of COMMON VARIABLE IMMUNODEFICIENCY.

persistent generalized lymphodenopathy (PGL). *See* HIV INFECTION.

pFc′ fragment. Fragment produced by digestion of IgG (or Fc FRAGMENT) with the enzyme pepsin. It consists of the two C_H3 domains (probably the carboxy-terminal 116 residues of both chains), which form a non-covalently bonded dimer.

Pfeiffer phenomenon. Rapid LYSIS of cholera bacteria by COMPLEMENT after these bacteria have been injected into the peritoneal cavity of an animal immune to cholera.

phage neutralization. Abolition of the activity of bacteriophage by antibodies, thereby preventing the infection of a bacterial host. The neutralizing activity can be quantitated by determining the reduction in number of plaques when phage are incubated with antibodies before plating on bacteria. It is a very sensitive assay for antibody activity.

phagocyte. Cell that ingests particulate material. NEUTROPHILS and MONONUCLEAR PHAGOCYTES are the principal phagocytes of the body.

phagocytosis. Ingestion of relatively large particles (e.g., bacteria or parts of a cell) by phagocytes (e.g., NEUTROPHILS, MACROPHAGES). The first event in phagocytosis is the binding of the particle to the plasma membrane of the phagocyte. Some particulate materials bind only when coated with specific antibody or COMPLEMENT (*see* OPSONIZATION). Following binding, the plasma membrane expands along the surface of the particle by means of actin-containing microfilaments that lie just under the cell surface. The particle is enveloped by the interaction of receptors on the surface of the phagocyte with ligands distributed on the particle's surface (called 'zipper interaction'). The invaginated membrane-enveloped particle is a large (1–2 μm) vesicle called a phagosome; this may fuse with a primary lysosome to form a phagolysosome (secondary lysosome), wherein the particle may be digested by hydrolytic enzymes. The fate of the intracellular particle varies depending on its nature and on the type of phagocytic cell. Some pyogenic bacteria are rapidly killed as a result of the oxidative processes that accompany phagocytosis. Some intracellular pathogens (e.g., *Mycobacterium leprae*, Leishmania, Toxoplasma, *Legionella pneumophilia*) remain viable inside the phagolysosome unless the macrophage is activated by INTERFERON-GAMMA. *See* ENDOCYTOSIS.

phagolysosome. *See* PHAGOCYTOSIS.

phagosome. *See* PHAGOCYTOSIS.

phenotype. Detectable characteristics of a cell or organism. The characteristics considered to be the phenotype may vary according to the methods used for detection. The phenotype results from the interactions of the GENOTYPE with the environment.

phenylbutazone (4-butyl-1,2-diphenyl-3,5-pyrazolidinedione). Drug used for the treatment of ANKYLOSING SPONDYLITIS and RHEUMATOID ARTHRITIS. It inhibits PROSTAGLANDIN synthesis and is a potent anti-inflammatory agent.

phenylbutazone

phorbol ester. Ester of myristic acid and phorbol alcohols. The most commonly used phorbol ester is 12-*O*-tetradecanoylphorbol-13-acetate (TPA), also called phorbol myristate acetate (PMA). TPA is a tumor promoter (substance that facilitates induction of tumors by carcinogens). TPA exerts pleiotropic effects on a number of cell types, including LYMPHOCYTES. TPA binds to and activates protein kinase C, resulting in the phosphorylation of serine and threonine residues in the cytoplasmic domains of transmembrane proteins (e.g., CD2, CD3). These biochemical reactions increase the expression of interleukin-2 receptors on T lymphocytes and stimulate their growth when INTERLEUKIN-1 is present in addition to TPA. TPA induces degranulation of POLY-

MORPHONUCLEAR LEUKOCYTES MAST CELLS AND PLATELETS

phylogenetic-associated residues. Amino acid residues found preferentially at certain positions in a protein of one or more species. The term has been used to describe such residues in IMMUNOGLOBULIN VARIABLE REGIONS.

pigeon breeder's lung. *See* HYPERSENSITIVITY PNEUMONITIS.

pinocytosis. *See* ENDOCYTOSIS.

plaque-forming assay. *See* HEMOLYTIC PLAQUE ASSAY.

plaque-forming cells. *See* HEMOLYTIC PLAQUE ASSAY.

plasma. Uncoagulated blood from which cells have been removed. *See* SERUM.

plasma cell. Terminally differentiated B LYMPHOCYTE that synthesizes and secretes immunoglobulin. Plasma cells are round or ovoid and have a mean diameter of 14 μm. The nucleus is eccentric and its chromatin is distributed in a pattern resembling the spokes of a wheel ('cartwheel nucleus'). Plasma cells have abundant cytoplasm with prominent rough ENDOPLASMIC RETICULUM and GOLGI COMPLEX. The cytoplasm stains red with pyronin ('pyroninophilic') due to its high content of RNA. Plasma cells do not divide and have a half-life of about two to four days. They are identified by reactions with fluorescein-labeled antibodies to immunoglobulin in the cytoplasm (*see* IMMUNOFLUORESCENCE). Plasma cells are usually found in SECONDARY LYMPHOID ORGANS (e.g., LYMPH NODES and SPLEEN). In contrast to B lymphocytes, plasma cells have no surface immunoglobulin or COMPLEMENT RECEPTORS.

plasma cell antigen (PC-1, PC-2). ALLOANTIGEN in the membranes of mouse PLASMA CELLS.

plasmapheresis. Procedure in which blood is removed from an individual, centrifuged, and the cells are then re-infused into the patient. Plasmapheresis is used in the treatment of autoimmune disease (e.g., GOODPASTURE'S SYNDROME) to remove the antibodies that cause the disease. It is also used in the treatment of MACROGLOBULINEMIA OF WALDENSTRÖM to remove the macroglobulin that, in excessive amounts, increases blood viscosity and causes symptoms.

plasmid. Extrachromosomal double-stranded circular DNA molecules found in most bacterial species and in some eukaryotes. Ordinarily, a plasmid is not essential to its host cell. However, many plasmids contain genes (e.g., for antibiotic resistance) that may be essential in certain environments. Plasmids range in size from 1 to 200 kilobases. Although plasmids are dependent on the replication machinery of the host cell, they contain their own genes for regulating the time of synthesis and the number of plasmid copies per cell. The replication of plasmids under stringent control is coupled to that of the host, and only one or a few copies of such plasmids are found per cell. Plasmids under relaxed control have copy numbers of 10–200; in such plasmids the copy number can be increased to several thousand per cell if host protein synthesis is shut off (e.g., by treatment with chloramphenicol).

Plasmids are frequently used as cloning VECTORS. To be useful for cloning, a plasmid should have the following properties: (1) small size and relaxed mode of replication; (2) presence of one or more selectable markers (e.g., antibiotic resistance) to allow identification of transformants and to prevent loss of the plasmid from the bacteria; (3) a single recognition site for one or more restriction enzymes in regions of the plasmid that are not essential for replication and into which foreign DNA can be inserted. If there are two or more genes for antibiotic resistance on the plasmid, it is useful if the site for DNA insertion is located within one of them, so that insertion inactivates the gene, allowing identification of bacteria containing the recombinant. Another useful marker is the *E. coli lac* gene, which may be inactivated as the result of insertion of exogenous DNA into the coding region. In this case, recombinants that do not produce β-galactosidase can be recognized by their failure to produce a colored product when the bacterial colonies grow on medium containing an appropriate chromogenic substrate.

platelet. Small (2–4 μm in diameter), spherical, colorless, refractile, non-nucleated particle of the blood that is derived from MEGAKARYOCYTES of bone marrow. Platelets are required for the clotting of blood. Platelets contain SEROTONIN and HISTAMINE; their release from platelets contributes to immediate hypersensitivity reactions (*see* PLATELET-ACTIVATING FACTOR). Mammalian platelets (except those of primates) bear COMPLEMENT RECEPTOR 1 on their surfaces and are important in IMMUNE ADHERENCE in these species.

platelet-activating factor (PAF). Phosphorylcholine derivative released from MAST CELLS, POLYMORPHONUCLEAR LEUKOCYTES and MACROPHAGES when antibodies bound to Fc RECEPTORS on these cells encounter antigen. PAF aggregates PLATELETS and releases intracellular platelet constituents (e.g., SEROTONIN, HISTAMINE). Administration of PAF causes transient THROMBOCYTOPENIA, hypotension, and increased vascular permeability. PAF is thought to play a role in IMMEDIATE HYPERSENSITIVITY reactions.

platelet activating factor

Pol I. *See* DNA POLYMERASE (*E. coli*).

polyacrylamide gel. Medium used for electrophoretic separation (*see* ELECTROPHORESIS) of proteins and nucleic acids. Acrylamide in solution is polymerized and cross-linked, and allowed to set into a gel in tubes or between glass plates. The porosity of the gel can be varied, allowing the separation of molecules in different size ranges. Separations are influenced by both size and charge. *See* POLYACRYLAMIDE GEL ELECTROPHORESIS IN SODIUM DODECYL SULFATE.

polyacrylamide gel electrophoresis in sodium dodecyl sulfate (SDS-PAGE). Technique for separating proteins according to their molecular weights. The protein or mixture of proteins is incubated in excess SDS, usually at an elevated temperature and in the presence of a reducing agent to ensure complete denaturation. Under these conditions, the amount of sodium dodecyl sulfate (SDS) bound to most proteins, per unit weight, is approximately constant. Therefore, different protein–SDS complexes have essentially identical charge-to-mass ratios and migrate in polyacrylamide gels of the correct porosity according to polypeptide size. Unlabeled proteins can be detected by staining with dye (e.g., Coomassie blue) and radiolabeled proteins by autoradiography. A plot of log molecular weight against mobility is approximately linear, and the molecular weight of an unknown protein can be estimated by comparison with standard proteins. However, some proteins (e.g., glycoproteins) bind relatively less SDS and others (e.g., membrane proteins) bind relatively more SDS than the proteins used as standards. Consequently, such proteins migrate anomalously in SDS gels, the apparent molecular weight of a glycoprotein being higher and that of a membrane protein lower than the true molecular weight. *See* ELECTROPHORESIS, POLYACRYLAMIDE GEL.

polyarteritis nodosa. Segmental VASCULITIS of small and medium-sized muscular arteries of all organs. In 30 percent of cases, hepatitis B antigen is found in the blood, and this suggests that the disease is caused by IMMUNE COMPLEXES. Affected blood vessel walls are infiltrated with NEUTROPHILS; ultimately NECROSIS of the arteries occurs. The male-to-female ratio among patients is 3:1. The disease may respond favorably to treatment with CYCLOPHOSPHAMIDE.

polyclonal. Related to or derived from many CLONES.

polyclonal activator. Substance that stimulates T or B LYMPHOCYTES, regardless of their antigen specificity. Polyclonal activators include plant lectins that activate T lymphocytes and/or B lymphocytes and bacterial products (e.g., LIPOPOLYSACCHARIDES) that activate B lymphocytes.

polyclonal antibodies. Antibodies, derived from many different CLONES of antibody-forming cells, all of which react with a particular antigen. This term is used to contrast to the term, MONOCLONAL ANTIBODIES. IMMUNIZATION usually results in a polyclonal antibody response.

polydeoxyribonucleotide synthase (ATP-requiring) (DNA ligase; EC 6.5.1.1). Enzyme that catalyses the formation of phosphodiester bonds between 5'-phosphoryl and 3'-hydroxyl groups in DNA and that requires ATP as a cofactor. Such enzymes have been isolated from a variety of sources including bacteriophage T4 and rat liver. DNA ligases seal single-stranded breaks in duplex DNA. *In vivo* they function in DNA replication and recombination and may play a role in DNA repair. It has been shown that the DNA ligase isolated from bacteriophage T4 can also catalyse blunt-end ligation of DNA (i.e., ligation between molecules lacking complementary single-stranded termini). This property makes the T4 DNA ligase useful in various manipulations of DNA *in vitro* (e.g. addition of synthetic linkers to duplex DNA). In the presence of high concentrations of any of several types of macromolecules (e.g., polyethylene glycol and bovine serum albumin), DNA ligase from rat liver has also been shown to catalyse blunt-end ligation. The T4 enzyme is a single chain of 487 amino acid residues and can be isolated from T4-infected *E. coli*. During catalysis, the cofactor is split to form an enzyme–AMP complex. *See* POLYDEOXYRIBONUCLEOTIDE SYNTHASE (NAD⁺-REQUIRING).

polydeoxyribonucleotide synthase (NAD⁺-requiring) (DNA ligase; EC 6.5.1.2). Enzyme that catalyses the formation of phosphodiester bonds between 5'-phosphoryl and 3'-hydroxyl groups and that requires NAD⁺ as a cofactor. Such an enzyme has been isolated from *E. coli*. Although under ordinary assay conditions, the *E. coli* DNA ligase does not catalyse blunt-end ligation, this activity can be demonstrated when the assay is carried out in the presence of high concentrations of macromolecules and may, therefore, occur in living cells. During catalysis, the cofactor is split to form an enzyme–AMP complex. *See* POLYDEOXYRIBONUCLEOTIDE SYNTHASE (ATP-REQUIRING).

polyimmunoglobulin receptor. Receptor for polymeric immunoglobulins, which mediates the TRANSCYTOSIS of polymeric IgA and IgM into external secretions. These receptors are found on the surfaces of epithelial cells and hepatocytes; in the gut, they are located on the basolateral surface of epithelial cells. After the polymeric immunoglobulin is bound, the receptor-ligand complex undergoes ENDOCYTOSIS and is transported across the cell in vesicles; EXOCYTOSIS of this complex occurs at the apical cell surface, releasing the immunoglobulin into the lumen of the gut. Similar processes occur in hepatocytes in some species, resulting in transport of IgA into the bile. Before release into the secretions the receptor is proteolytically cleaved close to the membrane and discharged while still bound to the polymeric immunoglobulin. Thus, the receptor is used for only one round of transport. The portion of the receptor bound to immunoglobulin and released with it into the secretions is called the SECRETORY COMPONENT.

The primary translation product of one form of rabbit polyimmunoglobulin receptor, deduced from the cDNA sequence, was found to consists of 773 amino acid residues: a SIGNAL SEQUENCE (18 residues), an extracellular portion (629 residues), most of which becomes the secretory component, a transmembrane segment (23 residues), and a long cytoplasmic segment (103 residues). There are two sites for N-LINKED OLIGOSACCHARIDES. Analysis of the primary structure indicates that the protein is composed of seven DOMAINS, each containing approximately 110 residues. The amino-terminal five domains have a high degree of homology with each other. As in immunoglobulin domains, each has a pair of cysteine residues that could form an intradomain disulfide bridge spanning 60–70 amino acid residues. The five amino-terminal domains have significant similarity in amino acid sequence to immunoglobulin VARIABLE REGIONS, especially to those of kappa chains, as well as to Thy-1. Thus, the polyimmunoglobulin receptor is a member of the IMMUNOGLOBULIN SUPERFAMILY. The sixth domain, which contains the membrane-spanning segment, also has some resemblance in sequence to immunoglobulin kappa variable regions, but it does not have a pair of cysteine residues positioned to form a loop of the size characteristic of immunoglobulin domains. The seventh (cytoplasmic) domain has no similarity in sequence to immunoglobulins.

Human secretory component is similar in amino acid sequence to the first five domains of the rabbit polyimmunoglobulin receptor; after appropriate alignment there is about 55 percent identity.

polymorphism. Occurrence, with appreciable frequency in a population, of two or more variants at a particular genetic locus. The variants may or may not code for a protein. In human populations, appreciable frequency is usually taken to be at least 1 percent. The existence of polymorphisms can be established by direct analysis of DNA (e.g., determination of RESTRICTION FRAGMENT LENGTH POLYMORPHISMS) or by analysis of gene products (e.g., by electrophoretic and/or immunological techniques). Examples of polymorphisms in human populations are the ABO and RH BLOOD GROUPS, molecules of the HLA complex (class I, II, and III), the Gm ALLOTYPES of IMMUNOGLOBULIN GAMMA CHAINS, and the Km ALLOTYPES of IMMUNOGLOBULIN KAPPA CHAINS.

polymorphonuclear leukocyte (PMN). White blood cell of myeloid (*see* MYELOID CELL) lineage (13 μm in diameter), characterized by a nucleus composed of three distinct lobes that are connected by thin strands of chromatin. PMNs are classified by the staining properties of the specific or SECONDARY GRANULES in the cytoplasm: EOSINOPHILS (5 percent), BASOPHILS (2 percent) and NEUTROPHILS (approximately 90 percent). All PMNs contain PRIMARY GRANULES. The term 'poly' (an abbreviation for polymorphonuclear leukocyte) is frequently used to mean neutrophil. *See* MYELOCYTE.

polymyositis. Inflammatory disease of muscle that is presumed to have an immunological cause. Patients experience muscle weakness and pain. Microscopically, the muscle is infiltrated with LYMPHOCYTES. Extracts of normal muscle are MITOGENS for T LYMPHOCYTES from patients with polymyositis. Serum of patients contains autoantibodies to some tRNA synthetases.

polynucleotide 5′-hydroxyl-kinase (polynucleotide kinase; EC 2.7.1.78). Enzyme, usually obtained from *E. coli* infected with bacteriophage T4, that catalyses the transfer of the γ-phosphate group from ATP to the 5′-hydroxyl terminus of DNA, RNA, oligonucleotides or even nucleoside-3′-phosphate. Since naturally occuring nucleic acids have 5′-phosphoryl, not 5′-hydroxyl groups, the 5′-phosphoryl group must first be removed, e.g., with ALKALINE PHOSPHATASE. When $[\gamma^{32}P]$-ATP is used, the label is incorporated at the 5′ end of the DNA or RNA strand. The enzyme is used for labeling 5′ ends of DNA, e.g., for sequencing by the Maxam–Gilbert technique and for S1 NUCLEASE MAPPING. The function of polynucleotide kinase *in vivo* is not known.

polyvalent. *Synonym for* MULTIVALENT.

polyvalent antiserum. *Synonym for* MULTIVALENT ANTISERUM.

polyvalent vaccine. VACCINE composed of several ANTIGENS, such as various strains of poliovirus, or pneumococcal polysaccharides, or DPT (diphtheria, pertussis, tetanus).

postcardiotomy syndrome. Fever, chest pain and pericardial effusion occurring days to weeks after cardiac surgery or any traumatic injury to the heart. Patients have AUTOANTIBODIES to antigens of the heart, detectable by IMMUNOFLUORESCENCE. The symptoms respond rapidly to CORTICOSTEROID therapy. A similar syndrome has been observed in patients who have had myocardial infarctions.

Prausnitz–Küstner reaction. Skin test in humans for IMMEDIATE HYPERSENSITIVITY to a particular allergen. Test serum is injected intracutaneously into a normal recipient who is challenged 24–48 hours later with a putative ALLERGEN. A positive reaction is indicated by a wheal and flare reaction (*see* URTICARIA) at the injection site within 20 minutes. The positive reaction results from the transfer of antibody. This reaction, which is named after the two physicians who were donor and recipient in the original test, is now only of historic interest. *See* PASSIVE CUTANEOUS ANAPHYLAXIS.

pre-B cell. Earliest cell in the B LYM-PHOCYTE lineage. Pre-B cells are identified by the presence of IMMUNOGLOBULIN MU CHAINS in the cytoplasm and by the absence of surface immunoglobulin. Pre-B cells are present in the bone marrow of adults and in the liver of the fetus at 10 weeks of gestation. Pre-B cells are found in normal numbers in the bone marrow of males with X-LINKED AGAMMAGLOBULINEMIA, but B lymphocytes do not develop. Studies of IMMU-NOGLOBULIN GENES show that the heavy chain *V*, *D* and *J* gene segments have become contiguous in pre-B cells. However the light chain genes segments are not rearranged. *See* IMMUNOGLOBULIN GENE REARRANGEMENT.

precipitation. *See* PRECIPITIN, PRECIPITIN REACTION.

precipitin. Antibody that forms precipitates with the appropriate antigen. At one time, it was thought that the ability to form precipitates was the property of a particular type of antibody, but it is now known that most antibodies are capable of precipitating with antigen.

precipitin curve. Plot of results of a set of PRECIPITIN REACTIONS in which increasing amounts of antigen are added to a constant amount of a mixture of antibodies (antiserum). The total amount of precipitate or the amount of antibody precipitated is plotted against the amount of antigen added. The curve is divided into three zones: ANTI-BODY EXCESS, EQUIVALENCE and ANTIGEN EXCESS, according to the presence or absence

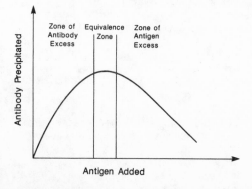

precipitin curve

of detectable antibody or antigen in the supernatant. *See* QUANTITATIVE PRECIPITIN REACTION.

precipitin reaction. Reaction in which antibodies combine with soluble antigen to form a precipitate. *See* QUANTITATIVE PRECIPITIN REACTION, PRECIPITIN CURVE.

primary agammaglobulinemia. *See* ANTI-BODY DEFICIENCY SYNDROME, PRIMARY IMMU-NODEFICIENCY.

primary biliary cirrhosis. Chronic disease of the liver, characterized by progressive destruction of intrahepatic bile ducts. The disease is seen predominantly in middle-aged women. Almost all patients (more than 90 percent) have antibodies to mitochondrial membrane antigens, as well as circulating IgM-containing immune complexes. The relationship of the immunological abnormalities to the pathogenesis of the disease is unclear.

primary granule. Cytoplasmic organelle (0.8 μm in diameter) of POLYMORPHONU-CLEAR LEUKOCYTES that stains blue (azurophilic) with Wright or Giemsa stains. Primary granules contain myeloperoxidase (*see* MYELOPEROXIDASE DEFICIENCY), collagenase and elastase. They constitute 10–20 percent of the cytoplasmic granules of polymorphonuclear leukocytes. *See* SECOND-ARY GRANULE, TERTIARY GRANULE.

primary immune response. IMMUNE RESPONSE that takes place following the first encounter with antigen. The rate of development and magnitude of this response depends upon the immunogenicity (*see* IMMUNOGENIC) of the antigen; it is usually slower and of smaller magnitude than the SECONDARY IMMUNE RESPONSE to the same antigen. In the primary response there is usually a lag period of several days between introduction of the antigen and the appearance of ANTIBODY or specific T LYMPHOCYTES in blood; the serum antibody is of low titer and usually of low affinity with a relative predominance of IgM. In contrast, the secondary antibody response has a short latent period and consists mostly of IgG antibodies. The distinction between primary and secondary immune response may be less apparent when highly immunogenic antigens, such as bacteria, viruses and particulate antigens, are used or after immunization with ADJUVANT.

primary immunodeficiency. Any failure or compromise of specific immunity caused by an intrinsic defect in B and/or T LYMPHOCYTES.

*Primary immunodeficiency diseases**

A. *Predominantly antibody defects*
1. **X-linked agammaglobulinemia**
2. **X-linked hypogammaglobulinemia with growth hormone deficiency**
3. Autosomal recessive agammaglobulinemia
4. **Immunoglobulin deficiency with increased IgM (and IgD)**
5. **IgA deficiency**
6. Selective deficiency of other immunoglobulin isotypes (*see* **IgG subclass deficiency**)
7. **Kappa chain deficiency**
8. **Immunodeficiency with thymoma**
9. **Transient hypogammaglobulinemia of infancy**

B. *Combined immunodeficiency*
10. **Common variable immunodeficiency**
    a. Predominant antibody deficiency
    b. Predominant cell-mediated immunity defect
11. **Severe combined immunodeficiency**
12. **Reticular dysgenesis**
13. **Adenosine deaminase deficiency**
14. **Purine nucleoside phosphorylase deficiency**
15. **MHC class I deficiency** ('bare lymphocyte syndrome')
16. **MHC class II deficiency**

C. *Immunodeficiency associated with other major defects*
17. **Wiskott–Aldrich syndrome**
18. **Ataxia-telangiectasia**
19. **Third and fourth pouch syndrome (DiGeorge's syndrome)**
20. **Transcobalamin 2 deficiency**
21. **Immunodeficiency with partial albinism**
22. **Immunodeficiency following hereditary defective response to Epstein–Barr virus**

*Words in boldface type are defined. This classification is modified from the WHO Committee on Immunodeficiency Diseases.

primary interaction. Binding of antigen and antibody. Primary interaction does not refer to subsequent events such as precipitation (*see* PRECIPITIN REACTION) or COMPLEMENT FIXATION. It can be measured by tests such as EQUILIBRIUM DIALYSIS, FLUORESCENCE QUENCHING and various radioimmunoassays.

primary lymphoid organ. LYMPHOID organ where T or B LYMPHOCYTES mature. In primary lymphoid organs, STEM CELLS mature in the absence of antigenic stimulation. The THYMUS is the primary lymphoid organ for T lymphocytes in all vertebrate species. The BURSA OF FABRICIUS is the primary lymphoid organ for B lymphocytes in birds. In adult mammals, the primary lymphoid organ for B lymphocytes is the bone marrow. *See* SECONDARY LYMPHOID ORGAN.

primary structure. Linear amino acid sequence of a polypeptide or protein. *See* QUATERNARY STRUCTURE, SECONDARY STRUCTURE, TERTIARY STRUCTURE.

primed lymphocyte. Lymphocyte from an immunized (*see* IMMUNIZATION) individual or lymphocyte that has been exposed to antigen *in vitro*.

private idiotypic determinant (IdI). IDIOTYPIC DETERMINANT that is unique to an antibody produced by a single individual. Typically, private idiotypic determinants reflect unique amino acid sequences in the HYPERVARIABLE REGIONS of antibody heavy and/or light chains. *See* PUBLIC IDIOTYPIC DETERMINANT.

private specificity. Antigenic determinant that is unique to one member of a family of proteins (e.g., a group of ALLOANTIGENS). The term is often used to refer to determinants on molecules in the MAJOR HISTOCOMPATIBILITY COMPLEX (e.g., a determinant associated with a single H-2 allele (H-2K or H-2D)). *See* PUBLIC SPECIFICITY.

privileged site. Tissue where ALLOGRAFTS are protected from rejection (e.g., the anterior chamber of the eye or the brain) perhaps because of poor lymphatic drainage. The slow diffusion of antigen from privileged sites to lymphoid organs appears to retard GRAFT REJECTION.

pro-C3. Single-chain polypeptide that is cleaved into the alpha and beta chains of C3. The beta chain is amino-terminal.

pro-C4. Single-chain polypeptide that is cleaved into the alpha, beta and gamma chains of C4. The beta chain is amino-terminal, the gamma chain is carboxy-terminal.

pro-C5. Single-chain polypeptide that is cleaved into the alpha and beta chains of C5. The beta chain is amino-terminal.

progressive systemic sclerosis. *Synonym for* SYSTEMIC SCLEROSIS.

progressive vaccinia. Relentless progression of a smallpox VACCINATION lesion, spreading from the initial site of vaccination, and resulting in death. This complication of smallpox vaccination occurs in children who have primary immunodeficiency of cell-mediated immunity (e.g., SEVERE COMBINED IMMUNODEFICIENCY). *See* ECZEMA VACCINATUM, GENERALIZED VACCINIA.

promoter. Region of DNA that plays an essential role in the initiation of transcription of a gene. In bacteria, it is the DNA segment(s) to which RNA POLYMERASE binds when transcription is initiated. Two hexamer sequences, centered at about 10 and 35 nucleotides upstream (5′) from the origin of transcription, appear to be particularly important. The sequence at −10 is called the 'Pribnow box' and its consensus sequence is TATAAT; the sequence at −35 has the consensus sequence TTGACA. Strong promoters (high levels of transcription) generally match the consensus sequence more closely than do weak promoters. Sequences further upstream may also influence promoter efficiency.

Initiation of transcription by the RNA polymerases of eukaryotes is considerably more complex than it is in the case of prokaryotes. For transcription by RNA polymerase II (*see* DNA-DIRECTED RNA POLYMERASE), there are important sequences in the region just 5′ to the transcriptional start site. The most conserved of these is the 'TATA' box, a conserved AT-rich segment centered about 25 base pairs upstream from the start site and usually flanked by G/C-rich sequences. Additional promoter elements may lie further upstream, e.g., a consensus sequence containing the nucleotides CAAT about 70 bases from the start site; there may also be more distant upstream sites. Genes transcribed by RNA polymerase III contain internal promoters downstream (~50–100 nucleotides 3′) from the transcriptional start site. For transcription by RNA polymerase I, a number of sequences surrounding the start site appear to be important. In addition to the RNA polymerases, a variety of 'transcription factors' (proteins that regulate transcription by interacting with specific promoter elements or that bind directly to polymerases) are required. Such factors may confer species, stage and tissue specificity on the promoter.

Transcription of IMMUNOGLOBULIN GENES depends on a 'TATA' box and also requires a promoter element, the octamer ATTTGCAT, which is 70 ± 10 nucleotides upstream from the start site of κ and λ transcription; the complement (ATGCAAAT) is found at the same location with respect to heavy chain genes. This octamer element is also found in other promoters. There are at least two proteins that bind to the octamer sequence, one of which is found only in lymphoid cells and probably confers tissue specificity. This octamer is also found in the heavy chain ENHANCER.

properdin (P). Protein of the ALTERNATIVE PATHWAY OF COMPLEMENT. Properdin binds to the alternative pathway C3 CONVERTASE (C3bBb) and stabilizes it. C3 NEPHRITIC FACTOR has similar activity.

Properdin is composed of a single polypeptide chain of 441 amino acid residues. There are two sites for attachment of N-linked oligosaccharides (asparagines at positions 370 and 400). By electron microscopy, properdin is seen to form cyclic oligomers (mainly dimers, trimers and tetramers) by interaction between the 30–40 amino acid residues at the amino- and carboxy-termini. Properdin contains six repeating motifs of approximately 60 amino acid residues (between positions 53 and 413). In these motifs, 11 of the positions are always occupied by the same amino acid residues: cysteine at positions 10, 14, 17, 48 and 54, tryptophan at 7, serine at 8 and 11, valine at 12, threonine at 13 and arginine at 23. The repeating motif is homologous to 60 amino acids at the amino- and carboxy terminal ends of C7, C8α and C8β and the amino terminal end of C9. This 60 residue motif is also found in three repeats in each chain of the homotrimer, thrombospondin, which binds fibrinogen, plasminogen, FIBRONECTIN and other matrix molecules. It is also found in a circumsporozoite protein of several species of malaria and is thought to facilitate entry of circumsporozoites into hepatocytes.

Properdin was the first protein described in the alternative pathway of complement, which was formerly called the properdin system.

properdin deficiency. Rare genetic deficiency inherited as an X-linked recessive. Affected males have less than 2 percent of the normal amount of PROPERDIN in serum and they are susceptible to neisserial infections. In one kindred, a mutant form of properdin has been found in serum of affected males. Heterozygous females have half-normal to normal amounts of properdin in serum and may also be susceptible to neisserial infections.

prophylactic   immunization. Protection against infections usually by active immunization (*see* ACTIVE IMMUNITY) and sometimes by passive immunization (*see* PASSIVE IMMUNITY).

prostaglandin (PG). Molecule derived from arachidonic acid by the action of an enzyme called cyclooxygenase. PGD_2 is released from MAST CELLS following IgE-mediated reactions; it causes dilation of small blood vessels and constriction of bronchi and blood vessels in the lung. PGE_2 is released from MONONUCLEAR PHAGOCYTES following binding of antigen–antibody complexes to Fcγ RECEPTORS. PGE_2 inhibits expression of CLASS II HISTOCOMPATIBILITY MOLECULES in MACROPHAGES and T LYMPHOCYTES and also inhibits the growth of T lymphocytes.

PGD_2 and PGE_2 (as well as PGI_2 or prostacyclin released from endothelial cells) inhibit platelet aggregation and thus antagonize the action of thromboxane A_2, the principal PG metabolite released from platelets.

ASPIRIN and INDOMETHACIN, two potent anti-inflammatory drugs, inhibit PG synthesis. Prostaglandins were so named because they were first found as a substance(s) in seminal fluid that contracts uterus and were thought to come from the prostate gland.

protein A (SpA).   Constituent of the cell wall of many strains of *Staphylococcus aureus* that binds to some IMMUNOGLOBULINS. Protein A has been used extensively as a reagent for identifying and isolating immunoglobulins and antigen–antibody complexes (e.g., IMMUNOBLOTTING). Protein A has also been used to remove antibodies and immune complexes from serum of patients by extracorporeal filtration. The usual source for protein A is the Cowan I strain of *S. aureus*.

Protein A binds to the Fc region (*see* Fc FRAGMENT) of human IgG subclasses (except IgG3), to mouse IgG subclasses, and to IgG of many other mammalian species; the strength of the interaction varies according to the immunoglobulin. Other classes of immunoglobulin (e.g., IgM, IgA) may also bind protein A, but these so-called alternative interactions appear to be mediated by the Fab region (*see* Fab FRAGMENT), and are weaker. Protein A can be used in soluble form or it can be coupled to insoluble matrices (e.g., AGAROSE); whole staphylococci (usually heat-killed and formalin-fixed) with protein A on their surfaces can also conveniently be used for immunoprecipitation.

Protein A is covalently linked to peptidoglycans in the bacterial cell wall. The gene encoding a precursor protein has been sequenced from strain 8325-4. The corresponding protein consists of 524 amino acid residues. There is a putative signal sequence of 36 amino acid residues, five repeats of a 58-residue unit, which display considerable (about 65–80 percent) identity in amino acid sequence and are responsible for IgG binding, 12 repeats of an eight amino acid unit and a carboxy-terminal region containing a hydrophobic stretch that may serve as a membrane anchor. Due to processing at the amino- and carboxy-terminal ends, the M_r of the protein isolated from the Cowan I strain is about 42,000 and its amino-terminus is blocked. Cleavage of the protein by trypsin releases four IgG-binding DOMAINS. The fifth domain encoded by the cloned gene may be specific to strain 8325-4 or may not bind IgG due to sequence differences. X-ray diffraction studies indicate that the main contacts between human IgG1 and protein A are formed by nine residues in C_H2 and C_H3 of Fc and eleven residues in each of the repeat-units of protein A. The inability of human IgG3 to bind protein A may be the result of a single amino acid substitution in C_H3.

The physiological function of protein A is not clear. It has been suggested that it may help the bacterium evade the immune response by covering its antigenic determinants with immunoglobulins, which are autologous or self-antigens (i.e., not foreign), and therefore not IMMUNOGENIC.

protein G. Constituent of the cell wall of group G streptococci that binds to the Fc region (*see* Fc FRAGMENT) of most IgG molecules. Protein G binds to all four sub-classes of human IgG (including IgG3 to which PROTEIN A does not bind). Compared to protein A, protein G reacts more strongly and with a wider range of IgGs from different mammalian species. (The only IgG to which protein A is reported to bind more strongly is that from the cat). Protein G does not appear to bind to other immunoglobulin classes (e.g., IgM and IgA) and is therefore a more versatile and specific reagent for complex formation with IgGs.

Like protein A, protein G is covalently attached to the bacterial cell wall. It has been solubilized by treatment with papain to yield a product of M_r 30,000. The gene encoding protein G has been cloned from several strains of streptococci. That from strain GX7809 encodes a protein of 448 amino acid residues including a putative SIGNAL SEQUENCE of 33 residues, two sets of repeated sequences, each occurring twice (A1 and A2, each of 37 residues; B1 and B2, each of 55 residues), a proline-rich section, five repeats of a highly-charged pentapeptide, and a carboxy-terminal segment that may function as a membrane anchor. The IgG binding activity has been localized to the B repeats. A protein G gene isolated from another streptococcal strain specifies three A and three B repeats, but is otherwise similar. Group C streptococci produce IgG-binding proteins that resemble those from group G in structure and function. Except for the putative signal sequence and membrane anchor, there is little if any significant similarity in sequence between protein G and protein A. However, in general organization, these proteins share some structural features (e.g., repeated immunoglobulin-binding segments).

protein S. Vitamin K-dependent plasma protein that acts as a cofactor for protein C in the clotting system. It is a single polypeptide chain (M_r 69,000) that, like other vitamin K-dependent clotting factors, contains approximately 10 gamma-carboxyglutamic acid residues. About half of plasma protein S is bound to the C4 BINDING PROTEIN; the bound form of protein S is inactive.

protoplast. Protoplasm of a cell, including the cytoplasmic membrane (cell membrane, plasma membrane), but excluding the cell wall that surrounds the cytoplasmic membrane. In Gram-positive bacteria, this cell wall consists of a thick (20–80 nm) layer of peptidoglycan. In Gram-negative bacteria, the cell wall is bipartite, consisting of a thin (~1 nm) peptidoglycan layer surrounded by the LIPOPOLYSACCHARIDE-containing outer membrane. Protoplasts are osmotically fragile, but can be protected from lysis by placing them in hypertonic solutions (e.g., 20 percent sucrose). Protoplasts can be prepared from Gram-positive cells either by inhibiting cell wall synthesis (with antibiotics such as penicillin) or by enzymatic digestion of the peptidoglycan layer (with LYSOZYME). Protoplasts of Gram-negative bacteria can be prepared by similar treatment although in this case the outer membrane limits access to the peptidoglycan layer and may require disruption (e.g., with EDTA) to allow protoplast preparation; such protoplasts usually contain remnants of the outer membrane and are often called spheroplasts.

protoplast fusion. Method for transfer (TRANSFECTION) of DNA from bacteria into other bacteria or into cultured animal cells such as MYELOMA cells. Protoplasts, which may be prepared by lysozyme–EDTA treatment of *E. coli* carrying an appropriate plasmid, are fused with myeloma cells by methods similar to those used in production of B cell hybridomas (e.g., treatment with polyethylene glycol).

prozone. Zone in a titration at which high concentrations of antibodies apparently fail to react even though less concentrated solutions of the same antibodies do react. In AGGLUTINATION reactions, cells in the prozone do not agglutinate but may have antibodies on their surfaces; the failure to agglutinate may be the result of saturation of each particle with antibodies so that no cross-linking occurs. In some precipitin reactions, the antigen–antibody complexes formed in antibody excess may be relatively small and remain soluble.

pseudoalleles. Distinct genes that are functionally related and so closely linked that they behave as if they are allelic.

pseudogene. DNA sequence that resembles a gene but that is not expressed because of one or more defects that impair some stage of gene expression (e.g., faulty promoter, deficient splice signal, in-frame stop signal). Once the normal gene product is no longer produced, there is no selective barrier to the further accumulation of mutations, so pseudogenes typically have a number of defects. Some pseudogenes, which resemble mRNA in that they have 3'-poly-A tracts and correctly excised INTRONS, are thought to originate from the insertion of reverse transcripts (possibly carried by a retrovirus) into the GENOME.

pseudoglobulin. Globulin that is sparingly soluble in water, as distinct from a EUGLOBULIN, which is insoluble in water.

public idiotypic determinant (IdX or CRI). IDIOTYPIC DETERMINANT that is found in many members of the same species, usually on antibodies specific for a particular antigen. However, such shared determinants can also occur on apparently unrelated antibodies. These determinants are also known as cross-reacting idiotypic determinants, hence the abbreviations IdX or CRI. Public idiotypic determinants reflect similarities in amino acid sequence of antibody heavy and/or light chains; they have been used as markers for the gene segments encoding VARIABLE REGIONS. *See* PRIVATE IDIOTYPIC DETERMINANT.

public specificity. Antigenic determinant that is shared by more than one member of a family of proteins (e.g., a group of ALLOANTIGENS). The term is often used to refer to determinants on molecules in the MAJOR HISTOCOMPATIBILITY COMPLEX. Public determinants may be shared by many proteins or by as few as two. *See* PRIVATE SPECIFICITY.

pulsed field gradient gel electrophoresis (PFGE). Technique for separating large pieces of DNA by application of alternating electric fields to an AGAROSE gel matrix. The field may be alternated in one dimension by reversing the anode and cathode (field inversion gel electrophoresis or FIGE) or it may be alternated in two directions (orthogonal field alternation gel electrophoresis or OFAGE). With present technology, molecules of several thousand kilobases (e.g., yeast chromosomes) can be resolved. PFGE is being used for studies of chromosomal organization in a variety of organisms including humans.

purified protein derivative (PPD). Soluble protein fraction precipitated by trichloroacetic acid from medium in which *Mycobacterium tuberculosis* has been grown. It is widely used in TUBERCULIN tests.

purine nucleoside phosphorylase deficiency. Form of SEVERE COMBINED IMMUNODEFICIENCY that results from the inheritance of mutant forms of purine nucleoside phosphorylase (EC 2.4.2.1) (PNP). The immunodeficiency is caused by accumulation of metabolites that are toxic for T LYMPHOCYTES; B LYMPHOCYTES are usually present in normal numbers. PNP, which is present in all mammalian cells, catalyses phosphorolysis of guanosine, deoxyguanosine and inosine. PNP deficiency results in increased intracellular concentrations of guanosine, deoxyguanosine, guanosine triphosphate (GTP) and deoxyguanosine triphosphate (dGTP). dGTP inhibits ribonucleoside-diphosphate reductase, an enzyme involved in DNA synthesis. Precursors of T lymphocytes are more vulnerable to destruction by the accumulation of these metabolites than are other cells. Unlike adenosine deaminase (*see* ADENOSINE DEAMINASE DEFICIENCY), PNP is not more abundant in lymphoid tissue compared with other tissue.

PNP is a trimer of M_r 32,000 subunits. The gene encoding PNP has been mapped to chromosome 14q13.1; it encodes a polypeptide chain of 289 amino acid residues. PNP deficiency is inherited as an autosomal recessive. Levels of PNP (usually measured in red blood cells) are half-normal in heterozygotes. PNP deficiency has been treated successfully with transplants of bone marrow cells.

purpura. Hemorrhage into the skin causing the appearance of a purple or purple–blue rash.

purpura hyperglobulinemia. Skin hemorrhages of the lower extremities, particularly about the ankles. The phenomenon is observed in patients with markedly elevated serum immunoglobulins as in SJÖGREN'S SYNDROME, MACROGLOBULINEMIA OF WALDENSTRÖM, MULTIPLE MYELOMA, etc.

pyogenic infection. Bacterial infection that induces the formation of pus. Bacteria causing pyogenic infections include *Staphylococcus aureus*, *Streptococcus pyogenes*, *Streptococcus pneumoniae* and *Hemophilus influenzae*. Susceptibility to pyogenic infections is found in patients with ANTIBODY DEFICIENCY SYNDROMES and in patients having defects in PHAGOCYTIC CELLS or COMPLEMENT components (e.g., C3 DEFICIENCY, FACTOR H DEFICIENCY, FACTOR I DEFICIENCY).

pyrogen. Substance that causes fever.

pyroglobulin. Monoclonal immunoglobulin (e.g., MYELOMA PROTEIN) that precipitates irreversibly at 56°C, in contrast to BENCE–JONES PROTEIN, which precipitates at 56°C but redissolves upon boiling. *See* CRYOGLOBULIN.

Q

Qa antigen. *See* TLA COMPLEX.

Qa region. *See* TLA COMPLEX.

quantitative precipitin reaction. Immunochemical reaction in which the amount of precipitate, formed as a result of mixing antigen and antibodies in various proportions, is determined quantitatively, usually by washing the precipitates and then measuring the amount of protein in each. The determination of protein content can be made by several procedures, e.g. micro-Kjeldahl analysis (to determine nitrogen content), measurement of the optical density (at approximately 280 nm) of the dissolved precipitin. *See* PRECIPITIN CURVE.

quaternary structure. Packing of two or more folded polypeptide chains into a higher-order structure. *See* PRIMARY STRUCTURE, SECONDARY STRUCTURE, TERTIARY STRUCTURE.

Quin-2. Quinoline derivative that increases in fluorescence intensity when it binds to free Ca^{2+}. Quin-2 is administered as an ester so that it can enter cells; subsequently it is de-esterified. The fluorescence intensity of B and T LYMPHOCYTES loaded with Quin-2 increases upon activation, an indication of an increase of free Ca^{2+} in the cytosol.

Quin 2

181

R

radial immunodiffusion. *See* SINGLE RADIAL IMMUNODIFFUSION.

radioallergosorbent test (RAST). Test to measure IgE antibody specific for an ALLERGEN. The allergen is bound to an insoluble carrier, such as DEXTRAN beads. The serum to be tested is reacted with the insolubilized allergen, the particles are washed and then reacted with a radiolabeled antibody to human IgE. The labeled antibody binds only to the IgE antibody in the test serum that has been taken up by the particle-bound allergen. The allergen must be in excess relative to the total antibodies (all classes) in the test serum to assure complete uptake of the antibodies. The anti-IgE antibody must be in excess relative to the bound IgE antibodies. The amount of radioactivity bound to the beads is then proportional to the amount of specific IgE antibody to the allergen in the test serum. *See* RADIOIMMUNOSORBENT TEST.

radioimmunoassay (RIA). Any method for detecting or quantitating antigens or antibodies utilizing radiolabeled reactants. RIA can be used to detect very small quantities of antigens or antibodies, even in complex mixtures. In one frequently used version of RIA for antigen detection, the antigen is radiolabeled and reacted with a limiting amount of specific antibody (Ab 1). The complex containing bound antigen is then separated from free antigen (e.g., by reaction with a second antibody (Ab 2) specific for Ab 1). Unlabeled antigen in a test sample is used to compete with the binding of labeled antigen. The amount of test antigen is determined from the extent of inhibition obtained with standards containing defined amounts of the same antigen. *See* RADIOALLERGOSORBENT TEST, RADIOIMMUNOSORBENT TEST.

radioimmunoelectrophoresis. Variant of IMMUNOELECTROPHORESIS in which radiolabeled antibody or antigen is used to react specifically with particular PRECIPITIN arcs, followed by autoradiography to localize the radiolabel.

radioimmunosorbent test (RIST). Test to measure total IgE concentration in serum. Anti-IgE is bound to an insoluble carrier such as DEXTRAN beads. The serum to be tested is reacted with a standard amount of radiolabeled IgE and the mixture is then reacted with the insolubilized anti-IgE. After appropriate incubation and washing, the amount of radiolabeled IgE adhering to the beads is determined. The IgE in the test serum competes with the radiolabeled standard IgE for binding to the beads. The decrease in amount of labeled IgE relative to a control (no unlabeled IgE) is a measure of the IgE concentration in the test serum. The assay can be made quantitative by determining the degree of inhibition obtained with known IgE standards. *See* RADIOALLERGOSORBENT TEST, RADIOIMMUNOASSAY.

ragweed Weed of the Ambrosiae family whose pollen contains the most common

IUIS nomenclature	Old nomenclature	Approx M_r
Amb a I	Antigen E*	38,000
Amb a II	Antigen K*	38,000
Amb a III	Ra3	10,000
Amb a IV	Ra4 (BPA-R)	28,000
Amb a V	Ra5S	5,000
Amb a VI	Ra6	11,500
Amb t V	Ra5G	4,400

*Antigens E and K are heterodimers, which share many antigenic determinants.

Source: *International Archives of Allergy and Applied Immunology,* **85**:194, 1988.

respiratory ALLERGENS in North America. The two common species are the short and giant ragweed: *Ambrosia artemisiifolia (eliator)* and *Ambrosia trifida*. Their characterized allergens are listed in the table. The amino acid sequences of Ra3 (101 amino acid residues), Ra5S (45 residues) and Ra5G (40 residues) have been determined.

Raji cell assay.   Test for immune complexes in human serum. Raji cells are a line of transformed human B LYMPHOCYTES that lack surface IMMUNOGLOBULIN, but have Fcγ RECEPTORS, COMPLEMENT RECEPTOR 1, COMPLEMENT RECEPTOR 2 and receptors for C1q. Test serum is mixed with Raji cells, and the amount of immune complex bound is quantitated with radiolabeled F(ab')$_2$ antibodies to IgG.

random breeding.   Random mating of individuals in a population. If the random-bred population is sufficiently large, it will remain genetically diverse. However, small closed populations, even if randomly bred, tend to become genetically uniform. *See* INBREEDING, OUTBREEDING.

Raynaud's phenomenon.   Sudden, painful vasospasm of the fingers usually upon exposure to cold that may occur alone or in many CONNECTIVE TISSUE DISEASES (e.g., SYSTEMIC LUPUS ERYTHEMATOSUS, SYSTEMIC SCLEROSIS) and in CRYOGLOBULINEMIA.

RCA locus (*regulator of complement activation locus*). Segment of DNA (750 kb) on the long arm of chromosome 1 (1q3.2) that contains the genes encoding COMPLEMENT RECEPTOR 1, COMPLEMENT RECEPTOR 2, DECAY ACCELERATING FACTOR and C4 BINDING PROTEIN, in that order. These proteins bind to C4b, C3b, or C3dg and thereby regulate COMPLEMENT activation. They are mainly composed of short and long consensus repeats (*see* CONSENSUS SEQUENCE OF C3/C4 BINDING PROTEINS). FACTOR H, which is homologous to the proteins encoded in the RCA locus, is encoded by a gene that maps to chromosome 1, approximately 7 centiMorgans from the RCA locus.

reaction of identity.   Reaction in two-dimensional DOUBLE IMMUNODIFFUSION in which a continuous precipitin line forms when two antigens, in adjacent wells, react with antibodies diffusing from a third well. Such a reaction demonstrates antigenic identity of the two antigens with respect to the antibodies. *See* Figure.

reaction of non-identity.   Reaction in two-dimensional DOUBLE IMMUNODIFFUSION in which two distinct precipitin lines form when two antigens, in adjacent wells, react with a mixture of antibodies to each of them diffusing from a third well. The precipitin line formed by each of the two antigen–antibody systems is not affected by the presence of the other; typically the two precipitin lines cross. Such a reaction demonstrates that the two antigens do not share any determinants that can be detected by these antibodies. *See* Figure.

reaction of partial identity.   Reaction in two-dimensional DOUBLE IMMUNODIFFUSION in which a continuous precipitin line plus a spur form when two antigens, in adjacent wells, react with antibodies diffusing from a third well. Such a reaction demonstrates that the two antigens are related but not identical. (Some of the antibodies react with both antigens, but other antibodies – those that

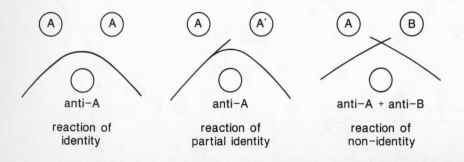

reaction of
identity

reaction of
partial identity

reaction of
non–identity

form the spur – react with only one of the antigens). *See* Figure.

reactive lysis.   Lysis of unsensitized red blood cells (not coated with antibody) initiated by complexes of C5b and C6 in the presence of C7, C8 and C9. Reactive lysis occurs as a bystander phenomenon when COMPLEMENT is activated.

reagin.   *See* IgE.

Rebuck skin window.   *See* SKIN WINDOW.

receptor-mediated endocytosis.   *See* ENDOCYTOSIS.

recombinant DNA.   DNA strand resulting from the physical joining of two or more pre-existing DNA strands. Traditionally, in eukaryotes, the term refers to the result of DNA exchange during meiosis or mitosis or by gene conversion. Recently, the term has come to be used to describe DNA constructs created *in vitro*.

recombinant DNA technology.   Methodology associated with the isolation, purification and replication of genes from one organism in another. It usually involves ligation of genomic or cDNA into a PLASMID or viral VECTOR in which the DNA can be replicated.

recombinant inbred (RI) **strain.**   Strain derived by INBREEDING two members of the F_2 generation of a cross between two INBRED STRAINS. A distinct line can be produced from each randomly chosen pair. This results in the genetic fixation of alleles present in the original F_2 pair. Recombinant inbred strains are useful in establishing genetic linkages. For this purpose, the distribution of genes among a group of different recombinant inbred lines is compared. To date, recombinant inbred strains are available only in the mouse.

Reed–Sternberg giant cells.   *See* HODGKIN'S DISEASE.

regional enteritis.   *See* INFLAMMATORY BOWEL DISEASE.

relapsing polychondritis.   Episodic, progressive inflammatory disease of cartilage, most frequently involving the external ears and presumed to have an immunological cause. Patients have antibodies to collagen in serum.

restitope.   In ANTIGEN PRESENTATION, the part of a T CELL RECEPTOR that interacts with a CLASS II HISTOCOMPATIBILITY MOLECULES. *See* AGRETOPE, DESETOPE, HISTOTOPE.

restriction endonuclease.   Bacterial endonuclease that recognizes and binds to a short sequence of DNA; binding is followed by cleavage, either within the recognition site or elsewhere, depending on the enzyme. In addition, for each restriction activity, a bacterial strain possesses a DNA methylase that recognizes the same sequence and 'modifies' it by adding methyl groups to either adenine or cytosine residues. As a rule, the methylation blocks binding of the restriction enzyme, rendering the DNA resistant to cleavage. However, certain restriction enzymes specifically cleave only methylated sequences. In either case, the effect of the restriction-methylase activities in a bacterial strain is to provide a mechanism for degrading foreign DNA molecules, while protecting the bacterium's own DNA.

The restriction–modification systems were originally discovered by their effects on bacteriophage DNA. Phage DNA can pass from one bacterium to another within the same strain because it has the same methylation pattern as that of the host DNA. When the phage DNA enters a new bacterial strain, it is subject to attack by the host endonuclease activity. Hence, the phage tends to be 'restricted' to one strain of bacteria. However, a small fraction of the phage DNA may escape cleavage in the new host. If such DNA survives one cycle of replication, it acquires the methylation pattern of the host since it has been replicated in the presence of host methylase. These phage can now continue to replicate efficiently in the new host. The non-heritable change (a specific methylation pattern) that confers on the phage the ability to grow on a new host is called modification.

The name of a restriction or methylation activity is derived from the first letter of the genus name and the first two letters of the species name of the bacterium (*Escherichia coli* = *Eco*; *Hemophilus aegyptius* = *Hae*);

Bacterial sources and target sequences for some representative restriction endonucleases

Bacterium	Name of Enzyme	Target Sequence and Cleavage Site
Bacillus amyloliquefaciens H	Bam HI	G$^\downarrow$GATCC C CTAG$_\uparrow$G
Escherichia coli RY13	Eco RI	G$^\downarrow$AATTC CTTAA$_\uparrow$G
Hemophilus aegyptius	Hae III	GG$^\downarrow$CC CC$_\uparrow$GG
Hemophilus gallinarum	Hga I	GACGC(N)$_5$ $^\downarrow$ CTGCG(N)$_{10\uparrow}$
Klebsiella pneumoniae	Kpn I	GGTAC$^\downarrow$C C$_\uparrow$CATGG
Moraxella bovis	Mbo I	$^\downarrow$GATC CTAG$_\uparrow$
Moraxella nonliquefaciens	Mnl I	CCTC(N)$_7$$^\downarrow$ GGAG(N)$_{7\uparrow}$
Nocardia otitidis-caviarum	Not I	GC$^\downarrow$GGCCGC CGCCGG$_\uparrow$CG
Serratia marcescens	Sma I	CCC$^\downarrow$GGG GGG$_\uparrow$CCC

N = any nucleotide

strain or type identification follows as an additional letter, which may be either lower or upper case (e.g., *Bam* HI). If a particular host has several different restriction-modification systems, these are identified by roman numerals (e.g., *Hae* I, *Hae* II, *Hae* III).

Restriction enzymes, all of which require Mg^{2+}, have been classified into three types. Type I restriction enzymes (EC 3.1.21.3) are large and complex proteins, consisting of three types of subunit, which carry both the restriction and methylation activities. These enzymes have an absolute requirement for ATP (or dATP) and *S*-adenosyl-L-methionine. They recognize bipartite asymmetrical DNA sequences (e.g., *Eco* B: TGAN$_8$TGCT) and cleave the DNA at sites that are probably random and at least 1,000 base pairs from the recognition site. Methylation occurs at the recognition site. Type II restriction endonucleases (EC 3.1.21.4) are relatively simple enzymes; the methylation activity is associated with a separate protein. For example, the *Eco* RI enzyme is a single polypeptide of 276 amino acid residues, which interacts with the recognition sequence as a dimer; the methylase is a somewhat larger polypeptide. The recognition sequences for type II enzymes are four to six (rarely eight) nucleotides long and usually, but not always, have a twofold axis of symmetry (i.e., a PALINDROME). The cleavage may be at the axis of symmetry, but is frequently 'staggered', yielding DNA fragments with protruding COHESIVE ENDS. For example, *Eco* RI makes single-stranded breaks four nucleotides apart in opposite strands, generating a 5' 'overhang', thus:

5' G$^\downarrow$AATT C 3'
3' C TTAA$_\uparrow$G 5'

The overlapping segments can associate by hydrogen bonding with other fragments having similar cohesive ends. Other type II restriction endonucleases generate protruding 3' termini; still others generate blunt-ended fragments with no cohesive ends. A few recently discovered type II restriction endonucleases (e.g., *Hga* I) cleave DNA at a measured short distance to one side of the asymmetric target sequence. Type III restriction enzymes (EC 3.1.21.5) consist of two different types of subunit. These enzymes require but do not hydrolyse ATP; S-adenosyl-L-methionine stimulates the reaction but is not absolutely required. Type III enzymes cleave the DNA 24–26 base pairs 3′ to the recognition sequence. Type II, but not types I or III, restriction endonucleases are extensively used in RECOMBINANT DNA TECHNOLOGY.

restriction fragment length polymorphism (RFLP). Polymorphism in the genome that is detected by comparing restriction maps (*see* RESTRICTION MAPPING) of DNAs from different individuals. Variations in positions of restriction sites (i.e., sites where restriction endonucleases cleave the DNA) may be detected as differences in lengths of restriction fragments, as revealed by SOUTHERN BLOTTING with suitable MOLECULAR HYBRIDIZATION PROBES. It is possible to find such polymorphisms in any type of DNA sequence (e.g., exons, introns, flanking sequences). The DNA sequence variations detected by this procedure display Mendelian inheritance and can be used as genetic markers in linkage studies. RFLPs are used in family studies to provide markers linked to defective genes that cause inherited diseases.

restriction mapping. Localization of the positions of RESTRICTION ENDONUCLEASE cleavage sites on a DNA molecule. The DNA is digested with one or a combination of restriction endonucleases, the fragments are separated by gel electrophoresis, and their sizes are determined by comparing their mobilities with those of DNA fragments of known size. The fragments in the gel can be visualized either by staining with ethidium bromide or, for end-labeled fragments, by AUTORADIOGRAPHY. It is often useful to start with an end-labeled fragment and carry out partial digestion so that, on average, only one cleavage occurs per molecule. From the sizes of the various fragments, the positions of the restriction sites can be deduced; e.g., the difference in size between a pair of adjacent fragments on the gel corresponds to the distance between neighboring sites.

reticular dysgenesis. Very rare form of SEVERE COMBINED IMMUNODEFICIENCY in newborns characterized by profound T LYMPHOCYTE and B LYMPHOCYTE deficiencies and an absence of NEUTROPHILS. The syndrome results in rapid death of affected infants, unless they are salvaged with a transplant of BONE MAROW. Reticular dysgenesis is inherited as an autosomal recessive.

reticuloendothelial blockade. Reduction in the rate of clearance of particles injected into the circulation as a result of a previous administration of particles (e.g., colloidal gold) that have an affinity for, or are taken up by, MACROPHAGES of the liver and spleen.

reticuloendothelial system (RES). Cells capable of taking up vital dyes and particles. The term was originally used to include a variety of cells that are highly active in ENDOCYTOSIS and/or PHAGOCYTOSIS (e.g., MACROPHAGES) or less active (e.g., fibroblasts and endothelial cells). The major function of the RES – the clearance of particles from the blood – is carried out by macrophages in the liver and, to a lesser extent, in the SPLEEN. The activity of the RES can be measured by the rate of elimination of radiolabeled ALBUMIN or of [^{51}Cr]-labeled red blood cells, sensitized with antibodies.

Rh blood group. ANTIGENIC DETERMINANTS of human red blood cells detected by ALLOANTIBODIES, usually obtained from women who have had a child with HEMOLYTIC DISEASE OF THE NEWBORN. The Rh alloantigens are proteins, which have not yet been biochemically characterized. The Rh locus is thought to consist of three closely linked pairs of alleles: *Dd, Cc* and *Ee*. In Caucasians the most common linkage groups are DCe and dce. The locus has been mapped to chromosome 1. Antibodies to the Rh antigens, but not specifically to the alloantigenic determinants, were first obtained by immunizing guinea-pigs and rabbits with red blood cells of *Macaccus rhesus* monkeys. Hence the designation Rh. Rh alloimmunization to the D antigen is the most frequent cause of hemolytic disease of the newborn. The alloimmunization of mothers occurs when Rh-positive red blood cells of the baby, which bear the D antigen, enter the circulation of a mother whose red blood cells are Rh-negative (i.e., do not bear the D antigen). The mother makes alloantibody of the IgG class to antigenic determinants of the D antigen. During a subsequent pregnancy with an Rh-positive baby the alloantibodies, which cross the placenta, cause HEMOLYSIS of the baby's red blood cells. Alloimmunization can be prevented by administration of $Rh_0(D)$ IMMUNE GLOBULIN in women whose red blood cells are Rh-negative and who have just given birth to a baby whose red blood cells are Rh-positive.

$Rh_0(D)$ immune globulin.   Preparation of human IMMUNE SERUM GLOBULIN from donors who have been hyperimmunized to the $Rh_0(D)$ antigen. It contains sufficient antibodies to suppress an immune response to 15 ml of packed $Rh_0(D)$-positive erythrocytes. It is given within 72 hours after delivery to prevent ALLOIMMUNIZATION of Rh-negative women by Rh-positive red blood cells from the baby. *See* Rh BLOOD GROUP.

rheumatoid arthritis (RA). Chronic disease presumed to have an immunological cause and characterized by symmetrical multiple joint swellings, particularly of the fingers and wrists. The disease tends to wax and wane in severity. The synovial membranes are infiltrated with NEUTROPHILS, MACROPHAGES, LYMPHOCYTES and PLASMA CELLS. Eventually, vascular granulation tissue, called a pannus, forms and erodes the cartilage of the joint, causing deformities. The disease is two to three times more common in women than in men. RHEUMATOID FACTOR occurs in approximately 70 percent of patients. The cause of rheumatoid arthritis is not known.

rheumatoid factor.   Autoantibody to IgG or IgA, usually of the IgM class, found most frequently in serum of patients with RHEUMATOID ARTHRITIS. These autoantibodies may be monoclonal or polyclonal. To detect rheumatoid factors, particles, usually of latex, are coated with IgG or IgA and their AGGLUTINATION by test serum is measured. The different reactivities of various individual rheumatoid factors define human allotypic determinants (e.g., Gm, Am and Km ALLOTYPIC DETERMINANTS).

rheumatoid nodule.   Subcutaneous nodule in a patient with RHEUMATOID ARTHRITIS that

usually forms at pressure points such as the elbow. Microscopically, the nodule has a central area of NECROSIS surrounded by palisading connective tissue cells and an outer mantle of infiltrates of LYMPHOCYTES.

rhodamine isothiocyanate.   *See* IMMUNOFLUORESCENCE.

ricin.   Highly potent TOXIN from the seeds of *Ricinus communis* plants. It is a HETERODIMER, in which each chain – A and B – has an M_r of 30,000. The B chain is responsible for binding to cells and the A chain is responsible for CYTOTOXICITY. The B chain binds to galactosyl residues on the cell surface, enabling the molecule to enter the cell in endocytic vesicles. The A chain then dissociates from the B chain, reaches the cytosol, binds to ribosomes and inhibits protein synthesis. Ricin or its A chain, coupled to an antibody, can be used in IMMUNOTOXINS.

ring test.   Qualitative test for detecting, by precipitation, the presence of antigens or antibodies. A solution containing antibodies (or antigen) is layered on top of a solution containing antigen (or antibodies) without mixing the two solutions. If the complementary reactants are present, a precipitate forms at the interface. The test, which can be carried out in test tubes or capillary tubes, is a simple way to establish the presence of a precipitating antigen–antibody system. *Synonym for* interfacial test.

R-loop.   Structure formed when RNA that is complementary to one strand of DNA in a duplex is hybridized to the denatured duplex under conditions in which the RNA–DNA hybrid is more stable than the original duplex. RNA displaces the DNA strand having the same sense and forms a double-stranded hybrid with the complementary DNA strand. This structure: an RNA–DNA hybrid and a displaced DNA strand form a loop (the R-loop), which can be detected by electron microscopy. When a gene containing an INTRON is hybridized with the corresponding mRNA, the DNA of the intron is not complementary to any part of the mRNA and is extruded as a double-stranded loop between two adjacent R-loops. This technique has been used to show that the coding sequences of many eukaryotic (e.g., IMMUNOGLOBULIN) genes are interrupted by introns.

RNA polymerase.   *See* DNA-DIRECTED RNA POLYMERASE.

RNA splicing.   Excision of specific segments from a primary RNA transcript and subsequent ligation of the resulting non-contiguous segments to form a mature RNA molecule (tRNA, rRNA or mRNA). Splicing reactions occur in the cell nucleus (or mitochondrion or chloroplast) and are extremely precise. In the formation of mRNA of higher eukaryotes, the INTRONS that are spliced out most always begin with the dinucleotide GU and end with the dinucleotide AG. An additional sequence, located 20–50 base pairs upstream of the 3′ splice site also appears to play a role in the splicing reaction. Typically, before splicing, the RNA is capped (addition of 7-methylguanylate and, usually, methylation of one or two terminal riboses) at the 5′ end and polyadenylated at the 3′ end. Small nuclear ribonucleoprotein particles (snRNPs) appear to be required for the splicing of mRNA precursors. (Antibodies to these particles are found in some patients with AUTOIMMUNE DISEASE such as SYSTEMIC LUPUS ERYTHEMATOSUS.) Sometimes, a primary transcript can be processed in more than one way to yield two or more different mature mRNAs (alternative splicing). This can occur by choice of different splice sites (e.g. as in synthesis of related forms of CLASS I HISTOCOMPATIBILITY MOLECULES, FIBRONEC-TIN and some viral proteins) or by competition between polyadenylation and splicing (as in the processing of immunoglobulin heavy chain transcripts that give rise to secreted and membrane forms of the protein).

RNA-directed DNA polymerase (reverse transcriptase; EC 2.1.7.7.49). DNA polymerase found in retroviruses (e.g., Rous sarcoma virus, avian myeloblastosis virus (AMV), HUMAN IMMUNODEFICIENCY VIRUS (HIV)) that can synthesize DNA from an RNA template. It requires a primer with a free 3′-hydroxyl group, which is base-paired with the template. The product of the reaction is a DNA–RNA hybrid. Despite its name, the enzyme also catalyses DNA synthesis from a DNA template. The reverse

transcriptase molecule also carries a ribonuclease H activity, which selectively degrades the RNA strands in DNA–RNA hybrids (therefore the designation H) in either the 5′→3′ or 3′→5′ direction.

The polymerase (pol) from AMV is derived from a larger precursor polyprotein (gag–pol); it consists of two subunits, alpha (M_r 60,000) and beta (M_r 92,000). The alpha subunit is generated by proteolytic cleavage of some of the beta subunits. The alpha subunit carries the polymerase as well as the ribonuclease H activity, the latter activity being associated with a M_r 24,000 domain that is probably derived from the carboxy-terminal portion of the chain. The remaining M_r 32,000 fragment of the beta subunit is a DNA endonuclease.

Reverse transcriptase is an important enzyme in RECOMBINANT DNA procedures as it is used for first-strand synthesis of cDNA. That from AMV is used most commonly. The enzyme can also be used in a 'filling reaction' to label the ends of DNA fragments having protruding 5′ ends.

rocket   immunoelectrophoresis.   Quantitative test to determine the concentration of an antigen in a test sample (usually serum). One of the reactants (usually ANTISERUM) is incorporated into an agarose gel; wells cut into the gel are filled with the second reactant (usually antigen). An electric current is applied so that the antigen migrates into the gel. The area of the resulting rocket-shaped zone of precipitation is proportional to the concentration of antigen. By comparison with a set of antigen standards, the concentration of antigen added to the well can be determined. Provided that the antiserum is specific, the antigen need not be pure. The major advantage of this technique, compared to SINGLE RADIAL IMMUNODIFFUSION, is speed; the migration of antigen into the gel is completed in hours instead of days.

rosette.   Cluster resembling a rose, such as is formed by ERYTHROCYTES (E) adhering to CD2 on T LYMPHOCYTES (i.e., E-ROSETTE) or by SENSITIZED erythrocytes (*see* EA or EAC) to Fc RECEPTORS or COMPLEMENT RECEPTORS of NEUTROPHILS.

Rot.   The product of RNA concentration (R_0) and incubation time (t) in an RNA-driven hybridization reaction. When a small amount of single-stranded DNA is hybridized with a large amount of RNA, the Rot value is a measure of the amount of RNA complementary to the DNA probe. *See* Cot.

runt disease   *See* THYMECTOMY.

Russell body   Globular mass in the ENDO-PLASMIC RETICULUM of normal PLASMA CELLS or MYELOMA cells. Russell bodies are composed of IMMUNOGLOBULINS and stain with eosin.

S

S protein. Protein in human serum that inhibits the formation of the MEMBRANE ATTACK COMPLEX of COMPLEMENT. S protein is a single polypeptide chain of 478 amino acid residues, including a signal sequence of 19 residues; it contains three sites for attachment of N-linked oligosaccharides. Three molecules of S protein bind to each nascent complex of C5b, C6 and C7, and prevent the insertion of the complex into cell membranes. S protein also prevents the polymerization of C9 on complexes of C5b, C6, C7 and C8.

S protein is identical to vitronectin (serum spreading factor), which is functionally similar to FIBRONECTIN. Vitronectin, so called because of its affinity for glass surfaces, binds to certain cell membranes and to complexes of thrombin and antithrombin III.

S region. Segment of the mouse MAJOR HISTOCOMPATIBILITY COMPLEX (MHC) in which the genes for complement components C2, FACTOR B, C4A (Slp) and C4B (Ss) are encoded. The term is also used to describe the homologous region of the human MHC, between HLA-B and HLA-D, where the genes for the four similar components are located. The products of the S region are called CLASS III MOLECULES.

S1 nuclease (EC 3.1.31.1). Endonuclease, from *Aspergillus oryzae*, that degrades single-stranded DNA or RNA to 5'-phosphomononucleotides or oligonucleotides. S1 nuclease (M_r 32,000) requires Zn^{2+} and is active at pH 4.0–4.5. It is used in S1 NUCLEASE MAPPING, in the removal of COHESIVE ENDS from restriction fragments, and to open the HAIRPIN LOOP generated during the synthesis of double-stranded cDNA. S1 nuclease has been found to cleave active genes in the region of the PROMOTER.

S1 nuclease mapping. Procedure for mapping the ends and splice points of RNA transcripts in relation to specific sites (e.g., positions of restriction endonuclease cleavage) in their template DNAs. Conditions are established that favor the formation of RNA–DNA hybrids (relative to DNA–DNA hybrids). The resulting structures are treated with S1 NUCLEASE, which degrades single-stranded RNA and DNA tails; the remaining RNA–DNA hybrid, which is resistant to digestion, is analysed by gel electrophoresis. If the DNA was first labeled with ^{32}P, it can be detected by AUTORADIOGRAPHY of the gel. If the DNA is unlabeled, it can be detected with an appropriate ^{32}P-labeled DNA or RNA probe after transfer to nitrocellulose (i.e., by SOUTHERN BLOTTING).

Sabin–Feldman dye test. Serological test for toxoplasmosis. Dilutions of heat-inactivated (*see* HEAT INACTIVATION) human test serum are mixed with Toxoplasma organisms in the presence of COMPLEMENT. If antibodies to the Toxoplasma are present in the serum, the Toxoplasma organisms are killed, as indicated by uptake of methylene blue. The titer refers to the serum dilution at which 50 percent of the test organisms are killed.

sacculus rotundus. Terminal portion of rabbit ileum, which is rich in LYMPHOID tissue. At one time it was thought to be the mammalian equivalent of the BURSA OF FABRICIUS. See GUT-ASSOCIATED LYMPHOID TISSUE.

sarcoidosis. Disease characterized by the occurrence of GRANULOMAS, with little or no NECROSIS. Sarcoidosis occurs most frequently in young adults and may affect any organ of the body, but most commonly the LYMPH NODES of the lungs. The disease is characterized by mild POLYCLONAL HYPERGAMMA-GLOBULINEMIA and ANERGY to skin test materials that elicit DELAYED-TYPE HYPERSEN-SITIVITY. Sarcoidosis is usually mild and approximately 60 percent of patients recover spontaneously or after treatment with CORTI-COSTEROIDS. The cause is not known. *See* KVEIM REACTION.

Scatchard equation. Equation used to describe the binding of a univalent LIGAND to a multivalent macromolecule (e.g., antibody): $r/c = Kn - Kr$. At equilibrium, r is the molar concentration of bound ligand divided by the molar concentration of antibody (i.e., the average number of ligand molecules bound per antibody molecule), c is the molar concentration of free ligand, n is the VALENCE OF the antibody molecule, and K is the ASSOCIA-TION CONSTANT. *See* SCATCHARD PLOT.

Scatchard plot. Plot of experimental binding data in which r/c is plotted against r (*see* SCATCHARD EQUATION). If all the binding sites are identical and independent, the plot should be a straight line with slope of $-K$ (negative value of the ASSOCIATION CON-STANT) and intercept on r axis of n (maximum value of r or number of sites per molecule). If the binding sites are not identical or not independent, the plot is not linear, the slope $(-K)$ varying with the extent of site occupancy. For the binding of LIGANDS to heterogeneous antibodies, an AVERAGE ASSOCIATION CONSTANT is often defined as the reciprocal of the free ligand concentration required for half-saturation of the antibody sites.

Schick test. Skin test for circulating antibodies to diptheria TOXIN. Diptheria toxin (0.2 ml) is diluted so as to contain about 1 ng and is injected into the skin. At another site, 0.2 ml of diluted toxin heated at 70°C for 5 minutes is injected as a control. A red, raised circular area (1–2 cm in diameter), appearing in four to seven days, indicates a lack of antibodies to diphtheria (i.e., susceptibility to diphtheria). A reaction occurring within 24 hours is called a 'pseudo reaction' and does not indicate whether the test subject is immune or susceptible.

schlepper. *Synonym for* CARRIER.

Schultz–Dale reaction. Contraction of isolated uterine or intestinal strips in a water bath upon addition of antigen. The tissue strips are either taken from a primed donor or from an unprimed donor followed by SENSITIZATION of the tissue by ANTISERUM *in vitro*. The contraction is due to release of HISTAMINE and other mediators of ANA-PHYLAXIS.

SCID mouse. Mouse of a mutant strain derived from BALB/C17 (CB-17/SCID) characterized by SEVERE COMBINED IMMU-NODEFICIENCY (SCID). The trait is autosomal recessive. SCID mice have no B LYM-PHOCYTES or T LYMPHOCYTES because of a selective defect in hematopoietic STEM CELLS

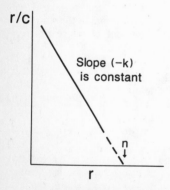

Homogeneous population of binding sites

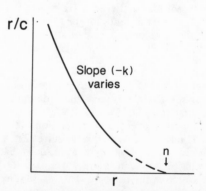

Heterogeneous population of binding sites

that generate LYMPHOCYTES. They have normal lymphoid stroma in lymph nodes and spleen, which can be repopulated by bone marrow stem cells from normal CB-17 mice. Bone marrow stem cells from CB-17/SCID mice will not generate lymphocytes after transplantation into X-irradiated CB-17 mice. SCID mice have normal numbers of MONONUCLEAR PHAGOCYTES, NATURAL KILLER CELLS and GRANULOCYTES. Serum of SCID mice lacks IMMUNOGLOBULINS and they do not manifest CELL-MEDIATED IMMUNITY. About 15 percent of SCID mice develop serum immunoglobulin late in life. SCID mice appear to lack a lymphocyte-specific DNA recombinase so that effective rearrangement of the T CELL RECEPTOR GENES and IMMUNOGLOBULIN GENES does not occur.

scratch test.   Skin test to ascertain the presence of IgE antibodies to particular ALLERGENS. A small abrasion is made in the skin with a needle. A drop of an aqueous solution of an allergen is placed on the abrasion and the site is observed for an immediate wheal and flare reaction (URTICARIA), which occurs when IgE antibodies to the allergen are present on MAST CELLS of the test subject.

secondary disease.   Chronic GRAFT-*VERSUS*-HOST DISEASE in mice

secondary granule.   Cytoplasmic organelle of POLYMORPHONUCLEAR LEUKOCYTES. In NEUTROPHILS, secondary granules contain lactoferrin, vitamin B12-binding protein and lysozyme. In EOSINOPHILS, secondary granules contain cationic peptides. In BASOPHILS, secondary granules contain HEPARIN, HISTAMINE and PLATELET ACTIVATING FACTOR. *See* PRIMARY GRANULE.

secondary immune response.   Accelerated, enhanced IMMUNE RESPONSE that develops upon encounter with an antigen for the second time. The secondary immune response can be detected within a few hours after antigen is introduced, whereas in the PRIMARY IMMUNE RESPONSE there is usually a lag period of several days after antigen administration. The secondary response is characterized by strong CELL-MEDIATED IMMUNITY and high titers of IgG antibodies often of high affinity. Antigens that induce a secondary immune response are proteins or glycoproteins that stimulate T cell reactivity.

Immunological memory denotes the capacity to develop a secondary immune response. The term secondary immune response is also used to describe the third, fourth, fifth or n^{th} response to an antigen; such responses are similar to the second response. *Synonym for* anamnestic reaction.

secondary immunodeficiency.   Any failure or compromise of specific IMMUNITY that is not due to an intrinsic defect in B or T LYMPHOCYTES. Secondary immunodeficiency results from loss of immunoglobulins or T lymphocytes, as occurs in INFLAMMATORY BOWEL DISEASE; from destruction of B or T lymphocytes by cytotoxic drugs or ionizing radiation; from displacememt of normal B or T lymphocytes by malignant cells as in MULTIPLE MYELOMA or CHRONIC LYMPHOCYTIC LEUKEMIA; from infection of B or T lymphocytes, as in ACQUIRED IMMUNODEFICIENCY SYNDROME.

secondary lymphoid organ.   LYMPHOID organ where mature T and B LYMPHOCYTES encounter antigen to initiate an IMMUNE RESPONSE. The secondary lymphoid organs include LYMPH NODES, SPLEEN, TONSILS and GUT-ASSOCIATED LYMPHOID TISSUE. The structure of all these organs is such as to maximize interaction between lymphocytes and antigen-charged ACCESSORY CELLS. *See* PRIMARY LYMPHOID ORGAN.

secondary structure.   Organization of the peptide backbone of a polypeptide or protein chain due to formation of hydrogen bonds between carbonyl oxygen and amide nitrogen atoms. The ALPHA HELIX, BETA-PLEATED SHEET and COLLAGEN HELIX are examples of secondary structures. *See* PRIMARY STRUCTURE, QUATERNARY STRUCTURE, TERTIARY STRUCTURE.

second-set rejection.   Accelerated rejection of a graft because of prior IMMUNIZATION of the recipient (e.g., by previous grafting). *See* GRAFT REJECTION.

secreted immunoglobulin.   IMMUNOGLOBULIN that is secreted by a PLASMA CELL. The secreted immunoglobulin is the form that accumulates in serum and other body fluids. *See* MEMBRANE IMMUNOGLOBULIN.

secretor.   Person whose secretions (e.g., gastric juice, saliva, tears, ovarian cyst mucin) contain ABO BLOOD GROUP substances. Secretors are homozygous (*Se/Se*) or heterozygous (*Se/se*) for the gene *Se*; they constitute approximately 80 percent of the population. *See* NON-SECRETOR.

secretory component (SC). Polypeptide chain (M_r 75,000) that is found in a variety of external secretions (e.g., tears, bile, colostrum) usually complexed to secreted polymeric immunoglobulins (IgA or, less frequently, IgM), but sometimes also found in free form. It is derived, by proteolytic cleavage, from the POLYIMMUNOGLOBULIN RECEPTOR on the surfaces of epithelial cells or hepatocytes.

Human SC contains about 550 amino acid residues and seven N-LINKED OLIGOSACCHARIDES. The polypeptide can be divided into five domains; these are the five amino-terminal (extracellular) domains of the polyimmunoglobulin receptor. As in immunoglobulin domains, each domain contains a disulfide bridge spanning 60–70 amino acid residues. The cysteine residues forming these disulfide bridges are in homologous positions to cysteines in the five extracellular immunoglobulin-like domains of the rabbit polyimmunoglobulin receptor. In addition, four of the domains of human SC have a smaller disulfide loop. In free secretory component, the fifth domain contains yet another intrachain disulfide bridge, which is labile to reduction and which may rearrange to form two interchain disulfide bridges to the alpha chain when SC becomes covalently bound to IgA. In humans, SC appears to be joined, by two disulfide bridges, to only one of the two monomer units of secretory IgA. In some varieties of IgA, SC may not be covalently bound to the immunoglobulin. Human SC is similar in amino acid sequence (55 percent identity) to the amino-terminal five domains of rabbit polyimmunoglobulin receptor and is a member of the IMMUNOGLOBULIN SUPERFAMILY.

For transport of polymeric immunoglobulins into external secretions, the immunoglobulin, secreted by a PLASMA CELL, binds to the polyimmunoglobulin receptor on the basolateral surface of an epithelial cell. During or after TRANSCYTOSIS of the resulting complex, proteolytic cleavage of the receptor occurs; most of the extracellular portion (called the secretory component) of the receptor remains bound to the immunoglobulin and this complex is released into the secretions. The carboxy-terminus of human SC is uneven, presumably due to variable proteolytic cleavage from the intact receptor. It is thought that binding of SC to IgA increases the resistance of IgA to cleavage by proteolytic enzymes found in external secretions.

secretory component deficiency. Very rare disorder in which no IgA is found in secretions due to the failure of SECRETORY COMPONENT synthesis by epithelial cells. The few reported cases have had prolonged diarrhea following infection of the gastrointestinal tract. It is not known if the POLYIMMUNOGLOBULIN RECEPTOR is absent or defective.

secretory IgA. *See* IgA (immunoglobulin A).

selective immunoglobulin deficiency. *See* IgA DEFICIENCY and IgG SUBCLASS DEFICIENCY.

selective theory. Theory that explains the SPECIFICITY of the IMMUNE RESPONSE by antigen selection of pre-existing antibodies or antibody-like cell receptors. Selective theories differ from INSTRUCTIVE THEORIES, which state that antigen is required to induce specificity of the antibody. An early form of selective theory was proposed by Paul Ehrlich (*see* SIDE-CHAIN THEORY). The current, widely accepted selective theory is the CLONAL SELECTION THEORY.

semisyngeneic graft. GRAFT from a member of one strain into an F_1 hybrid produced by mating any member of that strain with a member of another strain (e.g., A into A×B). Such a graft is usually accepted.

sensitization. Administering antigen (i.e., priming) so that a heightened response (i.e., SECONDARY IMMUNE RESPONSE) is obtained upon subsequent CHALLENGE with that antigen.

sensitized cell. (1) Cell that has been coated with antibodies and/or COMPLEMENT components. (2) Cell from a primed donor.

sequential determinant. ANTIGENIC DETERMINANT that is dependent on the sequence of a few contiguous residues in a macromolecule. The amino acid residues comprising the sequential determinant of a protein are clustered within a relatively small (about six residues) peptide segment. Such a determinant is not expected to be affected by denaturation of the protein. The binding of antibodies to a sequential determinant of a protein can often be inhibited by an appropriate peptide derived from the protein. *See* CONFORMATIONAL DETERMINANT.

seroconversion. Conversion from negative to positive reactivity in a test for serum antibodies.

serotherapy. Treatment of an infectious disease by the administrative of ANTISERUM in order to achieve PASSIVE IMMUNITY. Serotherapy was frequently practised for the treatment of pneumococcal infections before the introduction of antibiotics.

serotonin (5-hydroxytryptamine). Potent vasoconstrictor of large blood vessels, vasodilator that enhances permeability of small blood vessels, and constrictor of bronchi. Serotonin is widely distributed in animals and plants. In humans 90 percent of serotonin is in the enterochromaffin cells of the gastrointestinal tract; the remainder is in PLATELETS and the brain where it is a neurotransmitter. In rodents (e.g., rats, mice) and Bovidae (e.g., cows) serotonin is present in MAST CELLS and is a mediator of ANAPHYLAXIS. In humans, PLATELET-ACTIVATING FACTOR, released from mast cells during anaphylaxis, induces release of serotonin from platelets. However, serotonin is not thought to play a role in human anaphylaxis. Serotonin is synthesized from the amino acid tryptophan in two enzymatic reactions involving hydroxylation and decarboxylation. The activity of serotonin is inhibited by ergot alkaloids, such as lysergic acid diethylamide (LSD) and reserpine.

serotonin

serotype. Antigenic variant within a bacterial species identified with antibodies to surface antigenic determinants of the variants. Serotyping is used to classify Salmonella, Shigella and streptococci. *See* H ANTIGEN, O ANTIGEN, KAUFMANN–WHITE SCHEME.

serpin. Acronym for *ser*ine *p*rotease *in*hibitor (e.g., C1 INHIBITOR).

serum. Fluid remaining in blood after clotting. Serum is PLASMA from which fibrinogen and clotting factors have been removed. The major protein components in serum are: SERUM ALBUMIN (35–55 mg/ml), IMMUNOGLOBULINS of all ISOTYPES (~20 mg/ml in total), α1-antitrypsin (~3 mg/ml), transferrin (~3 mg/ml), α2-macroglobulin (~2.5 mg/ml), haptoglobin (~2 mg/ml).

serum albumin. The major protein component of SERUM OR PLASMA. Its concentration ranges from 35 to 55 mg/ml. Human serum albumin is a single chain of 585 amino acid residues crosslinked by 17 disulfide bridges. It is synthesized in the adult liver in a precursor form with a signal sequence of 18 amino acid residues and an additional basic precursor (i.e., 'propeptide') sequence of six residues, which is cleaved from proalbumin in the Golgi apparatus, thereby generating mature serum albumin. Serum albumin is important in maintaining the osmolarity of the blood and it binds a great many blood constituents including fatty acids, hormones, bilirubin and drugs. It is the most anionic (negatively charged) of the serum proteins.

serum amyloid A component (SAA). Serum protein (M_r 20,000) that is the precursor of the major component of amyloid deposits in secondary AMYLOIDOSIS. SAA is a single polypeptide chain of 114 amino acid residues. After peptides are cleaved from the amino- and carboxy-terminal ends of SAA the residual protein (M_r 8,000) forms fibrillar amyloid deposits. In INFLAMMATION, the serum level of SAA may rise 1000-fold to 1 mg/ml. *See* SERUM AMYLOID P COMPONENT.

serum amyloid P component (SAP). Serum protein of unknown function that is a minor component (10–15 percent) of amyloid deposits in secondary AMYLOIDOSIS. SAP is composed of two disk-like structures; each disk is a pentamer of identical subunits of 204 amino acid residues. Serum concentration of SAP is 30 μg/ml; the level does not rise during INFLAMMATION. The gene for SAP has been mapped to chromosome 1q2.1 and is linked to the gene for C-REACTIVE PROTEIN. *See* SERUM AMYLOID A COMPONENT.

serum sickness. IMMUNE COMPLEX DISEASE that may develop several days after the introduction of a large amount of foreign protein into the circulation. The usual signs and symptoms of serum sickness include fever, joint pains, skin rash and red blood cells and protein in the urine. These are the consequences of the deposition of ANTIGEN–ANTIBODY COMPLEXES that fix COMPLEMENT and attract neutrophils, which cause tissue injury upon degranulation. Serum sickness occurred frequently during SEROTHERAPY for infectious diseases. *See* ARTHUS REACTION.

severe combined immunodeficiency (SCID). Syndrome of infants that is caused by a profound deficiency of T LYMPHOCYTES and a variable deficiency of B LYMPHOCYTES. Infants with SCID are extremely susceptible to OPPORTUNISTIC INFECTIONS (e.g., with *Pneumocystis carinii*, adenovirus, *Candida albicans*) and die of these infections in infancy or early childhood. SCID may be inherited as an X-linked recessive or autosomal recessive. Of the latter group, half of the affected infants have ADENOSINE DEAMINASE DEFICIENCY or PURINE NUCLEOSIDE PHOSPHORYLASE DEFICIENCY. In all cases of SCID, regardless of the cause, the THYMUS has few or no lymphocytes and Hassell's corpuscles. SCID is treated with transplants of BONE MARROW CELLS. *See* SCID MICE.

sex-limited protein. *See* SLP.

Shine–Dalgarno sequence. A short sequence in bacterial mRNA, lying 4–9 bases 5′ to the initiator triplet AUG, which is complementary to a sequence in 16 S ribosomal RNA. It promotes binding of the mRNA to the ribosome and the initiation of translation. The consensus Shine–Dalgarno sequence is 5′ UAAGGAGGU 3′.

short homologous repeats. *See* CONSENSUS SEQUENCE OF C3/C4 BINDING PROTEINS.

Shwartzman reaction. Hemorrhagic lesions induced by LIPOPOLYSACCHARIDES (LPS). In the local Shwartzman reaction, LPS is injected intradermally, followed by a second injection intravenously; hemorrhage occurs at the site of the first injection. In the systemic or generalized Shwartzman reaction, both injections are given intravenously, resulting in acute tubular NECROSIS of the kidney and hemorrhagic lesions in lung, liver and other viscera. Contrary to earlier opinion, the Shwartzman reaction has no immunological basis.

sialophorin (CD43). Major cell surface glycoprotein on all T LYMPHOCYTES, thymocytes, some B LYMPHOCYTES, PLATELETS, MONOCYTES and NEUTROPHILS, detected by monoclonal antibodies. Sialophorin from lymphocytes and monocytes (M_r 115,000), or from neutrophils and platelets (M_r 135,000) is a single polypeptide chain; the two forms differ only in carbohydrate content. Twenty-seven percent of the amino acid residues are threonine or serine, to almost all of which are attached O-LINKED SACCHARIDES, containing galactose β1-3 galactosamine. In mature T lymphocytes and medullary thymocytes sialic acid is attached to the galactose and galactosamine; the cortical thymocytes are only partially sialylated. The adherence of cortical thymocytes, but not of medullary thymocytes or T lymphocytes, to peanut lectin is due to this incomplete sialylation. Completely sialylated O-LINKED SACCHARIDE structures do not adhere to peanut lectin.

Human sialophorin consists of 400 amino acid residues, including a signal sequence of 19 residues, an extracellular domain of 235 residues, a putative transmembrane segment of 23 residues and a cytoplasmic domain of 123 residues. Sialophorin contains one site for N-LINKED OLIGOSACCHARIDES. The gene encoding sialophorin is on chromosome 16.

Antibody to sialophorin activates T lymphocytes; during activation of T lymphocytes, the cytoplasmic domain is phosphorylated. This glycoprotein is defective in the membrane of T lymphocytes from males with the WISKOTT–ALDRICH SYNDROME. The equivalent protein in the rat is called leukosialin.

side-chain theory. Form of SELECTIVE THEORY proposed by Paul Ehrlich in 1900 to explain the presence of ANTITOXIN in serum after IMMUNIZATION with bacterial TOXINS. Ehrlich postulated that cells contained surface extensions of their protoplasm (haptophores) that bind to the ANTIGENIC DETERMINANTS of the toxin (toxophores); after the cell is stimulated, the haptophores are shed into the circulation and become the antitoxin. Proposed at a time when there was no understanding of the cellular basis of immunity, this theory was a remarkably prescient explanation of cellular recognition of antigen.

signal peptide.   *See* SIGNAL SEQUENCE.

signal sequence.   Sequence of 16 to 30 amino acid residues that is thought to initiate transport of secreted proteins across the membrane of the ENDOPLASMIC RETICULUM. Signal sequences typically contain a core of 4 to 12 hydrophobic residues, which may facilitate interaction with the membrane. Transmembrane proteins may also have signal sequences; these proteins usually also contain a 'stop-transfer' sequence of about 20 hydrophobic residues, which stops translocation of the growing polypeptide and anchors it in the phospholipid bilayer. The signal sequence of most secreted and many transmembrane proteins is at the aminoterminus and is removed by enzymatic cleavage of the nascent chain in the endoplasmic reticulum. Some membrane proteins and a few secreted proteins (e.g., ovalbumin) have uncleaved internal signal sequences that facilitate membrane insertion. The interaction of secreted and some integral membrane proteins with the endoplasmic reticulum is mediated by a signal recognition particle (6 distinct polypeptides and a 300-base RNA) and its receptor, known as 'docking protein', which is an integral membrane protein (single chain of M_r ~72,000) of the rough endoplasmic reticulum. *Synonym for* signal peptide, leader sequence, leader peptide.

simple allotype.   ALLOTYPE that varies from another allotype in amino acid sequence at only one or a few positions. Simple allotypes (e.g., Km) are usually products of ALLELES at a single genetic locus. *See* COMPLEX ALLOTYPE.

single immunodiffusion.   Type of IMMUNODIFFUSION in which one reactant (e.g., ANTISERUM) is incorporated into a gel and the second reactant (e.g., ANTIGEN) is introduced onto the surface of a gel-filled tube (method of Oudin), or into a well of an agar plate (method of Mancini, *see* SINGLE RADIAL IMMUNODIFFUSION). The antigen diffuses into the gel and forms a precipitate when the antigen concentration reaches EQUIVALENCE with the antibodies, forming a line or ring of precipitation (*see* PRECIPITIN CURVE). Single immunodiffusion can be used to quantitate either the mobile or stationary reactant.

single radial immunodiffusion.   Quantitative IMMUNODIFFUSION test (method of Mancini). One of the reactants (usually ANTISERUM) is incorporated into a gel (e.g., AGAROSE) before it solidifies. The other reactant (usually antigen) is placed into a well made in the gel. When the antigen diffuses from the well into the gel, it precipitates with the antiserum. As antigen continues to diffuse from the well, the precipitate comes into ANTIGEN EXCESS, dissolves and reforms further from the well. At the EQUIVALENCE ratio of antigen and antibody (*see* PRECIPITIN CURVE), a ring or halo of precipitate is finally formed; the area within this ring is proportional to the antigen concentration. By comparison with a set of antigen standards, the concentration of antigen added to the well can be determined. Provided that the antiserum is specific, the antigen need not be pure.

single-hit theory.   Theory that complement-mediated HEMOLYSIS is brought about by a single lesion produced in the ERYTHROCYTE membrane as a result of the activation of COMPLEMENT.

Sips distribution.   Distribution, originally used to describe the adsorption of gases to (heterogeneous) catalyst surfaces, that has been applied to the distribution of ASSOCIATION CONSTANTS in a heterogeneous population of antibody sites. The Sips distribution resembles closely the normal (Gaussian) distribution. As applied to antibody sites, the logarithms of the association constants (log K) are distributed about a mean, which is denoted log K_0; the dispersion about this mean is described by a parameter, a, that varies from 0 to 1 and that is inversely related to the width of the distribution (i.e., the smaller a, the greater width). The explicit function for the distribution is $\log r/(n-r)$ $= a \log c + a \log K_0$, where r is the molar concentration of the bound ligand divided by the molar concentration of antibodies, n is the valence of the antibodies and c is the molar concentration of free ligand. The values of a and $\log K_0$ are estimated from the linear plot of $\log r/(n-r)$ against $\log c$. By convention, K_0 (the antilog of the mean of the distribution, $\log K_0$) is called the 'AVERAGE ASSOCIATION CONSTANT'. However, this is a misnomer because, although $\log K_0$ is the mean of all the $\log K$, K_0 is *not* the mean of all the K. Nevertheless, for symmetrical distributions, such as the Sips and normal distributions, K_0 will be the *median* association constant.

When the antibody sites are half-saturated with ligand, $r = n-r$, $\log K_0 = -\log c$, and $K_0 = 1/c$. Again, by convention, the 'average association constant' has been taken to be the reciprocal of the free ligand concentration resulting in half-saturation of the sites. However, as discussed above, this value is not actually the mean of the association constants and, only in an ideal symmetrical distribution, will it be the median value of these constants.

If the population of antibody sites is homogeneous, $a = 1$ and the Sips equation reduces to the SCATCHARD EQUATION $r/(n-r)$ $= Kc$.

Sips plot. Plot of data obtained in measuring the binding of LIGAND to a population of antibodies, in which $\log r/n-r$ is plotted against $\log c$ (*see* SIPS DISTRIBUTION). If the plot is a straight line (i.e., the data conform to the Sips equation), the slope, a, is a measure of the heterogeneity of the antibodies with respect to AFFINITY.

Sjögren's syndrome. AUTOIMMUNE DISEASE characterized by keratoconjunctivitis sicca (dry eyes) and xerostomia (dry mouth), and usually accompanied by CONNECTIVE TISSUE DISEASE such as RHEUMATOID ARTHRITIS. The salivary glands are enlarged and heavily infiltrated with LYMPHOCYTES. There are numerous AUTOANTIBODIES, both organ non-specific (e.g., RHEUMATOID FACTOR and a variety of antibodies to uridine-rich nuclear RNA) and organ-specific (e.g., to ductal epithelium of the lacrymal and salivary glands). Sjögren's syndrome has been observed in recipients of bone marrow transplants who have GRAFT-*VERSUS*-HOST DISEASE. Pathology similar to Sjögren's syndrome has been observed in NZB × NZW F_1 mice (*see* NEW ZEALAND MICE).

skin test. Any test carried out by injecting or applying substances to the skin to ascertain the state of IMMUNITY of the host. *See* DICK TEST, PATCH TEST, SCRATCH TEST, TUBERCULIN TEST, SCHICK TEST.

skin window. Technique for observing the evolution of INFLAMMATION. Skin is injured by scraping. Cover slips are successively placed on the abrasion and stained upon removal to ascertain the types of cells responding to the injury. For the first four hours, neutrophils are mainly found on the cover slips; subsequently, increasing numbers of monocytes and decreasing numbers of neutrophils are found. Skin window is also called Rebuck window after the physician who developed the technique.

skin-sensitizing antibody. Antibody that binds to mast cells in skin and thus prepares a skin site for an IMMEDIATE HYPERSENSITIVITY reaction. *See* HETEROCYTOTROPIC ANTIBODY, HOMOCYTOTROPIC ANTIBODY, IgE, PASSIVE CUTANEOUS ANAPHYLAXIS and PRAUSNITZ–KÜSTNER REACTION.

skin-specific histocompatibility antigen. MINOR HISTOCOMPATIBILITY ANTIGEN found in the skin of mice. The existence of this antigen is demonstrated by the following experiment. Spleen cells from an F_1 offspring of two INBRED STRAINS are transplanted into a heavily irradiated parent. Subsequently (three months later) various tissues are transplanted from the opposite parent onto the CHIMERA. Skin grafts are rejected, albeit at a low and inconsistent rate. However, tissues other than skin are not rejected. The spleen cells of the F_1 mouse are initially tolerant to the tissues of both parents but eventually lose TOLERANCE to the skin of one parental strain when residing in the other parent. The putative gene encoding the sensitizing antigen has been named *Sk*.

slow reacting substance of anaphylaxis (SRS-A). LEUKOTRIENES C4, D4 and E4, thought to be responsible for many of the symptoms of ANAPHYLAXIS. SRS-A was first identified as a biological activity in extracts of guinea-pig lung following anaphylaxis induced by cobra venom. The activity contracted guinea-pig ileum, but at a slower rate than HISTAMINE and was not inhibited by ANTIHISTAMINES.

slp. Sex-limited protein of mice (found normally only in males and inducible in females by androgens). It is the product of the COMPLEMENT locus, *C4A*, and is not hemolytically active. *See* Ss PROTEIN.

Snell–Bagg mouse. Mouse belonging to a mutant strain (dw/dw), characterized by pituitary dwarfing. The *dw* mutation is an autosomal recessive trait. These mice have a small THYMUS and depressed CELL-MEDIATED IMMUNITY.

solid-phase immunoassay. Any immunoassay in which antigens or antibodies are attached to an insoluble matrix. For example, in a typical assay for antibodies, an antigen is attached to the matrix and a test sample, containing antibodies to the immobilized antigen, is added. There should be an excess of antigen relative to the antibodies. After a suitable interval, the matrix is washed and radiolabeled antibodies directed to CONSTANT REGION determinants of the bound antibodies (e.g., anti-Fc) are then added in excess. Unbound radiolabeled antibodies are washed away and the residual radioactivity adhering to the matrix is determined. The assay can be standardized by adding known amounts of antibodies to the antigen. The insoluble matrix may be beads (e.g., Sepharose) or wells in a polystyrene or polyvinyl chloride tissue culture plate to which proteins (e.g., antigens) adhere nonspecifically. Care must be taken so that excess sites on the plate (i.e., sites not containing the immobilized antigen) are saturated with unrelated protein before addition of the test antibody.

soluble complex. Antigen–antibody complex that is soluble (i.e., not precipitated). Such complexes usually contain excess antigen. *See* PRECIPITIN CURVE.

somatic mutation. MUTATION in a somatic cell, which is inherited only by its descendants. Accelerated somatic mutation (called somatic hypermutation) is thought to be important in generating diversity in the VARIABLE REGIONS of the light and heavy chains of antibodies. Evidence for the occurrence of somatic mutations can be obtained by comparing sequences of expressed variable regions with germline *V*, *J* (and *D*) GENE SEGMENTS. Somatic mutations are found more frequently in IgG and IgA antibodies than in IgM antibodies.

Southern blotting. Technique, described by and subsequently named after E.M. Southern, for detecting particular sequences in a mixture of DNA fragments, usually obtained by digestion with one or more RESTRICTION ENDONUCLEASES, that have been separated, according to size, by gel ELECTROPHORESIS. The resulting fragments are denatured (by soaking the gel in sodium hydroxide) and 'blotted' onto a sheet of nitrocellulose or nylon that is laid on top of the gel. The relative positions of the DNA fragments are preserved during the transfer. The DNA in the filter is then hybridized with an appropriate labeled probe (e.g., radiolabeled DNA or RNA) which hybridizes to complementary sequences in the fragments. Unbound probe is washed away, and the location of the hybridized probe is revealed by AUTORADIOGRAPHY. The technique can be used both to detect specific sequences in cloned DNA and in digests of genomic DNA. It is sufficiently sensitive to detect single-copy genes in the total mammalian genome. Strictly speaking, 'blotting' refers to the method for transferring DNA from the agarose gel to the nitrocellulose, but the term is often used to describe the entire procedure: electrophoresis, transfer and hybridization. *See* NORTHERN BLOTTING, IMMUNOBLOTTING.

specific granule. *Synonym for* SECONDARY GRANULE.

specificity. Ability of antibodies or lymphocytes to discriminate among different LIGANDS.

spectrotype. Pattern of bands on an ISOELECTRIC FOCUSING gel. The spectrotype can serve as a marker for a single protein (that may appear as a cluster of bands because of post-translational modifications) or a group of proteins. A spectrotype of secreted antibody can be used as a marker for a CLONE of antibody-producing cells.

spheroplast. Type of PROTOPLAST prepared from Gram-negative bacteria and hence retaining remnants of the outer membrane.

spleen. Major SECONDARY LYMPHOID ORGAN located in the upper abdomen in direct communication with the main arterial circulation. In contrast to LYMPH NODES, which filter LYMPH, the spleen filters blood. The spleen consists of lymphoid tissue around arterioles (white pulp) surrounded by lakes of blood (red pulp). The periarteriolar lymphoid sheath consists of small masses of B LYMPHOCYTES (FOLLICLES) interspersed among T LYMPHOCYTES. The arterioles terminate in specialized venules that lie between the white pulp and the red pulp – the so-called marginal sinus. B and T lymphocytes traverse the marginal sinus, circulate through the white pulp for about six hours, and return to the venous circulation via the red pulp. The spleen traps blood-borne antigens and IMMUNE RESPONSES to them are initiated there. The red pulp scavenges old red blood cells and is a reserve site for hemopoiesis. Individuals lacking a spleen are very susceptible to some blood-borne bacterial infections (e.g., with pneumococci and *Hemophilus influenzae*).

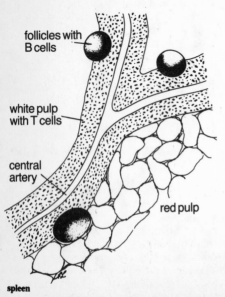

follicles with
B cells

white pulp
with T cells

central
artery

red pulp

spleen

split tolerance. Form of partial TOLERANCE in which there is tolerance to some ANTIGENIC DETERMINANTS and an IMMUNE RESPONSE to other antigenic determinants of ALLOGENEIC cells.

Ss protein. Product of the COMPLEMENT locus, *C4B* in mice. Unlike the product of the *C4A* locus, SLP, Ss is hemolytically active.

suicide. In immunology, the death of cells that have specifically taken up highly radio-labeled antigen.

suppressor macrophage. Highly activated MACROPHAGE from infected or tumor-bearing animals that inhibits *in vitro* immune reactions by releasing products of arachidonic acid metabolism (e.g., PROSTAGLANDINS) and/or oxygen radicals.

suppressor T lymphocyte. T lymphocyte involved in the inhibition and/or termination of an IMMUNE RESPONSE and perhaps in the induction and maintenance of immunological TOLERANCE. It is thought that the outcome of an immune response is the result of the opposing effects of HELPER T LYMPHOCYTES and suppressor T lymphocytes. It is also thought that the activity of suppressor T lymphocytes predominates in situations where some molecules of antigen are not processed. Suppressor T lymphocytes bear CD8 molecules on their surface. The identity of suppressor T cells as a separate subset is seriously questioned. *See* CYTOTOXIC T LYMPHOCYTE.

suramin (Antrypol, 8,8'-(carbonylbis(imino-3,1-phenylenecarbonylimino))bis-1,3,5-naphthalene trisulfonic acid). Drug used in the treatment of trypanosomiasis (African sleeping sickness). Suramin is of interest to immunologists because it binds to C3b thereby preventing the binding of FACTOR H and FACTOR I. Suramin also inhibits complement-mediated lysis by inhibiting the binding of the MEMBRANE ATTACK COMPLEX to cell membranes.

SV40. Oncogenic animal virus, member of the polyoma family. SV40 was discovered as an agent that multiplied in rhesus monkey kidney cultures (used for propagating polio

suramin sodium

virus) and was subsequently found to produce cytopathic changes in cell cultures from African green monkeys. It was then shown that this virus produces sarcomas when it is injected into newborn hamsters. The genome of SV40 is a small covalently closed circular duplex DNA of 5243 base pairs. The virus can enter two types of life cycle depending on the host cell. In permissive cells (usually permanent cell lines derived from the African green monkey), virus replication results in lysis of the cells and release of a large number of viral particles. In non-permissive cells (usually mouse, hamster or human cell lines), there is no lytic infection but oncogenic transformation of the cells can occur. In such cells, DNA sequences of the SV40 genome are integrated into the host genome. Transformed cells have distinctive morphology and growth characteristics (e.g., ability to grow in suspension in soft agar).

SV40 was the first animal virus to be developed as a cloning VECTOR. Requirements for assembly of SV40 virions impose a strict limitation on the amount of foreign DNA that can be packaged. Therefore, strategies to circumvent this size limitation have had to be developed. In one such strategy, a region of the viral genome is removed and replaced with an equivalent amount of foreign DNA; the recombinant can replicate and be packaged into virions in permissive cells. A helper virus must be supplied to provide the genetic functions lost by removal of native virus sequences. In a second strategy, recombinants are constructed but are not packaged into virions and produce no lytic infection. They are maintained in host cells transiently as high copy number plasmid-like DNA molecules, which are not integrated into the host chromosome.

Svedberg unit. Unit for expressing sedimentation coefficients; one Svedberg unit (S) equals 10^{-13} second. IgG antibodies sediment at 7 S, IgM antibodies at 19 S.

switch (S) region. Region of DNA that mediates the recombination events that lead to CLASS SWITCHING. Switch regions are approximately one to six kilobases in length and lie about one to four kilobases upstream (5′) to each heavy chain C GENE SEGMENT, except C_δ. These regions are composed of tandem repetitions of short (<80 base pairs) DNA sequences. S_μ contains tandemly repeated blocks of two pentameric sequences: GAGCT and GGGGT, which are contained in other switch regions, although not in the form of precise tandem repeats as in S_μ. In the other switch regions, the pentamers are embedded in larger repeat units. The four S_γ are homologous to each other and are based on an approximately 50 base pair repeat; their similarity to S_μ diminishes with distance, i.e., $S_{\gamma 3}$ is most similar and $S_{\gamma 2a}$ least similar to S_μ. However, S_ϵ and S_α, the 3′-most switch regions, are more similar to S_μ. Sequences unique to a particular switch region may be important for mediating isotype-specific switching. See IMMUNOGLOBULIN GENES, IMMUNOGLOBULIN GENE REARRANGEMENT.

syngeneic. Possessing almost identical GENOTYPES (e.g., individual mice of an INBRED STRAIN). See ISOGENIC.

synthetic antigen. Molecule synthesized in the laboratory and used for IMMUNIZATION. Synthetic polypeptides have been used to study the molecular basis of IMMUNOGENICITY. Immunogenicity of synthetic polypeptides is enhanced by the presence of a variety of amino acid residues and, in particular, by aromatic and charged amino acid residues.

systemic lupus erythematosus (SLE). Common AUTOIMMUNE DISEASE in which there are inflammatory destructive changes in many organ systems and many ANTINUCLEAR ANTIBODIES. A combination of signs and symptoms and laboratory findings are characteristic of SLE; a rash of fixed erythema forming a butterfly pattern on the face and exacerbated by exposure to sunlight, oral ulcers, pain in the joints, INFLAMMATION of the pleural and/or pericardial sacs, seizures or psychosis, antinuclear antibodies, protein in the urine, leukopenia, THROMBOCYTOPENIA and HEMOLYTIC ANEMIA. SLE is ten times more common in women than in men. The symptoms tend to wax and wane in severity. The immunological basis of SLE appears to be an uncontrolled differentiation of B LYMPHOCYTE clones, many of which produce autoreactive antibodies. The most characteristic antibodies in SLE are to double- and single-stranded DNA and to soluble ribonucleoproteins (Sm). Deposits of immune complexes containing DNA have been found in the kidney and in other organs. Serum COMPLEMENT is decreased. The use of CORTICOSTEROIDS and immunosuppressive drugs (e.g., CYCLOPHOSPHAMIDE) has markedly improved the survival of patients with SLE, which was almost invariably fatal in the past. SLE also occurs in NZB × NZW F_1 mice (*see* NEW ZEALAND MICE) and other INBRED STRAINS of mice, as well as in dogs. SLE can be induced by drugs (e.g., hydralazine). The serum of patients with drug-induced SLE contains antibodies to histones, which are usually not found in other forms of SLE A mild form in which the only symptom is the butterfly rash of the face, is called 'discoid lupus'.

systemic sclerosis. Disorder of connective tissue, characterized by induration and thickening of the skin (scleroderma), that may affect only the fingers and face or that may be extensive and involve the viscera, notably the gastrointestinal tract, heart, lungs and kidneys. When it affects only the skin it is called 'scleroderma'. Patients have HYPERGAMMAGLOBULINEMIA, CRYOGLOBULINEMIA, RHEUMATOID FACTOR, ANTI-NUCLEAR ANTIBODIES and antinucleolar antibodies. Antinucleolar antibodies react with a degradation product (M_r 70,000) of DNA topoisomerase I, which is found in the nucleolus. The disease is presumed to have an immunologic cause; the systemic form is usually fatal. *See* CREST SYNDROME.

T

T cell growth factor-1. *Synonym for* INTERLEUKIN-2.

T cell growth factor-2. *Synonym for* INTERLEUKIN-4.

T cell leukemia. *See* ADULT T-CELL LEUKEMIA–LYMPHOMA.

T cell receptor (TcR). Protein on the surface of T LYMPHOCYTES that specifically recognizes molecules of the MAJOR HISTO-COMPATIBILITY COMPLEX (MHC), either alone or in association with foreign antigens (*see* CLASS I HISTOCOMPATIBILITY MOLECULES and CLASS II HISTOCOMPATIBILITY MOLECULES). The nature of the T cell receptor remained elusive for many years; it was eventually identified by highly specific antibodies to individual T cell CLONES and also by examination of unique gene rearrangements in T lymphocytes. Since different T cell clones express TcR that vary in binding specificity and IDIOTYPE, the receptors are also sometimes called Ti, i denoting idiotype. In the cell membrane, the TcR is closely associated with the CD3 complex. The CD3 chains are believed to mediate signal transduction when the T cell receptor is engaged.

There are two types of TcR; both consist of two distinct membrane-embedded polypeptide chains, either alpha and beta ($\alpha\beta$ TcR) or gamma and delta ($\gamma\delta$ TcR). The first TcR to be described was the $\alpha\beta$ receptor. This receptor is widely distributed on mature T lymphocytes, usually on CD4+ or CD8+ T cells, but it has also been reported to occur on a subpopulation of thymocytes that lack CD4 and CD8. Another TcR, the $\gamma\delta$ receptor, is found on a small fraction of thymocytes and peripheral T cells (~0.2 percent of adult THYMUS and 0.2–1 percent of peripheral blood cells). Most cells bearing the $\gamma\delta$ TcR are CD4−, CD8−. DENDRITIC EPIDERMAL CELLS in mouse skin and cells in mouse and chicken intestinal epithelium also bear $\gamma\delta$TcR. Like IMMUNOGLOBULINS, the TcR polypeptide chains are encoded by gene segments that are assembled by somatic rearrangements (*see* T CELL RECEPTOR GENES). However, unlike immunoglobulins, the $\alpha\beta$ TcR recognize antigens only when these are presented in association with major histocompatibility molecules, usually on the surface of a cell (e.g., MACROPHAGE, B LYMPHOCYTE, TARGET CELL) (*see* MHC RESTRICTION). The $\alpha\beta$TcR on CD4+ cells recognize class II MHC molecules (non-self (allogeneic) class II or self class II + antigen); the $\alpha\beta$TcR on CD8+ cells recognizes class I MHC molecules (non-self (allogenic) class I or self class I + antigen). The specificity of the $\gamma\delta$ TcR is not yet clear.

The $\gamma\delta$ TcR appears in the mouse thymus at about 14 days of gestation, at least three days before the appearance of the $\alpha\beta$ TcR. It has not been established whether T lymphocytes that express the $\gamma\delta$ receptor are precursors of those expressing the $\alpha\beta$ receptor, or whether the two cell types represent distinct lineages but the weight of evidence favors the latter possibility.

Most information about the TcR polypeptide chains has been derived from the analysis of cDNA and genomic clones. These chains resemble immunoglobulin heavy and light chains in overall structural features. The M_r of the primary translation product (before glycosylation and cleavage of the signal peptide) is approximately 30,000; the M_r of the mature chain varies from 32,000 to 55,000. Each chain consists of a SIGNAL SEQUENCE, a variable DOMAIN and a constant domain that are each similar in size to an immunoglobulin domain and that also contain a centrally-placed disulfide bridge spanning about 50–60 amino acid residues, a short connecting peptide, a hydrophobic transmembrane region, and a short hydrophilic cytoplasmic tail. (Each of the putative transmembrane segments contains a conserved lysine residue that has been proposed to form a salt bridge with an acidic residues (aspartic or glutamic acid) in the transmembrane segments of the CD3 gamma, delta and epsilon chains). With the exception of one isotype of mouse gamma chain, the TcR chains contain one or more acceptor sites for attachment of N-LINKED OLIGOSACCHARIDES. The chains of $\alpha\beta$ receptors in both mouse and humans are cross-linked by disulfide bridges (between the connecting peptides); the chains of mouse, but of only some human, $\gamma\delta$ receptors are also cross-linked by disulfide bonds. The TcR are members of the IMMUNOGLOBULIN SUPERFAMILY. The constant domains of the beta and gamma chains are substantially similar in amino acid sequence to immunoglobulins; those of the alpha and delta chains show less similarity to immunoglobulin chains.

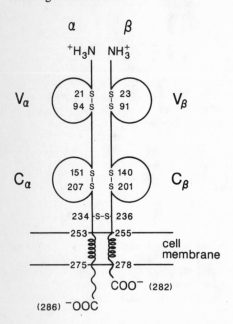

T cell receptor

T cell receptor genes. Genes that encode the VARIABLE REGIONS and the CONSTANT REGIONS of the polypeptide chains of the T CELL RECEPTOR (TcR). In the mouse, the genes for the alpha, beta and gamma chains are on separate chromosomes. In both mice and humans, genes encoding the delta chain have recently been located within the alpha gene complex. The human beta and gamma

chains are on the long and short arms, respectively, of chromosome 7 (*see* Table). There are many similarities between the structure, organization, and rearrangements of genes encoding T cell receptors and those encoding immunoglobulins (*see* IMMUNOGLOBULIN GENES, IMMUNOGLOBULIN GENE REARRANGEMENT). Both families of genes exist in two configurations, germ line and rearranged.

Chromosome map locations of T cell receptor genes

Gene	Human	Mouse
α	14q11-12	14
β	7q32-35	6
γ	7p15	13
δ	14q11-12	14

In the germ line, the DNA encoding a TcR polypeptide chain is found on distinct segments of DNA that are rearranged in thymocytes before the gene encoding the complete polypeptide chain is expressed. Different portions of the variable regions are encoded by two to four gene segments that are brought together by the rearrangement: a V GENE SEGMENT (encoding the signal sequence and first ~95–100 amino acid residues of the variable region), a J gene segment (encoding the last 13–21 residues of the variable region) and, in the case of the beta and delta chains, one or two D GENE SEGMENTS that encode a few amino acids between the V REGION and J REGION. In the rearranged DNA, these segments form the V–J or the V–D–J (or V–D–D–J) exon. Additional nucleotides may be inserted, by a non-template directed mechanism, on either side of D gene segments and, probably, also at V–J junctions (*see* N REGION). As in the case of immunoglobulin heavy chain gene rearrangements, a D_β may rearrange to a J_β without rearrangement of a V_β; such a rearranged gene may be transcribed, but corresponding translated polypeptides have not been identified.

The structure of the V gene segment of the TcR genes resembles that of the immunoglobulin genes. Most of the signal sequence and an untranslated region are encoded in an exon at the 5' end of the segment; the rest of the signal sequence as well as the bulk of the variable region are encoded at the 3' end of the segment. The two coding regions in the

V gene segment are separated by an INTRON of 100–400 base pairs. The constant region of each TcR chain is usually encoded by three or four exons, which are located downstream (3') from one or more J gene segments. In contrast to the immunoglobulin C GENE SEGMENTS, these exons do not correspond exactly to the presumed functional domains of the constant regions of the TcR (e.g., the connecting peptide of the beta chain in both mice and humans is encoded on three separate exons).

Two C_β gene segments in both mice and humans, separated by about 6 and 8 kilobases, respectively, have been described; each of these gene segments contain four exons. The amino acid sequences of the two constant regions differ by four (mouse) or five (human) amino acid residues. In mice, there are two clusters of seven J_β gene segments, each located 2–3 kilobases 5' to one of the C_β gene segments; the J_β in each cluster, six of which are functional, are separated by 36–421 base pairs. (An additional exon of 72 base pairs, $C_\beta 0$, is located between the $J_\beta 1$ cluster and $C_\beta 1$; this sequence is found in some beta chain transcripts.) About 500–600 base pairs 5' to each J_β cluster, there is a single D_β segment either 12 or 14 base pairs in length. The number and organization of J_β and D_β in humans is very similar to that in mice. The number of V_β gene segments in mice is probably relatively small (less than 30); 20 of these gene segments have recently been localized within a span of 250 kilobases of DNA 5' to the two $D_\beta J_\beta C_\beta$ clusters. The distance from the 3' end of this cluster to the $D_\beta J_\beta C_\beta$ is about 320 kilobases. One V_β segment ($V_\beta 14$) is located 10 kilobases 3' to the $D_\beta J_\beta C_\beta$ clusters; although it is in reverse transcriptional orientation, it is known to be utilized by a functional T cell clone. The V_β have been divided into different families, the members of each family being at least 75 percent identical in DNA sequence. In the V_β of mice most families seem to have only one member. Humans appear to have a similar number of families of V_β but fewer have only one member; accordingly, the total number of V_β is greater than in mice. In mice, the complete T cell receptor beta locus has been estimated to span 700 to 800 kilobases.

There is only a single C_α gene segment, containing four exons, in both mice and humans. An unusual aspect of the alpha gene family is the presence of many J gene segments spread over a large region of the chromosome. In the mouse, there are probably 50 or more J_α located 3–63 kilobases 5' to the single C_α; the different J_α are separated from one another by at least 500 base pairs. Presumably, when a V_α rearranges to one of the more 5' J_α, the resulting primary transcript is very long, including an intron of up to 63 kilobases. No D elements have been identified in the alpha gene complex. There seem to be 75–100 V_α; their location is not known but they are thought to be 5' to the J_α. The V_α have also been grouped into families and most of these contain more than one member. Therefore, the potential exists for many $V_\alpha–J_\alpha$ combinations. The organization of the alpha-chain genes in human genes seems to be similar to that in mice.

There are four C_γ gene segments in mice; one of these is a pseudogene in some strains and deleted in others. There are two C_γ in humans, separated by about 10 kilobases. Three of the mouse C_γ contain three exons (the detailed structure of the fourth is not yet determined); one of the human C_γ has three exons and the other has four or five exons. Two of the functional mouse C_γ and both human C_γ contain sites for N-LINKED OLIGOSACCHARIDES. One of the human C_γ does not encode a cysteine residue that ordinarily participates in interchain disulfide bridging, presumably accounting for the non-covalent association of some gamma-containing TcR heterodimers. In mice, one J segment has been found upstream to each of the four C_γ. In humans, one of the two C_γ has two upstream J_γ segments and the other C_γ has three such segments. No D segments have been identified in the mouse or human gamma locus. The number of V_γ gene segments appears to be relatively limited. Seven V_γ have been identified in mice, and they have been grouped into five families: four single-member families and one three-member family. Six of the V_γ have been linked in pairs; one of these pairs is in head-to-head orientation. In humans, fourteen V_γ have been found, but not all are functional. The V_γ and C_γ are interspersed in mice but not in humans. An unusual feature of the gamma gene family is that gene rearrangement and expression of mRNA frequently occurs without expression of the protein product on the cell surface. The TcR gamma locus in humans appears to span about 150 kilobases and that in mice at least 200 kilobases.

Recently, gene segments encoding the delta chain have been identified nested within the alpha chain locus. In mice, a single C_δ gene segment is located about 10 kilobases 5′ to the J_α cluster. Two J_δ and two D_δ gene segments have been identified upstream of the C_δ. The V gene segments used for alpha and delta chains are largely distinct, but there is some overlap. Some rearranged delta genes seem to contain both D_δ segments. The arrangement of alpha and delta genes is consistent with other evidence that the delta chain is expressed before the alpha chain since V_α to J_α rearrangement results in deletion of the D, J and C segments of the delta gene complex.

The ways in which diversity is generated by the TcR genes resemble the generation of diversity by the immunoglobulin genes, but there are some differences. The relative contribution of germline diversification may be relatively less than that due to gene rearrangements. Different variable-region sequences are generated, from a relatively limited repertoire of gene segments in the germ line, by combinatorial joining (utilization of different combinations of V, J and D segments), JUNCTIONAL DIVERSITY (variation in the position of the recombination point between two gene segments) and the addition of N nucleotides, which occurs in all four T cell receptor polypeptides (but only in the heavy chains of immunoglobulins. Thus, much of the potential variability, especially of gamma and delta chains, is concentrated near the $V–(D)–J$ junctions. Somatic hypermutation does not appear to occur in the TcR (in contrast to the immunoglobulins).

T cell subset. Subpopulation of T LYMPHOCYTES usually defined by a reaction with MONOCLONAL ANTIBODIES (e.g., CD4 subset). *See* CLUSTER OF DIFFERENTIATION.

T cell-conditioned medium. Medium from cultures of T LYMPHOCYTES that were stimulated with LECTINS, ANTIGENS or ALLOANTIGENS in a MIXED LYMPHOCYTE REACTION. The medium contains a variety of LYMPHOKINES.

t haplotype. Variant of the proximal region (~20 centiMorgans) of chromosome 17 of mice (*see* T/t complex.). These variants are defined by the occurrence of: (1) chromosomal inversions. Two such inversions have been identified; the major histocompatibility complex is included in the distal inversion. (2) Suppression of recombination between t haplotypes and wild-type chromosomes; presumably, recombination is suppressed as a result of the chromosomal inversion. (3) male transmission distortion. Up to 99 percent of the offspring of a male heterozygote inherit the t haplotype. Most t haplotypes contain at least one recessive lethal mutation. These mutations affect embryonic development at different stages. Different t haplotypes, containing different mutations, can complement each other. Thus, heterozygotes t^x/t^y are viable although both homozygotes t^x/t^x and t^y/t^y are not; (t^x/t^y males are sterile, but females of this genotype are completely fertile). At least 16 complementation groups have been identified. The t haplotypes were originally identified because they carry a mutation that enhances the effect of the T mutation (*see* T LOCUS), i.e., a mouse carrying T/t has no tail; a mouse carrying $T/+$ has a short tail. The male transmission distortion is believed to be responsible for maintaining the t haplotype at high levels in natural populations, despite its deleterious features.

T locus. Locus near the centromere of chromosome 17 of mice. The dominant mutation, T, was the first gene to be identified in the T/t complex. Heterozygotes for T and wild-type $(T/+)$ have a short tail. Homozygotes (T/T) die as embryos because the notochord is not formed. Heterozygotes for T and a t haplotype (T/t) are tailless. The T locus is also known as the brachyury locus. *See* T/t COMPLEX, T HAPLOTYPE.

T lymphocyte. Lymphocyte that matures in the THYMUS and is responsible for CELL-MEDIATED IMMUNITY and the regulation of growth and differentiation of other immunologically competent cells (e.g., B LYMPHOCYTES, MONONUCLEAR PHAGOCYTES). Mature T cells leave the thymus and recirculate in blood, LYMPH and SECONDARY LYMPHOID ORGANS. In LYMPH NODES, the T lymphocytes are localized to the deep cortex. T lymphocytes circulating in blood bind to specialized endothelial cells in the post-capillary venules of lymph nodes or the marginal sinus of the SPLEEN. They then traverse the venules into the deep cortex of the lymph node or white pulp of the spleen where they remain for about 12–24 hours and leave by the efferent LYMPHATICS to reach the major lymphatic circulation and the blood.

Mature T lymphocytes can be divided into two subsets that differ in function on the basis of surface antigenic determinants – CD4 and CD8. CD4+ cells recognize antigen associated with CLASS II HISTOCOMPATIBILITY MOLECULES, and CD8+ cells recognize antigen associated with CLASS I HISTOCOMPATIBILITY MOLECULES. Most CD4+ cells are HELPER T LYMPHOCYTES or responsible for DELAYED-TYPE HYPERSENSITIVITY reactions. Most CD8+ cells are cytotoxic and/or suppressor cells. Mature T lymphocytes in humans and mice bear CD3 and a TRANSFERRIN RECEPTOR. All human and many mouse T cells also have CD2, which is the E-rosette receptor. T lymphocytes also bear an antigen-specific receptor (see T CELL RECEPTOR).

T lymphocyte clone. Progeny of a single T LYMPHOCYTE. T lymphocytes from human blood or mouse SPLEEN are suspended in medium and stimulated with antigen. T lymphocytes that have responded to antigen by blast transformation are separated on density gradients from resting T lymphocytes. The activated T lymphocytes are appropriately diluted and aliquots are added to the wells of a tissue culture plate, and then stimulated with antigen and INTERLEUKIN-2. The dilution is such that usually, no more than a single T lymphocyte is added to each well (see LIMITING DILUTION ANALYSIS). Therefore, single clones are obtained. See B LYMPHOCYTE HYBRIDOMA, T LYMPHOCYTE HYBRIDOMA.

T lymphocyte hybridoma. CLONE resulting from the fusion of a mouse spleen T LYMPHOCYTE and a THYMOMA cell, BW5147, derived from the AKR strain of mice. The cells are fused by polyethylene glycol. The hybrid cells proliferate continuously and produce INTERLEUKIN-2 when stimulated with the appropriate antigen on an antigen-presenting cell. Unlike a T LYMPHOCYTE CLONE, T lymphocyte hybridomas grow in the absence of growth factors (e.g., interleukin-2).

Tac (CD25). Antigenic determinant of the INTERLEUKIN-2 (IL-2) RECEPTOR of human T LYMPHOCYTES. It is defined by a mouse monoclonal antibody, anti-Tac, which blocks the binding of IL-2 to the receptor and inhibits the proliferation of T lymphocytes.

Takayasu's arteritis. Severe, usually fatal, disease involving the aortic arch and its branches. All layers of the walls of involved arteries are inflamed and infiltrated with mononuclear cells. IMMUNOGLOBULIN deposition in the arteries can be detected by IMMUNOFLUORESCENCE. Intimal proliferation results in stenosis (marked narrowing) of the arterial lumen. Aneurysms (local dilatation of artery) may form and rupture. This rare disease occurs predominantly in young women. It is presumed to have an immunological cause.

target cell. Cell that is killed by CYTOTOXIC T LYMPHOCYTES, by ANTIBODY and COMPLEMENT, or by LYMPHOKINES, such as LYMPHOTOXIN.

T–B cell collaboration. Interaction between B LYMPHOCYTES and HELPER T LYMPHOCYTES that results in the growth and differentiation of B lymphocytes into antibody-secreting cells (PLASMA CELLS). In T–B cell collaboration, membrane IMMUNOGLOBULIN on B lymphocytes interacts with protein antigen, which, after ENDOCYTOSIS, is processed and presented (see ANTIGEN PRESENTATION) to helper T cells. The T CELL RECEPTOR recognizes the processed antigen plus CLASS II HISTOCOMPATIBILITY MOLECULES on the surface of the B lymphocyte; this results in the secretion by helper T cells of LYMPHOKINES that are essential for the growth and differentiation of the B lymphocytes into antibody-secreting cells. T–B cell collaboration is required for immunoglobulin CLASS SWITCHING. The antigens recognized by B and T lymphocytes are usually different. Ordinarily, B lymphocytes recognize native protein antigens, but they can also recognize denatured proteins or peptide fragments. However, T lymphocytes have an absolute requirement that the antigen (usually a peptide) be presented in association with class I or class II histocompatibility molecules.

The collaboration between B and T lym-

First injection	Second injection	Anti-DNP response
DNP–BSA	DNP–BSA	+
DNP–BSA	DNP–OVA	0
DNP–BSA + OVA	DNP–OVA	+
DNP–BSA	DNP–OVA + BSA	weak

phocytes has been demonstrated with model antigens consisting of HAPTEN–protein complexes. After an animal has been immunized initially (i.e., 'primed') with a hapten (e.g., the DINITROPHENYL (DNP) group) coupled to a 'carrier' protein (e.g., bovine serum albumin (BSA)) a second injection of the same hapten–carrier complex elicits a strong secondary response. However, if the second injection consists of the same hapten attached to a *different* protein carrier (e.g., ovalbumin (OVA)), there is a much weaker response, unless the animal had also been primed with the second carrier (OVA). This requirement for recognition of the original carrier is known as the 'carrier effect'. It can be shown that B lymphocytes in the primed animal recognize the hapten and T lymphocytes the carrier (after processing). The hapten and carrier must be physically linked to elicit the maximum response.

terminal transferase. *See* DNA NUCLEO-TIDYLEXOTRANSFERASE.

tertiary granule. Cytoplasmic organelle of NEUTROPHILS that contains acid hydrolases, gelatinase and the precursor of COMPLEMENT RECEPTOR 3. Tertiary granules are poorly characterized. *See* PRIMARY GRANULES, SECONDARY GRANULES.

tertiary structure. Folding of a protein chain by virtue of interactions among the side-chains of its constituent amino acid residues. The tertiary structure may be stabilized by disulfide bridges. *See* PRIMARY STRUCTURE, QUATERNARY STRUCTURE, SECONDARY STRUCTURE.

tetraparental mouse. *Synonym for* ALLO-PHENIC MOUSE.

theophylline (1,3 dimethylxanthine). Drug used in the treatment of ASTHMA; it dilates bronchi because it is a potent relaxant of bronchial and other smooth muscle. Theophylline is rendered more soluble by com-

plexing it with ethylenediamine; the complex is called aminophylline.

theophylline

thoracic duct. Duct that returns LYMPH to the blood. It leads from the cisterna chyli to the left subclavian vein. The cisterna chyli is a dilated chamber at the origin of the thoracic duct in the lumbar region. Lymph from the abdomen, chest and retroperitoneum collects in the cisterna chyli.

thoracic duct drainage. Prolonged drainage of LYMPH from the THORACIC DUCT. This technique is used to deplete lymphocytes from an animal or patient.

thrombocyte. *Synonym for* PLATELET.

thrombocytopenia. Decrease in the number of PLATELETS in the blood to less than 100,000/mm^3 (normal: 150,000–300,000/mm^3).

thrombocytosis. Increase in the number of PLATELETS in the blood to greater than 600,000/mm^3 (normal 150,000–300,000/mm^3).

Thy-1. Glycoprotein that is an abundant cell surface molecule on thymocytes of mice and rats and is also a major constituent of the membrane of neuronal brain cells and of fibroblasts from a number of species. Thy-1 was first identified as the theta (ϑ) ALLOAN-TIGEN of mouse thymocytes and was found to occur in two allelic forms: Thy-1.1 (ϑ-AKR) and Thy-1.2 (ϑ-C3H). The Thy-1 glycoprotein isolated from rat brains consists of

111 amino acid residues with two disulfide bridges linking cysteine 9 to cysteine 111 and cysteine 19 to cysteine 85; there are three N-LINKED OLIGOSACCHARIDES. Thymocyte Thy-1 has the same amino acid sequence but different carbohydrate structures. The amino acid sequence is related to VARIABLE REGION sequences of immunoglobulins. The smaller disulfide loop is similar in position to the conserved intradomain disulfide bridge of immunoglobulin domains. The larger disulfide loop is similar in position to extra disulfide bridges found in a few immunoglobulin domains. Thus, Thy-1 is a member of the IMMUNOGLOBULIN SUPERFAMILY.

A glycosyl phosphatidyl inositol anchor is attached to the carboxy-terminal cysteine residue via ethanolamine and this forms the hydrophobic site for membrane attachment. An additional stretch of 31 hydrophobic amino acid residues, predicted from the cDNA sequence, is not present in the mature protein. Mouse Thy-1 is very similar in structure to rat Thy-1, except it has one additional amino acid residue. A single amino acid substitution, arginine or glutamine at position 89, distinguishes Thy-1.1 from Thy-1.2. In the mouse, but not in the rat, Thy-1 is present on mature T lymphocytes as well as on thymocytes. It has been widely used as marker for mouse T LYMPHOCYTES. Treatment of lymphocytes with antibodies to Thy-1, in the presence of COMPLEMENT, leads to selective lysis of T lymphocytes and abrogation of T-dependent reactions. Thy-1 has been mapped to mouse chromosome 9.

Human Thy-1 is expressed on only a very small percentage of lymphocytes but is a major surface component of neurons and fibroblasts. The function of Thy-1 is not known. Mouse T lymphocytes cultured with phorbol myristic acid can be triggered to divide by cross-linking of Thy-1 with antibodies.

thymectomy. Surgical removal of the THYMUS. Clinically, thymectomy is used to treat MYASTHENIA GRAVIS. In newborn mice, this procedure is used to deprive the animal of T LYMPHOCYTES and therefore CELL-MEDIATED IMMUNITY and antibody responses to THYMUS-DEPENDENT ANTIGENS. Neonatally thymectomized mice do not gain weight and have atrophy of their lymphoid tissue. This is called runt disease or wasting disease.

thymic epithelial cell. Cell derived from the endoderm of the third and fourth pharyngeal pouches and having the characteristics of an epithelial cell. These cells express CLASS I HISTOCOMPATIBILITY and CLASS II HISTOCOMPATIBILITY MOLECULES and are thought to influence thymocyte differentiation. Fewer epithelial cells are found in the thymic medulla than in the cortex. Large thymic epithelial cells in close contact with thymocytes are called thymus nurse cells.

thymic hormone. Peptide (e.g., thymopoietin, thymosin) extracted from the thymus that has been proposed to regulate T cell differentiation. Thymic hormones have been assayed by diverse methods such as incubation of hormone with SPLEEN cells from NUDE MICE to induce expression of Thy-1 antigen.

thymocyte. LYMPHOCYTE in the THYMUS.

thymoma. Tumor of thymocytes. Thymomas, which usually grow slowly, are found in the mediastinum and may be associated with MYASTHENIA GRAVIS or immunodeficiency. *See* IMMUNODEFICIENCY WITH THYMOMA.

thymus. PRIMARY LYMPHOID ORGAN for T LYMPHOCYTE development. The thymus is located in most mammals in the superior anterior mediastinum (chest). It consists of epithelial cells derived during embryogenesis from cells of the third and fourth branchial (or pharyngeal) pouches, thymocytes (T lymphocytes in various stages of differentiation), MACROPHAGES and dendritic cells (*see* LANGERHANS CELLS). The thymus is divided into a cortex rich in immature T lymphocytes tightly packed between the epithelial cells and a medulla containing mature T lymphocytes and macrophages. At birth the weight of the thymus, relative to body weight, is maximal and the cortex is the site of intense mitotic activity. However only 5 percent of thymocytes emigrate from the thymus into the circulation. The thymus increases in absolute size until puberty; it then begins to decrease in size and may atrophy in later life. *See* HASSALL'S CORPUSCLE, NUDE MOUSE, THYMECTOMY, THYMIC EPITHELIAL CELL, THYMUS CELL DIFFERENTIATION.

thymus cell differentiation. Process of maturation of STEM CELLS into mature T LYMPHOCYTES that occurs in the THYMUS. The differentiation of stem cells involves the sequential acquisition and loss of cell surface markers that demarcate various stages of maturation. In humans, stem cells bearing CD38 (*see* list of CD antigens) become early thymocytes when they express CD2 and CD7 and then the TRANSFERRIN RECEPTOR. Early thymocytes subsequently express CD1, which is the marker of common thymocytes at mid-stage of differentiation. During this stage, the genes for the gamma and delta, and subsequently those for alpha and beta chains of the T CELL RECEPTOR rearrange (*see* T CELL RECEPTOR GENES). The thymocytes then express CD3, CD4 and CD8; the CD1 marker is progressively lost at this stage. Finally two distinctive subsets of mature T lymphocytes appear: the helper/inducer subset that is CD3+4+8− and the cytotoxic/suppressor subset that is CD3+4−8+.

In mice, a similar maturation process occurs. The stem cells can be identified by antibodies to Ly5. Mouse thymocytes express TL molecules (*see* Tla COMPLEX) that, like CD1 in humans, are lost in the late stages of differentiation. Thy-1 is expressed by mouse thymocytes in all stages of differentiation and by mature T lymphocytes.

During differentiation, thymocytes are in intimate contact with epithelial cells, which bear both CLASS I and CLASS II HISTOCOMPATIBILITY MOLECULES. With bone marrow transplants into irradiated mice, it has been possible to show that the ALLELES of class I and class II molecules in the stromal cells influence T cell recognition. For example, marrow stem cells from a mouse of haplotype A × B transplanted into an A recipient will develop helper T lymphocytes that recognize antigen in the context of antigen-presenting cells of haplotype A; when A × B cells are transplanted into a B recipient, the helper T lymphocytes will recognize antigen + B. How this process of acquisition of receptors restricted by the MAJOR HISTOCOMPATIBILITY COMPLEX allele develops is not yet understood. Overall, thymus cell differentiation is an inefficient process since about 90 percent of thymocytes die in the thymus.

thymus cell education. *See* THYMUS CELL DIFFERENTIATION.

thymus-dependent antigen. Antigen that requires interaction with HELPER T LYM-PHOCYTES in order to stimulate B LYM-PHOCYTES to produce antibodies. Thymus-dependent antigens must be presented to T lymphocytes by cells bearing CLASS II HISTOCOMPATIBILITY MOLECULES. All proteins and polypeptides are thymus-dependent antigens (*see* T–B CELL COLLABORATION).

thymus-independent antigen. Antigen that does not require interaction with T LYM-PHOCYTES in order to stimulate B LYM-PHOCYTES to produce ANTIBODIES. T-independent antigens include polysaccharides with repeating ANTIGENIC DETERMINANTS and LIPOPOLYSACCHARIDES from Gram-negative bacteria. Such antigens induce production of IgM and lead to little, if any, immunological memory (*see* SECONDARY IMMUNE RESPONSE). Whether or not any antigen is completely thymus-independent is not clear.

thymus nurse cell. *See* THYMIC EPITHELIAL CELL.

thymus-replacing factor (TRF). *See* INTERLEUKIN-5.

titer. Estimate of amount of antibody activity. The antibody-containing fluid (e.g., serum) is diluted serially until an end-point (e.g., failure to agglutinate red blood cells) is reached. The titer is often expressed as the reciprocal of the end-point dilution.

Tla complex. A segment of DNA, about 1.5 centiMorgans in length, on the telomeric side of the H-2 complex, and consisting of two regions called Qa and Tla.

The Qa region (220 kilobases) encodes the alpha chains of certain tissue-restricted CLASS I HISTOCOMPATIBILITY MOLECULES; these chains associate noncovalently with BETA-2 MICROGLOBULIN. The eight to ten genes in the Qa region of various INBRED STRAINS are designated *Q1, Q2, Q3, Q4, Q5, Q6, Q7, Q8, Q9* and *Q10*. Three molecules, encoded in the Qa region, have been characterized: Qa-1, Qa-2 and Q10. Qa-1 and Qa-2 are expressed on lymphoid cells; Q10 is expressed on liver cells. The genes in the Qa region exhibit very little polymorphism.

The Tla region (155 kilobases) encodes the alpha chains of other class I histocompatibility molecules; these chains also associate noncovalently with beta-2 microglobulin. There are 13 to 18 genes (depending on the inbred strain). The molecules encoded in the Tla region are called TL and are found on thymocytes of certain inbred strains and on some leukemia cells, the origin of the designation TL. TL+ leukemias may occur in mice that do not express TL on their thymocytes. The Tla region molecules also exhibit very little polymorphism. The function of Qa and TL molecules is not known.

tolerance. Immunological phenomenon consisting of the acquired incapacity of an individual to respond to a particular ANTIGEN. Tolerance can be induced by introducing an antigen into an individual at a very early stage in life, either during fetal or early postnatal life. Such an individual will not respond when challenged with the same antigen during adulthood. In contrast, the response to unrelated antigens is normal (i.e., there is selective loss of the response to the antigen that had been introduced in early life, TOLEROGEN).

Tolerance was discovered in non-identical twin cattle in which there had been exchange of blood *in utero* that resulted in a chimeric state (*see* CHIMERA) (i.e., each twin has hemopoietic cells from the other). In adulthood, each cow can accept grafts from its twin. Tolerance can be induced in fetal/ neonatal mice by injections of foreign cells or purified proteins. Immunological tolerance can also be induced in adult individuals by giving weak protein antigens either in repeated small doses or in large amounts (i.e., low-zone tolerance or high-zone tolerance, respectively).

The mechanisms involved in tolerance are complex. Three possibilities have been proposed: (1) inactivation or deletion of B LYMPHOCYTES (which apparently occurs if B lymphocytes are exposed to antigen in the absence of interactions with T LYMPHOCYTES); (2) inactivation or deletion of HELPER T LYMPHOCYTES; and (3) induction of SUPPRESSOR T LYMPHOCYTES. The lack of immunological response to AUTOLOGOUS proteins is self-tolerance.

tolerogen. Substance that is capable of inducing TOLERANCE. In general, tolerogens are also IMMUNOGENS. Whether tolerance or IMMUNITY follows antigen administration depends on a number of factors: dose, route of administration, immunological status of the recipient. For example, foreign cells are strong immunogens when given to an adult, but may be tolerogens when given to a fetus. Heterologous immunoglobulins are usually strong immunogens when aggregated, but are often tolerogens in the monomeric form.

tolerogenic. Capable of inducing TOLERANCE.

tolmetin (1-methyl-5-*p*-toluoylpyrrole-2-acetic acid). Drug used in the treatment of RHEUMATOID ARTHRITIS, JUVENILE RHEUMATOID ARTHRITIS and ANKYLOSING SPONDYLITIS because of its anti-inflammatory effects.

tolmetin

tonsil. Mass of LYMPHOID tissue in the oropharynx. The palatine tonsils lie between the palatoglossal and palatopharyngeal arches; the lingual tonsils are at the base of the tongue; the pharyngeal tonsils, also called adenoids, are at the back of the pharynx. Tonsils are SECONDARY LYMPHOID ORGANS and are composed mostly of B LYMPHOCYTES. *See* GUT-ASSOCIATED LYMPHOID TISSUE.

toxin. Poison, usually of high molecular weight, that is produced by a living organism and that is usually immunogenic. *See* LIPOPOLYSACCHARIDE, VENOM.

toxoid. TOXIN treated (e.g., with formalin) so that it retains its immunogenicity (*see* IMMUNOGENIC), but loses its toxicity. Diphtheria and tetanus toxoids are routinely used to immunize infants.

Tp44 (CD28). Membrane glycoprotein of T LYMPHOCYTES identified by a mouse monoclonal antibody. Tp44 is a HOMODIMER, M_r 74,000–92,000 (depending on cell source and probably due to variations in glycosylation);

under reducing conditions the M_r is 39,000–50,000. In the presence of PHORBOL ESTERS, anti-Tp44 causes T lymphocytes to proliferate. The function of Tp44 is not known. Tp44 is composed of 220 amino acid residues, including a signal sequence of 18 residues, an extracellular domain of 134 residues, a transmembrane segment of 27 residues and a cytoplasmic domain of 41 residues; there are five sites for attachment of N-LINKED OLIGOSACCHARIDES. Tp44 is a member of the IMMUNOGLOBULIN SUPERFAMILY. The amino-terminal 119 residues of the mature protein are homologous to variable region-like domains.

transcobalamin 2 deficiency (TC2 deficiency).　Deficiency of the principal vitamin B12 transport protein, transcobalamin 2. Affected infants have megaloblastic anemia and AGAMMAGLOBULINEMIA. Vitamin B12 is required for terminal differentiation of B LYMPHOCYTES. The anemia and agammaglobulinemia are corrected by administration of large doses of vitamin B12. TC 2 deficiency is inherited as an autosomal recessive.

transcytosis.　Process whereby ligands, which have been internalized by receptor-mediated ENDOCYTOSIS, are directed to the surface of the cell opposite to that at which they entered. The best-characterized examples of transcytosis involve transport of IMMUNOGLOBULINS across epithelia. The POLYIMMUNOGLOBULIN RECEPTOR on the basolateral surface of epithelial cells bind IgA or IgM; the complex is internalized (receptor-mediated endocytosis), transported across the cell, and released at the apical surface by EXOCYTOSIS. In transcytosis of IgA or IgM, the receptor is cleaved, and the ligand-binding portion, known as SECRETORY COMPONENT, remains bound to the polymeric immunoglobulin, which is released into secretions. Other epithelial cells transport monomeric IgG via Fc receptors (e.g., maternal IgG is transported from the small intestine of suckling rats into the circulation, in the direction opposite to that of IgA in adult intestine).

transduction.　Transfer of genetic information by a virus. Originally, the term described the transfer of genes from one bacterium to another by bacteriophage. Transduction is now also used to describe the transfer of genes by other viruses. For example, transducing retroviruses acquire proto-oncogenes (c-*onc*) from normal cells and transfer these genes (as ONCOGENES or v-*onc*) to other cells.

transfection.　Hybrid of TRANSFORMATION and infection, originally used to describe the introduction of phage DNA into bacteria. Subsequently, its use was broadened to include the introduction of viral (i.e., infectious) DNA into any cell, bacterial or eukaryotic. Presently, the term transfection is used quite loosely. In the context of eukaryotic cell biology, the transfer of any type of DNA (viral, cellular or plasmid) into an animal cell is often called transfection. This terminology was developed because the term transformation also has another meaning (i.e., malignant transformation). Some workers use the term transfection to describe the process whereby DNA is introduced into a cell, transformation being the relatively rare event of stable incorporation of DNA into the genome such that the cell is permanently altered. Several methods are used for the transfection of DNA into a variety of cells including LYMPHOID cells (e.g., coprecipitation of DNA with calcium phosphate, treatment with DEAE–dextran, PROTOPLAST FUSION, ELECTROPORATION).

transfectoma.　Stable line of antibody-producing cells created by the transfer of genetically engineered antibody genes into myeloma cell lines. Usually, genomic DNA (rather than cDNA) is used in order to facilitate expression by virtue of inclusion of unique regulatory sequences (e.g., PROMOTERS, ENHANCERS). The immunoglobulin heavy and light chain genes may be introduced one at a time in separate VECTORS or they may be cloned into the same vector.

transfer factor.　Substance in dialysates of lysates of human peripheral blood LEUKOCYTES that may be capable of transferring DELAYED-TYPE HYPERSENSITIVITY from one individual to another.

transferrin receptor (T9).　Cell membrane receptor for transferrin, a serum protein (M_r 76,000) that transports Fe^{3+}. The transferrin receptor is detected in humans with a mouse monoclonal antibody, anti-T9. Although the transferrin receptor is found on many cell types, it is most prominently expressed on the surface of activated T LYMPHOCYTES (about 250,000 molecules per cell). It is absent or barely detectable on resting T lymphocytes. The transferrin receptor is also expressed by early thymocytes. It is a glycoprotein, composed of two identical polypeptide chains (M_r 100,000) which are linked by disulfide bonds. When T lymphocytes are stimulated with MITOGENS or ANTIGENS, the transferrin receptor is expressed before the onset of DNA synthesis. Monoclonal antibodies to T9 inhibit DNA synthesis in activated T lymphocytes. The gene encoding the transferrin receptor has been mapped to chromosome 3p12-ter in humans.

transformation. Inherited change in a cell as the result of some experimental treatment. The term is used in three different contexts. (1) Transformation by DNA (genetic transformation): acquisition of a heritable altered phenotype as a result of the incorporation of exogenous DNA into a bacterial or eukaryotic cell (*see* TRANSFECTION). (2) Neoplastic (cellular) transformation: conversion of cultured animal cells to a state of unrestrained growth such that these cells come to resemble malignant cells. (3) LYMPHOCYTE transformation: activation of a resting lymphocyte so that it grows, divides and differentiates, i.e., becomes a BLAST CELL. The degree of blast transformation can be quantitated by measuring the incorporation of [³H]thymidine into the cell's DNA. Blast transformation can be induced by stimulation with LECTINS, LYMPHOKINES, alloantigens (e.g., in the MIXED LYMPHOCYTE REACTION) and, in the case of cells from IMMUNE individuals, by antigen.

Genetic transformation was discovered in bacteria when it was shown that living nonvirulent pneumococci could acquire the property of virulence from dead bacteria in the same culture. Subsequently, the material responsible for the 'transformation' was shown to be DNA.

transfusion reaction. Untoward immunological reactions observed in the recipient of a transfusion of blood or blood products. Such reactions are usually due to ALLO-ANTIBODIES that cause HEMOLYSIS of donor red blood cells. The reaction is characterized by pain in the extremities and back, shortness of breath and falling blood pressure, which may lead to shock. The patient sustains a brief period of hypothermia followed by fever. Hemoglobin appears in the urine.

transgenic organism. Organism carrying an exogenous gene in its GENOME. For example, in mice, the gene is usually introduced by microinjection into one of the two pronuclei of a recently fertilized egg. To allow the egg to develop, it is placed into the oviduct of a pseudopregnant female. The gene may become integrated into a chromosome; this occurs at a random position. If the DNA is integrated, it is transmitted through the germ line to subsequent generations and will be present in every cell; all tissues, at any developmental stage, can be analysed for expression of the inserted gene. Retroviruses may also be used to introduce foreign DNA into a mouse; in this case, infection is usually initiated at a later developmental stage (i.e., four to eight cell stage) and the resulting transgenic animal will be a mosaic; if germ line cells are infected, the exogenous DNA will be transmitted to progeny.

transient hypogammaglobulinemia of infancy. Self-limited disease of infants, characterized by a delay in the capacity to synthesize antibodies normally until 30–36 months of age. Although affected infants have normal numbers of B LYMPHOCYTES, their HELPER T LYMPHOCYTE function appears to be defective.

transplantation antigen. *See* CLASS I HISTOCOMPATIBILITY MOLECULES, CLASS II HISTOCOMPATIBILITY MOLECULES and MINOR HISTOCOMPATIBILITY ANTIGEN.

T/t complex. Proximal region of chromosome 17 of mice in which recombination is suppressed between t HAPLOTYPES and the wild-type chromosome. The region of recombination suppression spans about 20 cM and includes the T LOCUS and the MAJOR HISTOCOMPATIBILITY COMPLEX. There is about 5–11 cM of normal chromosome between the centromere and the beginning of the recombination-suppressed region. The T/t complex contains genes involved in early embryonic development.

tuberculin. Mixture of proteins from culture filtrates of *Mycobacterium tuberculosis*. It is employed in skin tests for DELAYED-TYPE HYPERSENSITIVITY to this organism. The term includes OLD TUBERCULIN and PURIFIED PROTEIN DERIVATIVE.

tuberculin test. Intradermal test for DELAYED-TYPE HYPERSENSITIVITY to TUBERCULIN. Positive reactions are presumptive evidence of CELL-MEDIATED IMMUNITY to *Mycobacterium tuberculosis*. See HEAF TEST, MANTOUX TEST and VOLLMER TEST.

tumor-associated antigen. Membrane or nuclear antigen of tumor cells that is not found – or found in lesser amounts – in normal cells of the type from which the tumor was derived. Tumor-specific transplantation antigens (TSTA) have been found in methylcholanthrene-induced skin tumors of mice. When such tumors are transplanted to a SYNGENEIC MOUSE, the recipient becomes immune to the tumor and rejects it and is resistant to the successful engraftment of a second tumor from the same source. Each tumor appears to have a distinct antigen. Oncogenic viruses can also induce expression of tumor-associated antigens. For each virus, the same antigen is expressed regardless of the tissue of origin of the tumor or the animal species in which the tumor is induced. These tumor-associated antigens are actually host antigens whose expression is induced by the virus. ONCOFETAL ANTIGENS are also considered to be tumor-associated antigens.

tumor enhancement. Prevention, by antibodies, of cell-mediated destruction of tumors. Two mechanisms that have been invoked to account for this phenomenon are: (1) antibody molecules cover TUMOR-ASSOCIATED ANTIGENS and block the induction of CELL-MEDIATED IMMUNITY; (2) antibodies cover tumor-associated antigens, thereby preventing their destruction by CYTOTOXIC T LYMPHOCYTES.

tumor necrosis factor (TNF). MONOKINE that induces leukocytosis, fever, weight loss, the ACUTE PHASE REACTION and necrosis of some tumors (e.g., methylcholanthrene-induced sarcomas in mice). TNF was first found in serum of animals primed with BACILLE CALMETTE-GUERIN (BCG) and then challenged with LIPOPOLYSACCHARIDE. A molecule identical to TNF, and named cachectin, was isolated from serum of animals with heavy parasitic infestations. Cachectin was found to have profound effects on general cellular metabolism and to be responsible for weight loss during infection or from neoplasia. Synthesis of TNF can be induced in MONONUCLEAR PHAGOCYTES by a variety of agents including lipopolysaccharides and PHORBOL ESTERS; secretion of TNF is maximal 8 to 24 hours later.

TNF (also called TNF–α)is a single polypeptide chain of 157 amino acid residues; it is not glycosylated. The gene for TNF has been mapped to the H-2 region of mouse chromosome 17 and the HLA region of human chromosome 6. The gene encoding TNF is closely linked to the gene encoding LYMPHOTOXIN (LT), a lymphokine that is also called TNF-β. TNF and LT are homologous proteins having approximately 30 percent amino acid sequence identity. They bind to the same receptor and have common biological activities: (1) inducing differentiation of myeloid cells; (2) activating neutrophils; (3) killing of RNA and DNA viruses by macrophages in synergy with INTERFERON-GAMMA. Both TNF and LT are assayed by their capacity to kill a mouse fibroblast line (L-929). In contrast to the other major monokine, INTERLEUKIN-1, TNF does not induce synthesis of INTERLEUKIN-2.

tumor promoter. *See* PHORBOL ESTERS.

tumor-specific transplantation antigen. *See* TUMOR-ASSOCIATED ANTIGEN.

type II interferon. *Synonym for* INTERFERON-GAMMA.

U

ubiquitin. Polypeptide of 76 amino acid residues that is present in all eukaryotes, but apparently not in prokaryotes. Ubiquitin is highly conserved, differing in only three amino acid residues from yeast to mammals. Ubiquitin exists either free or covalently bound to many cellular proteins, thereby marking them for selective degradation. Ubiquitin is also present in chromosomes, where it forms covalent complexes with histones; the functional role of ubiquitin in chromosomes is not known. Ubiquitin was originally found in extracts of THYMUS and was erroneously believed to be one of the 'THYMIC HORMONES'. It is found on the lymphocyte HOMING RECEPTOR (gp90MEL-14) and other cell surface receptors.

ulcerative colitis. *See* INFLAMMATORY BOWEL DISEASE.

unidentified reading frame (URF). OPEN READING FRAME (ORF) that does not correspond to a known protein.

unitarian hypothesis. View that the multiple functions of antibodies (e.g., AGGLUTINATION, COMPLEMENT FIXATION, LYSIS, PRECIPITATION) are all results of the same type of antibody molecule reacting with different LIGANDS. The opposing view is that each activity is associated with a distinct type of antibody molecule. Today, it is known that neither of these views is entirely correct, since different IMMUNOGLOBULIN CLASSES and subclasses do vary in their activities, but a particular activity (e.g., precipitation) is usually manifested by more than one class.

univalent. Having one binding site.

urticaria. Intensely itchy, patchy rash consisting of a raised, irregularly shaped wheal with a blanched center surrounded by a red flare. Urticaria is caused by HISTAMINE released from MAST CELLS due to immunological reactions or to chemical or physical agents. Among the immunological reactions causing histamine release are interactions between antigens and IgE antibodies bound to mast cells or generation of ANAPHYLOTOXINS by activation of COMPLEMENT. *Synonym for* hive.

uveitis. INFLAMMATION of the uveal tract (uvea, iris, ciliary body and choroid) of the eye. Uveitis is found in several immunological diseases, such as SARCOIDOSIS, BEHÇET'S DISEASE and JUVENILE RHEUMATOID ARTHRITIS.

V

V gene segment. Segment of DNA encoding most (i.e. the first ~95–100) amino acid residues of the VARIABLE REGIONS of IMMUNOGLOBULIN and T CELL RECEPTOR polypeptide chains. The V gene segment contains two coding regions, separated by an intron of 100–400 base pairs. The first (5′) of these coding regions is an exon that encodes a short untranslated region of mRNA as well as the first approximately 15–18 residues of the signal peptide. The second coding region, at the 3′ end of the segment, is part of an exon; it usually encodes the last four residues of the signal peptide and 95–100 residues of the variable region. The remainder of the variable region is encoded by a J GENE SEGMENT, and, in the case of immunoglobulin heavy chains and T cell receptor beta and delta chains, a D GENE SEGMENT. Before transcription, the V gene segment is juxtaposed to the 5′ end of a J or a D–J gene segment. (In PREB-CELLS an unrearranged V gene may be transcribed.) As a result of this rearrangement, an exon is formed, which encodes the end of the signal peptide and the entire variable region. *See* IMMUNOGLOBULIN GENES, IMMUNOGLOBULIN GENE REARRANGEMENT, T CELL RECEPTOR GENES.

V region. *See* VARIABLE REGION.

V_κ. VARIABLE REGION of an IMMUNOGLOBULIN KAPPA CHAIN; sometimes used to denote only that portion of the variable region encoded by the V_κ gene segment.

V_λ. VARIABLE REGION of an IMMUNOGLOBULIN LAMBDA CHAIN; sometimes used to denote only that portion of the variable region encoded by the V_λ gene segment.

vaccination. Production of ACTIVE IMMUNITY by administration of a VACCINE. Vaccination was introduced by Edward Jenner.

Jenner showed that immunity against smallpox could be induced by inoculating with cowpox, a virus that is not pathogenic for humans but that shares ANTIGENIC DETERMINANTS with smallpox virus.

vaccine. Pathogenic microorganisms or materials derived from such organisms that contain ANTIGENS in an innocuous form. When inoculated into a non-immune individual, the vaccine will provoke ACTIVE IMMUNITY to the microorganisms, but will not cause disease.

vaccinia. Virus, *Pox virus officinale*, originally derived from cowpox and used in VACCINATION to produce ACTIVE IMMUNITY to smallpox.

vaccinia gangrenosa. *Synonym for* PROGRESSIVE VACCINNIA.

valence. Number of binding sites on an antibody or antigen molecule. The antibody valence corresponds to the maximum number of antigen molecules that can bind to one antibody molecule (barring steric hindrance). Antigen valence is more difficult to define. An antigen typically has a number of distinct determinants, each of which may bind a different population of antibody molecules; these determinants may be overlapping.

variability plot. *See* WU–KABAT PLOT.

variable (V) region. In a set of equivalent proteins, that portion of each protein (or constituent polypeptide chain) that varies in sequence from one molecule to the next. In the IMMUNOGLOBULINS, the variable region is the segment of a heavy or light chain that varies in sequence in chains of the same ISOTYPE and ALLOTYPE: the amino-terminal DOMAIN of light chains (~110 amino acid residues) or of heavy chains (115–120 residues) (*see* IMMUNOGLOBULIN LIGHT and HEAVY CHAINS). The variable regions of heavy and light chains combine to form the binding site for antigen and, therefore, determine the SPECIFICITY of the antibody molecule. The portion of the chain encoded by the V GENE SEGMENT is sometimes also referred to as the variable or V region. By this definition, the V region would include the signal peptide, but not the portions of the variable region encoded by the J gene segment and, in the case of the heavy chain, the D gene segment. Thus the term 'V region' is sometimes ambiguous. Variable regions encoded by the V, J and sometimes D GENE SEGMENTS are also found in T CELL RECEPTORS.

The term variable region is also used to refer to those domains of CLASS I or CLASS II MAJOR HISTOCOMPATIBILITY MOLECULES that are most variable when equivalent molecules obtained from different members of the same species are compared: the α_1 and α_2 domains of class I molecules and the α_1 and β_1 domains of class II molecules. *See* CONSTANT REGION, HYPERVARIABLE REGION, FRAMEWORK REGION and COMPLEMENTARITY-DETERMINING REGION.

variolation.   Inoculation of pustular material from smallpox lesions into the skin of non-immune recipients with the aim of inducing IMMUNITY to smallpox. Variolation was difficult to control and frequently produced severe smallpox infection. Variolation was superseded by VACCINATION.

vasculitis.   INFLAMMATION and NECROSIS of blood vessels, as may occur in IMMUNE COMPLEX DISEASE.

vector.   DNA element used as a vehicle for cloning a fragment of foreign DNA (*see* CLONE). A vector should have the following properties: (1) capacity for autonomous replication in a host cell (i.e., it should contain an origin of replication); (2) presence of one or more selectable markers (e.g., antibiotic resistance); (3) presence of sites for RESTRICTION ENDONUCLEASES in non-essential regions, allowing foreign DNA to be inserted into the vector or to replace a segment of the vector. Major types of cloning vectors are PLASMIDS (e.g., pBR322), bacteriophages (e.g., LAMBDA or M13 BACTERIOPHAGE), COSMIDS, animal viruses (e.g., SV40, retroviruses). *See* EXPRESSION VECTOR.

veiled cell.   *See* LANGERHANS CELL.

venom.   Poison secreted by some animals (e.g., snakes, arthropods), delivered in bites and stings, and used for taking prey.

V$_\text{H}$.   VARIABLE REGION of an IMMUNOGLOBULIN HEAVY CHAIN; sometimes used to denote that portion of the variable region encoded by the V_H gene segment.

virus neutralization test.   Test to determine the TITER of antibodies to a virus. The infectivity of the test virus (e.g., for tissue culture cells or susceptible animals) is neutralized by antibodies.

V$_\text{L}$.   VARIABLE REGION of an IMMUNOGLOBULIN LIGHT CHAIN; sometimes used to denote the segment encoded by the V_L gene.

VLA (*very late appearing antigens*).   Five distinct HETERODIMERS of cell membranes that share a common beta chain (M_r 130,000) but have different alpha chains (M_r 130,000–210,000). VLAs were first found on membranes of LYMPHOCYTE that had been in culture for several days. Subsequently, one or more VLAs were found on all types of nucleated cells. VLAs may function as cell matrix adhesion receptors. For example, VLA-5 is the FIBRONECTIN receptor. *See* INTEGRIN FAMILY.

Vollmer test.   Skin PATCH TEST using TUBERCULIN.

W

wasting disease. *See* THYMECTOMY.

Wegener's granulomatosis. Disease characterized by GRANULOMAS and VASCULITIS with NECROSIS of the upper and lower respiratory tracts and GLOMERULONEPHRITIS. The disease is thought to have an immunological cause. The disease process responds favorably to CYCLOPHOSPHAMIDE treatment.

Western blotting. *See* IMMUNOBLOTTING.

white graft. Skin GRAFT that is rapidly rejected prior to vascularization and lymphocytic infiltration, possibly because of the presence of pre-existing antibodies to the graft. Presence of a white graft is a manifestation of so-called hyperacute graft rejection.

wild mouse. Unconfined mouse that has not been raised under laboratory or domestic conditions and whose reproduction is not controlled.

Winn test. Procedure to evaluate whether or not LYMPHOCYTES are sensitized to ALLOGENEIC cells or tumors. The allogeneic or tumor cells, together with the test lymphocytes, are injected into the skin of X-irradiated mice and the growth of the cell mass is evaluated. Sensitized T LYMPHOCYTES will diminish the multiplication of the allogeneic cells or tumors. The test is frequently used to study IMMUNITY to tumors.

Wiskott–Aldrich syndrome (WAS). X-linked IMMUNODEFICIENCY disease, characterized by a low number of small PLATELETS in the blood (THROMBOCYTOPENIA), eczema and defective CELL-MEDIATED IMMUNITY. Affected males have small plate-

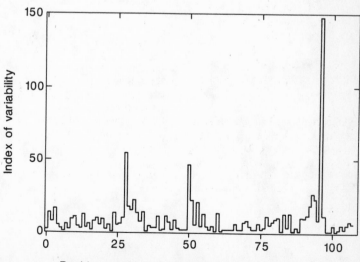

Wu-Kabat plot
From Wu, T.T. and Kabat, E.A. J. Exper. Med. 132:210, 1970.

lets, which are less than 1.8 μm in diameter (normal: 2.8–3.5 μm), and which lack surface glycoprotein Ib. The serum concentrations of IgA and IgE are elevated, that of IgM is decreased, but serum IgG concentration is usually normal. Patients have a markedly diminished antibody response to polysaccharide antigens (e.g., pneumococcal polysaccharides). Cell-mediated immunity declines progressively with age. T LYMPHOCYTES are abnormal when examined by scanning electron microscopy; they appear to have bald surfaces in contrast to the richly fimbriated appearance of normal T lymphocytes. The SIALOPHORIN of T lymphocytes is abnormal. The defect in WAS can be completely corrected by transplants of normal bone marrow cells.

Wu–Kabat plot. Bar graph to illustrate the degree of variability at each amino acid residue position in the VARIABLE REGIONS of IMMUNOGLOBULINS and T CELL RECEPTORS. An index of variability is defined as the number of different amino acids found at a given position divided by the frequency of the most common amino acid at that position. Since 20 amino acids are utilized in the polypeptide chains, the index ranges from 1 to 400. (Suppose that at a particular position, valine occurs in 50 out of 100 chains, leucine occurs in 25 chains, and isoleucine in the remaining 25 chains. In this case, there are three different amino acids and the frequency of the most common (valine) is 0.5; therefore, the variability at this position is 3/0.5 or 6.) To display the variability graphically, the index is plotted (in bar graph form) at each residue position. The resulting plot shows the degree of variability at each position and has been used to localize the HYPERVARIABLE REGIONS of the polypeptide chains of immunoglobulins and T cell receptors. *See* COMPLEMENTARITY-DETERMINING REGION, FRAMEWORK REGION.

X

xenograft. GRAFT to a member of a different species. Xenografts are usually rejected within a few days by antibodies and CYTOTOXIC T LYMPHOCYTES to histocompatibility antigens. *Synonym for* HETEROGRAFT.

X-linked agammaglobulinemia (XLA). Failure of immunoglobulin synthesis of all ISOTYPES that results from an absence of B LYMPHOCYTES. Affected males have recurrent PYOGENIC INFECTIONS. Their bone marrow contains a normal number of PRE-B CELLS in which CONSTANT REGIONS of IMMUNOGLOBULIN MU CHAINS can be discerned in cytoplasm by IMMUNOFLUORESCENCE. There may be faulty V_H–D–J_H gene rearrangement. The gene for X-linked agammaglobulinemia has been mapped to chromosome Xq21.3–22.

X-linked hyper-IgM immunodeficiency. *See* IMMUNOGLOBULIN DEFICIENCY WITH INCREASED IgM.

X-linked hypogammaglobulinemia with growth hormone deficiency. X-linked recessive form of HYPOGAMMAGLOBULINEMIA. Affected males have no B LYMPHOCYTES, and they are of short stature from failure of growth hormone synthesis. The gene for this deficiency does not map to Xq21.3–22, the location of the gene for X-LINKED AGAMMAGLOBULINEMIA.

Z

zidovudine (3'-azido-3'-deoxythymidine, AZT). Analogue of thymidine that inhibits REVERSE TRANSCRIPTASE. It has been used in the treatment of the ACQUIRED IMMUNODEFICIENCY SYNDROME. AZT is phosphorylated *in vivo* to 3'-azido-3'-deoxythymidine triphosphate, which binds to the reverse transcriptase of HUMAN IMMUNODEFICIENCY VIRUS and other retroviruses, thereby terminating elongation of DNA.

zymosan. Dried cell walls of yeast. Zymosan is a complex polysaccharide that has been used to study the activation of the ALTERNATIVE PATHWAY OF COMPLEMENT.

zidovudine

thymidine